The Art
of LIVING YOGA

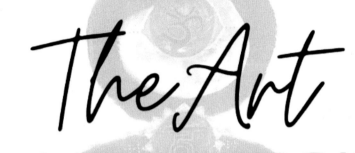

The Art
of LIVING YOGA

HONORING YOGA'S ROOTS
IN PHILOSOPHY & PRACTICE

CHRISTINE LILY KESSLER

First Electronic Edition: May 2022
First Print Edition: July 2022

D. D. Scott's
LetLoveGlow
Author Services

Photo Credits: All photo credits belong to the author unless otherwise noted.

For the curious Seekers.

Always keep learning to fly higher.

Contents

*Yoga is like an ancient river with countless rapids,
eddies, loops, tributaries, and backwaters, extending over
a vast, colorful terrain of many different habitats. So, when we
speak of Yoga, we speak of a multitude of paths and
orientations with contrasting theoretical frameworks
and occasionally incompatible goals.*

~ Georg Feuerstein

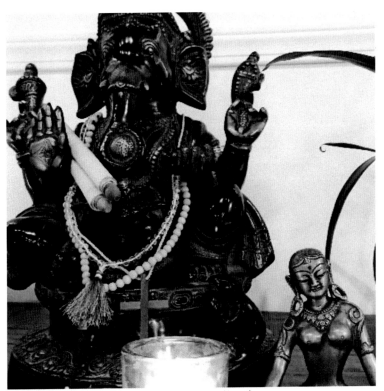

Om Gam Ganapataye Namaha

An Invitation

"The Art of Living Yoga" - I whispered these words to myself a few times when my colleague and friend Christine Lily Kessler first shared with me the title of this timeless book. The truth of these words immediately echoed with a truth in me, with the same Universal truth that also birthed me. A knowing that says we are all in this life together, interconnected, generous, creative, interdependent, yet solitary with the responsibility recommended to make our own choices, to be the needle of the compass, the brush and the paint and the canvas all in one. The reminder to walk my talk and to take the instruction manual of integrous living everywhere into my daily tasks settled in my heart as I tuned in to the rhythm of The Art of Living Yoga.

In the author's words:

The Art of Living Yoga explores the why behind the how in various yoga practices, from japa mala to other philosophy-based physical embodiment applications. Ultimately, this book is a peace offering to the world. I feel very called to honor yoga's roots and connect readers to the vastness and interconnection of our shared human history. I hope readers feel connected to our brothers and sisters who have come before us, as they, too, sought then taught ways to have a divine life worthy of breath while being in the thick of their humanness. In turn, our inner work and what we reflect from shared/innate knowledge honors and strengthens the trajectory of those who will come after us, who are fortified and nourished by our voices and experiences which have led to Grace. I want folks to claim their non-dominating power to be their own Guru, and to trust in that.

Messages support people in examining/questioning/discerning the culture in which they live, and to open into the bravery to feel into their bodies and glean intuitive wisdom that supports their unique, authentic life experience. The Hero's Journey is a biggie. I've included pieces of yogic history in nearly each chapter but have related it to my own personal examples that help make 'dusty history' come alive, potent with ancient tools and modern perspectives for personal growth.

The intricate care and immense knowledge in this book, the transparency, vulnerability and richness, all make it a treasure chest of references and tools. It is also a tribute of gratitude and honor to gurus, teachers, and masters in spirit or still walking this Earth. This blended collection of history and testimonials through the eyes, ears, and posture of Christine Lily Kessler is for student, teacher, or the curious observer to map out a brilliant blueprint for growth and change. Above all for peace. Within ourselves. And in this world.

Over the course of our collaboration, Lily and I repeatedly realize and celebrate the commonalities that we share that blend our differences. We see the beauty of our colors and the essential essence of our combined perspectives. Both of us are teachers and students, ongoing. More so, we are alchemists, always flirting with miracles and the potential for greatness through simplicity and the simplicity and loyalty of truth. The most basic and most powerful of our commonalities is the breath. The guru of all gurus is the breath. With pure breath comes clarity, and with clarity a channel of wisdom, and with wisdom come far-reaching influence and progress. Pure breath commands posture, integrity, resiliency. It invokes truth, creativity, and accountability. Breath is life. It is our conduit for all possibilities. Breath tempers and guides our emotions, suggests harmony to our egos. It is serious. It is funny. It is art. It is free.

Being our own guru is a very personal, necessary, and intimate journey, one based on the expression of perceptions and sometimes misperceptions that evolve over time. However, this journey of authenticating self weaves with truths that are universal and unifying with every manifestation of creation, visible and invisible, with every breath that is our own and of our sisters' and brothers' and every stranger and every tree, animal, and star. It is a given that we are delicately interconnected. The focus then is on the quality and purification of this union of inner journey and the external one; it is about the choreography of inner alignment and the dance with our brethren, with history and prophecy; it is about the practice and refinement of technique and science of living with its artistic and mystical expression, always soothing and freeing the bruised ego along the way.

The Art of Living Yoga is a key to this journey of discovery. It is a golden, brilliant, shining key to this mystical doorway of our ascending humanity toward peace. It is a compass with its pages a sacred guidance for the covenant of our souls and spirits to be true to ourselves and loyal to our collective exploration. *The Art of Living Yoga* is our honoring for wholeness as the marriage of self with life through the practice of Yoga and its richness of ancient traditions in a modern-day initiative.

We are all entrusted to honor the legacy of yoga in one way or another and to advance humanity. I invite you to explore the content of this glossary of history, personal stories, and tools. This book will carry you to greater heights as you also mark its pages with your wisdom and experiences.

May we join in this dialogue for peace.

With deepest gratitude -

Iva Nasr

Mentor, Speaker, Author
From Rifles to Roses: Memories and Miracles

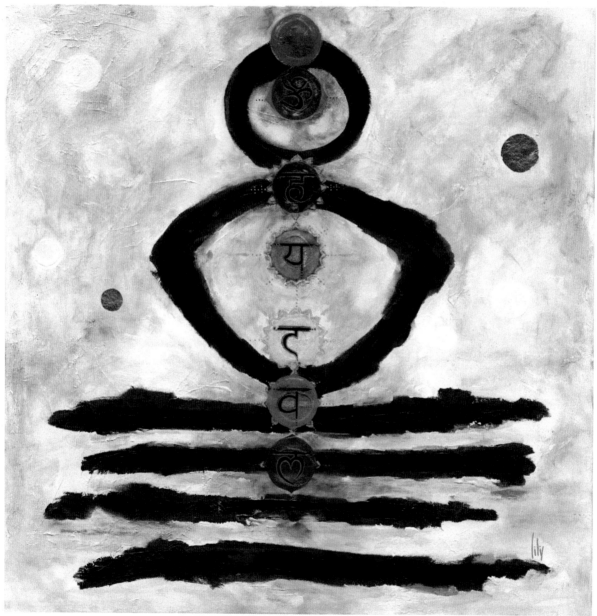

Mirror Within, painting by Lily Kessler

Unifying Mantra for Learning

We are all students, for all our lives.

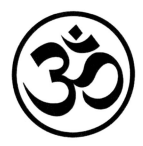

Oṁ Saha nāvavatu
Saha nau bhunaktu
Saha vīryam karavāvahai
Tejasvi nāvadhītamastu
Mā vidviṣāvahai

May we all be protected
May we all be nourished
May we work together with great energy
May our intellect be inspiring and unifying
Om, peace (in spirit), peace (in mind), peace (in body)

~ Also known as 'The Teaching Mantra'

The Art of Living Yoga: An Introduction

Yoga: Equanimity; Duality; Merging; Standing Within One's Self

Yoga is often misunderstood. Many people think of it only as a sequence of physical poses expressed on a mat. Culturally in the West, Yoga may be experienced as a means to weight loss, mindfulness, therapy, health, liberation, fashion, companionship; the list goes on. In addition, the many doorways of Yoga often lead to a greater personal journey in which the ego-self wends its way to a deeper understanding of the Higher Self and the interconnection to All.

Yoga's essence has existed since the dawn of humanity and has enriched the lives of millions around the planet. With its recent widespread popularity in the West people question if it is a physical practice, a religion, or a philosophy. Yoga can be a purely spiritual practice, and it can also be a psycho-physical one, uninhibited by religious dogmas. There is no one answer that can be provided in response to the question - *What is Yoga?* Your individual experience with the tradition is your personal key to what it is. And thus, the question becomes - *What is Yoga to you?*

The Yoga Tradition, in all its various forms, is manifested through a combination of holistic practices. By studying Yoga history and philosophy, homage is paid to those who have contributed to the tradition. Modern Yoga practitioners can then recognize their unique place in that lineage, contributing, in turn, to honoring the tradition by exploring its deep and tangled historical roots. Yoga offers the opportunity for complete transformation through various traditions, depending on personal tendencies.

Yoga is essentially awareness that everything is a teacher; all of your human experiences - joy, sadness, anger, frustration, unfulfillment - all contribute to your growth and understanding of your Divine Self. Only through unique, direct experience can transcendental knowledge - *supraconscious illumination* - be achieved. The Practice unfolds your ability to 'return home' through the process of introspection and involution; uncovering, recovering, and re-identifying your highest Self. *Asana* (Yoga poses), *pranayama* (control of the breath), meditation, and philosophical teachings allow Yoga to rise naturally within you so you may live fully in the present time and in the present space. The synergy of knowledge and experience is what the practice of Yoga is all about.

As you engage in the time-honored study of the Yoga Tradition, you recognize that individuals will not only interpret and embody its teachings uniquely but will also contribute to the tradition's growth in ways small and large. A Sanskrit word for philosophy is *darshan*, meaning sight and the personal experience of Truth. Many *Vedic* (relating to the *Vedas*, a large body of religious texts from ancient India) philosophies are comprised of unique but universal concepts. *The Upanishads*, an ancient, seminal text which distills the essence of the *Vedas* says, "Follow that advice of mine which is good and helpful for your progress and neglect even my own advice which is not."

In that spirit, I'm looking forward to this adventure with you.

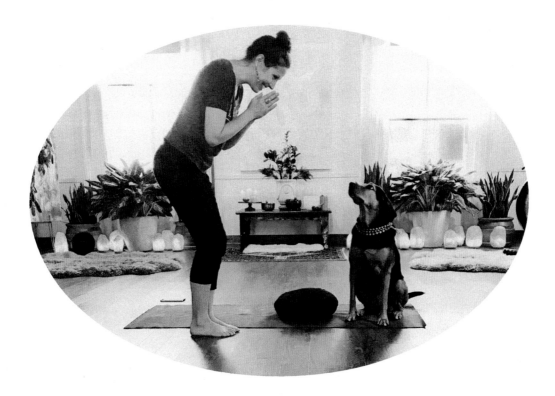

How to Approach This Book

The Yoga Tradition is growing rapidly in the West. Though its expansion is beautiful, important yogic history is being lost. It is my Calling to examine and compile the seeds and multitudes of paths within this tradition through the lens of my personal experiences. In doing so, I hope to offer you a starting point to explore the richness and beauty of the timeless teachings of this tradition.

Understanding the conceptual and philosophical *why* behind the methodological *how* has been a priority for me. I have traveled extensively around the planet in search of the most potent yogic teachings and teachers to complement my curiosity. In my vulnerable quest, I have learned to trust that I am my own guru. I wish to impart that *you*, too, are your own teacher and healer. Though I recommend you find teachers, scholars, and social communities who are inspirations for your yogic exploration, I also encourage you to remain keenly faithful to your own inner and sacred guru and guide.

Untangling the often complex and esoteric concepts of Yoga history and making them relatable to my daily life has been the root of my personal journey. As I continue my own study, my understandings will be refined. Yet, this book is a glimpse into how I relate to the Yoga Tradition, here and now.

Yoga's historical development is complex and often contradictory. Scholars and practitioners of the Yoga tradition often disagree about dates, translations of texts, and the significance of various influences. Therefore, it is impossible to make a conclusive timeline of Yoga's history or accurately give a comprehensive overview of the tradition. Keep in mind that Yoga's rich history of various philosophies, religions, and dates simply overlap. That said, I strive to compare, condense, and refine the influences into a tangible historical overview and timeline of Yoga's development.

Ultimately, this book is meant to be explored with the support of teacher-guidance in a group discussion format.

I have included multitudes of concepts, with each piece building upon another. Jargon will be unpacked throughout this book with a brief definition the first time each word/concept appears. There is also a glossary at the back of the book.

Please keep in mind that every concept I include, often repeated again and again, can be a life-long study within itself. So, please approach this book as a buffet of concepts, insights, and tools which are learned only through personal examination, experience, and dedication.

Question everything and take only what serves you but also be willing to change your mind and beliefs. It is my hope that you continue to deepen and refine your own study long after you've completed this training, bringing your integration of the information into your community. Keep learning … so you can continue teaching.

I understand that every person approaches Yoga uniquely. Regardless of your background and experience, or your intention to utilize this work either personally or professionally, you have the opportunity to explore your Authentic Self. With deep dedication and playful self-inquiry, you honor the practice by being a living torchbearer of this timeless tradition.

Be Nourished.

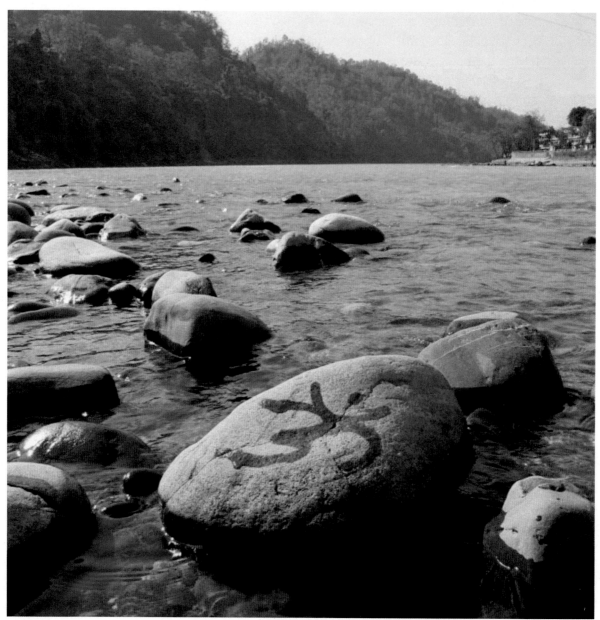

Mother Ganges

The River, She is flowing, flowing and growing. The River, She is flowing back to the Sea. Oh Mother, won't you carry me, your child I will always be, oh Mother, won't you carry me back to the Sea? I am the Ancient One. I am the Rising Sun. I am the True Light inside of You.

I learned this song in my first-ever yoga class.

While attending Highline Community College in Washington State, I registered for a one-credit Yoga course. Yoga wasn't as culturally popular in the 1990's as it is today, and I didn't know what I was getting into. On the first day of class I wore a long broom skirt and combat boots and was horrified when I realized I should be barefoot. I initially resisted the appropriate *Yoga dress code*, but my growing willingness to show my teacher respect was greater. He was an elderly man who dressed in simple cotton clothes with wildly bushy eyebrows. Yet he had a gentle and kind presence and was patient and supportive of everyone. His good energy was palpable by all and was such a rare delight to experience.

He sang this version of the song *The River Is Flowing*, which became a potent seed of Yoga that was planted into my heart on that very first day. It took years for that seed to sprout and grow, and even longer for me to consciously recognize Yoga for what it is. *This book reflects my current understanding.*

I now teach Yoga at Butler University in Indianapolis, Indiana. As I end my classes, I often sing this song in recognition of a completed Circle. Ultimately, it's a mantra that connects me to deeply appreciate my life's journey and see that sacred journey revealed in others. When I sing, I press my hands over my heart and I feel the song welling from a timeless, holy space within me. I feel alight as a Torchbearer of the Yoga Tradition, just as you are.

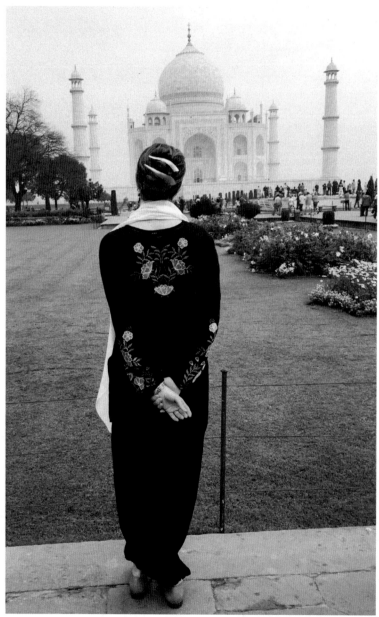

Present

Historical Timeline

PRECLASSICAL YOGA ERA

INDUS-SARASVATI AGE: 6500-4500 BCE
- SANATANA DHARMA: "ETERNAL LAW"
- INDUS RIVER VALLEY & SEALS

VEDIC AGE: 4500-2500 BCE
- CONSCIOUSNESS EXPLORED
- VIBRATION OF INTENTION & CAUSATION
- CAUSE & EFFECT: MANTRA & KARMA

SAMKHYA YOGA: 8000-100 BCE
- REALITY EXPLORED: PRAKRITI/PURUSHA
- BODY'S CONSTITUTION: DOSHAS
- AYURVEDA

UPANISHADIC AGE: 2000-1500 BCE
- NON-DUALISM OF ATMAN/BRAHMAN
- DISTILLATION OF VEDAS
- MEDITATION

BHAKTI YOGA: 1000-500 BCE
- ADORATION
- HINDU EPICS / UNIVERSAL INSIGHTS
- 3 BRANCHES OF YOGA

BUDDHISM: C. 500 BCE-PRESENT
- INDIVIDUALITY / MONASTIC TRADITION
- MIDDLE WAY
- FOUR NOBLE TRUTHS / EIGHT-FOLD PATH

CLASSICAL YOGA ERA

CLASSICAL YOGA: 75 BCE-100 CE
- THE YOGA SUTRA'S OF PATANJALI
- EIGHT-LIMBED PATH
- HARNESSING THE MIND

ESOTERIC AGE

TANTRA: 600-1300 CE
- 6 + 1 CHAKRA SYSTEM
- WESTERN NOTION OF EMBODIMENT
- SUBTLE BODY (NADIS, CHAKRAS, ETC.)

HATHA YOGA: C. 1300-1400 CE
- MIND V. BODY
- HATHA YOGA PRADIPIKA
- ASANA / BREATH / BANDHAS / MUDRAS

RISE OF MODERN YOGA

SWAMI VIVEKANANDA: 1872-1950
- INFLUENCED RISE OF MODERN YOGA
- INTRODUCED YOGA TO THE WEST

SRI T. KRISHNAMACHARYA: 1891-1989
- YOGA'S EXPANSION
- FATHER OF MODERN YOGA
- MODERN CONTRIBUTORS

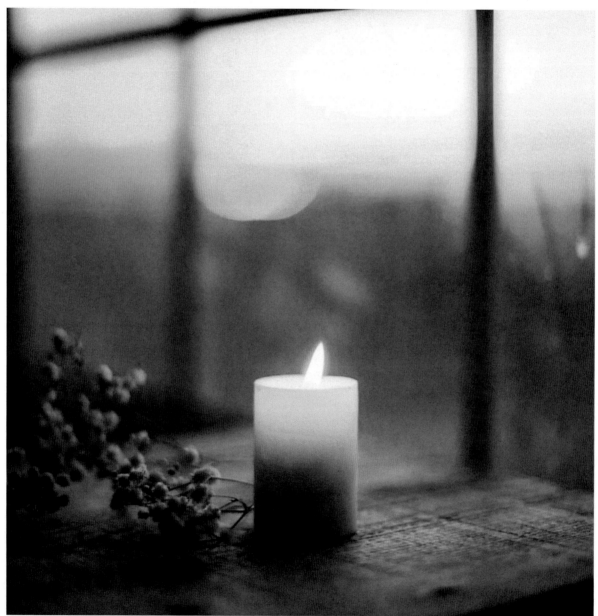

Sacred Spaces

Chapter 1

Yoga Off the Mat: Creating Sacred Space

Sweetness. This entire universe is filled with sweetness.
God wants us to experience this sweetness by having sweet thoughts,
by speaking sweet words, by performing sweet actions,
by letting the sweetness from our soul flow into other hearts.
Every heart is made of sweetness.
Sweetness is another name for the heart.

~ Swami Chidvilasananda

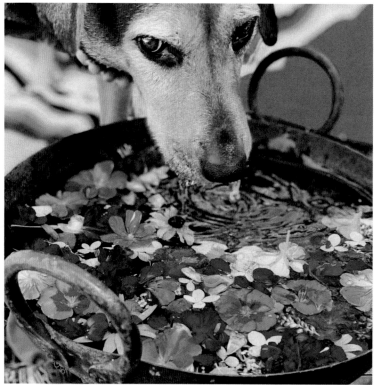

Sweet Shanti Ro

16

Chapter 1

Yoga Off the Mat: Creating Sacred Space

1. Overview

Chapter 1 introduces Yoga-off-the-mat and the value of creating and honoring Sacred Spaces. Different ways to create a unique altar space are explored, as well as the connection between Yoga as a philosophy and as a physical practice. Interconnectedness and responsibility in food choice is explained. Labels and their effects, personally and within society, are also explored.

2. Learning Objectives: I will …

a) Identify my labels and belief systems with WHY
b) Contemplate my use of prana
c) Understand the importance of Sacred Space
d) Explore and identify ways to create my own Sacred Space
e) Understand my relationship with food

3. Pre-lecture Assignment

a) List your labels for discussion

4. Reflection: *found at the end of the chapter*

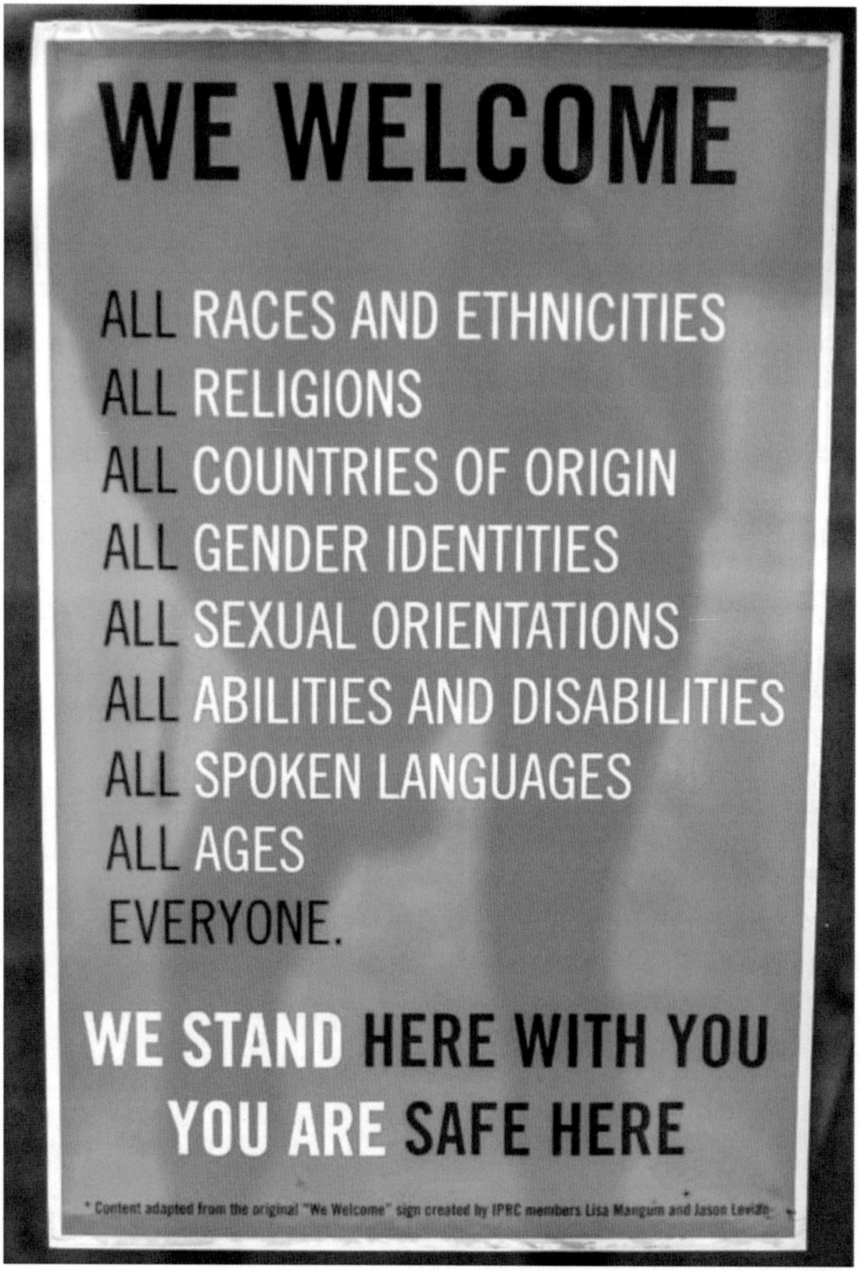
WE WELCOME
ALL RACES AND ETHNICITIES
ALL RELIGIONS
ALL COUNTRIES OF ORIGIN
ALL GENDER IDENTITIES
ALL SEXUAL ORIENTATIONS
ALL ABILITIES AND DISABILITIES
ALL SPOKEN LANGUAGES
ALL AGES
EVERYONE.
WE STAND HERE WITH YOU
YOU ARE SAFE HERE

Where is Your Seat?

**When you begin to study Yogic Traditions, you must be aware
of the *seat* in which you view yourself, other people, and perspectives.
You must become aware of the depths of your own conditioning and your
own cultural disposition and identification labels; your own situatedness.
It's what I call your *Yoga Off the Mat.***

The questions to ask yourself as we begin are this – ***How am I situated in relation to***:

My own cultural disposition?
The food I ate this morning?
My family make-up?
My partner?
My work environment?
Other?

All these factors intersect to create the conditioning of your unique collection of labels and of your individuality, at this particular moment. Packed in all this is the concept of worthiness – how worthy you believe you are based on WHAT and WHO is of importance and of value to you. And then, taking it a step further, you must consider WHY this is so for you.

One could argue that the goal of Yoga is to experience and to gain enough distancing from your personal conditioning to see it for what it is, rather than to be controlled and agitated by your own presumptions, prejudices, addictions, forms of identification – all these things which contribute to your situatedness; your seat.

Yoga offers tools for you to witness and then understand your conditioned patterns, then offers you the tools to dismantle the effects of your conditioning on an individual and collective level. To begin the sacred journey into the Tradition, you must be ready to change.

I am a CEO.
I am a traveler.
I am tattooed.
I am a divorcee.
I am an artist.
I am a yogi.
I am a father.
I am an activist.
I am poor.
I am new here.
I am thin.
I am Pro-Choice.
I am a graduate.
I am a woman.
I am tall.
I am vegan.
I am tough.
I am funny.
I am disabled.
I am retired.
I am Black.
I am popular.
I am Pro-Life.
I am anti-vaccine.
I am an author.
I am athletic.

I am middle-class.
I am short.
I am a victim.
I am fragile.
I am a student.
I am a Muslim.
I am rich.
I am Brown.
I am a Republican.
I am straight.
I am pro-vaccine.
I am a man.
I am gluten free.
I am an atheist.
I am misunderstood.
I am vegetarian.
I am a drug user.
I am Christian.
I am a survivor.
I am Goth.
I am a virgin.
I am a prisoner.
I am fat.
I am White.
I am stressed.
I am Indigenous.

I am young.
I am Pro-Gun.
I am an author.
I am an athlete.
I am weird.
I am a winner.
I am a veteran.
I am a Democrat.
I am an addict.
I am retired.
I am a teacher.
I am in charge.
I am lonely.
I am dependable.
I am old.
I am a doctor.
I am homeless.
I am Queer.
I am an illegal.
I am fashionable.
I am a theatre kid.
I am a minimalist.
I am a cheerleader.
I am a minimalist.
I am an Influencer.
I am shy.

What Are Your Labels?

… Gender, Sexual Orientation, Weight, Religion, Race, Income, Interests, Intelligence, Fashion …

Labels help categorize people into "safe" boxes that can be identified. Labels can be self-imposed or given to you by society, and you often agree to carry these labels, whether you identify with them or not.

Some of the most beautiful aspects of community are tied to common beliefs and interests. People in communities share a sense of pride, belonging, and contribution. Yet, institutions and environments demand certain behaviors. Bigotry and racism are born from community beliefs and interests, using labels as weapons, to keep people divided, often in the name of God and Country.

Those who don't fit into a category are often seen as odd or dangerous. Judgements of another person's worthiness are based on labels. Labels bind people together while excluding others. When bound to a label, interconnection with the larger world feels unsafe. Others (different than you) may seem *weird*. Ultimately, labels limit personal growth and transformation, which often leads to anger, distrust, and depression. The more labels are upheld and protected, personally or by society, individual perspectives become smaller, as does the ability to empathize with others outside a particular label. In turn, the more controlling and righteous social groups become.

I encourage you to identify the labels in every aspect of your life. When frustration or anger arises in a situation, ask yourself if you are categorizing that person with a label and then open yourself to a new aspect of freedom by examining what label of yours did the judging. Then ask if you can loosen the power your label has over you by not taking it so seriously. This is a step toward freedom. Freedom is given only when you give others room to fly without tethering them to a label.

Patterns, Consciousness and Truth

**And the day came when the risk to remain tight in a bud
was more painful than the risk it took to blossom. ~ Anaïs Nin**

Duality. Me and you. Light and dark. Bad and good. Love and fear. Sadness and joy. Blame and acceptance. Ultimately, Yoga is the merging of dualities. This requires your recognition of the great *Both/And* – in other words, you extinguish the labels (by which you have operated) by acknowledging them.

To merge dualities, you must first be willing to step outside the norm of your day-to-day perspectives. By doing so, you naturally begin to question things. You up-level in consciousness, allowing yourself to question who and why you are.

Who am I? Who was I? Why was I that way? Why do I feel this way?
What do I feel here in my body and mind, here and now?
Who taught me to be/think/respond/react in the ways that I do?
Who am I transforming into? When did I form my opinions?
Who taught me that this way of living and thinking is the only way?
Are my beliefs from the safety and comradery of an agreed-upon space,
or are they from the feeling of anger and the act of bravery of a rebellious space?

These are lifelong questions for you to ponder, and finding the answers takes courage and honesty. Each question and answer are acts of homecoming into yourself, loving the human you have been and are, here and now, regardless of any past agreement or situation you may have encountered.

The situations you uncover may be experienced as a "heaviness" in your life, often found in the most bitter of stories. But what can be learned from these experiences are the greatest gifts you can provide to both yourself and others. The things you might consider the most devastating can also provide the fertilizer that will help heal, enrich, and expand your life. The gifts can be found when you rise above these stories (and labels) and see a larger perspective, and in turn share with others what you have learned from your experience(s).

Question what your passions are and why.

Question what your repulsions are and why.

Most of your perspectives and beliefs are taught to you by your environment. As you get older, however, you may question if you wish to continue to emulate these teachings, or if you wish to rebel against them. Both have consequences.

Humans are designed to live in patterned ways of thinking with patterned belief systems. There is the conscious mind and the subconscious mind, and the subconscious mind holds these repetitive patterns and belief systems. Patterns offer you a false sense of safety. And they're safe because that which doesn't change is predictable. But this sense of safety provides you with only a very limited definition of yourself. In unknown situations, for example, invoking your patterns and belief systems, you act and react based on your previous actions and reactions rather than responding in a new way with perhaps more empowerment than you have exercised in your past.

The word *pattern* has a Yogic term, which is called a *samskara*. In the book *The Four Agreements*, Don Miguel Ruiz refers to this as the "Dream of the Planet", resulting from the domestication of humans. The very act of domestication is, in effect, forging our commonly held patterns of activity and belief systems. In other words, we act and believe as we've been "programmed" and/or taught to act and believe.

Embodiment of Patterned Energetics

Yoga allows you to address the current seats in which you sit and the labels you've identified with by teaching you tools to engage in a conscious response rather than an unconscious reaction. Unconscious reactions are generated from head-based emotional memories rather than a gut or intuition-based, in-the-now, holistic perspective. Emotional responses often spin you deep into a story from your past, entrapping you in a patterned way of thinking. For example, you may experience a feeling of friction, or nervous butterflies, a sinking feeling of despair or sadness, or a void of anxiety. A myriad of these patterns comprises your perspective of your life. You must learn to recognize these patterns, to dissect the stories creating them, and then lean into the new feelings you're generating to live an expansive life.

Practice

When you find yourself in a situation that is generating stress or anxiety or heavy emotions, pinpoint the exact area in your body in which you are experiencing these feelings. Each area of the body responds to a specific emotion. So, your physical sensations offer a key (in the form of an embodiment of an emotion-based pattern) to help you unlock the origin of the emotions you're feeling.

If your hand is on a hot surface, the brain senses this and tells the body to move. Likewise, if you need to change a situation in your life, the Universe will tell you to move in other sensory ways that are also felt in your body. These feelings you're experiencing are invitations presenting themselves to you to help you find your Truth.

To expand into being able to identify what your Truth *feels like* for you, you must first recognize what is happening externally in your world, without labeling yourself as playing any role in the story unfolding. This is the Hero's Journey. This is dissolving who you think you are so you can become who you truly are. When you usurp the power-hold of your patterned emotional states, inquiring into the why they're occurring, you are engaging in your own liberation. You are claiming your consciousness.

... this inquiry is your Yoga.

The Tale of Two Wolves

Where the mind goes, Prana flows.

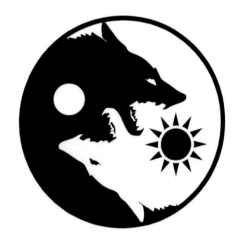

One evening, an elder told his grandson about a battle that goes on inside people.

He said: *"My son, the battle is between two wolves inside us all.*

One is Evil. It is anger, envy, jealousy, doubt, sorrow, regret, greed, arrogance, self-pity, resentment, inferiority, lies, false pride, superiority, and ego.

The other is Good. It is joy, peace, love, hope, serenity, humility, kindness, benevolence, empathy, generosity, forgiveness, truth, compassion, and faith.

The grandson thought about it for a minute and then asked his grandfather, "Which wolf wins?"

His grandfather simply replied, "The one you feed."

25

Prana and the Power of Visualization

Yearning for a new way will not produce it. Only ending the old way can do that.
You cannot hold onto the old all the while declaring that you want something new.
The old will defy the new; the old will deny the new; the old will decry the new.
There is only one way to bring in the new. You must make room for it.

~ Neal Donald Walsch

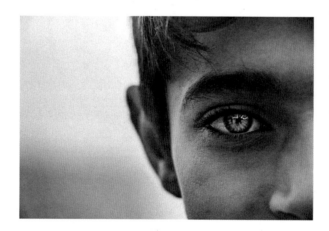

Prana is an ancient Sanskrit term that is a foundational concept in the Yoga Tradition. Prana is vital life force energy. (*Pra-* means "constant" and *-na* means "motion".) There are five types of Prana called Prana Vayus. They were first explored in the ancient Vedas, are outlined in the seminal text of *The Upanishads*, and are the basis for *Ayurveda, the Science of Life*.

Prana is known as *chi/qi/spirit* in Chinese Medicine, and it is ultimately moved through breath work, Reiki, asana, and other movement practices. In Eastern traditions, Prana centers are concentrated in the *nadis* (the channels through which the energies of the physical body flow), chakras, and meridians. Pranic energy is naturally always in motion.

Prana relies on the integrity of your breath to nourish your holistic body. It can be increased through joyful, connective activities that move the body such as Yoga, dancing, singing, other exercise modalities, and play! The more movement you generate, the more expansive your Prana, and thus the more your physical, emotional, mental, and spiritual bodies are in harmony with both your inner and outer worlds.

When Prana is not moving through your system, healing is more difficult. Lack of Prana results in the stagnation of your emotions and your organs, which results in further physical and emotional disharmony. The key is to become aware of your stagnant areas and use breath-based tools to infuse these areas with Prana. Prana, as a healing modality, is enhanced by visualization.

The power of visualization ~ and the belief in the REALITY of that visualization ~ is vital in all yogic practices.

Many practitioners invoke the imagination of colors and directional movement of breath to heighten the power of Prana. For example, visualize breath as a stream of white light pulled up through the earth into your body, exiting out through your skull, and/or reverse the direction. Pranic visualization can also bring awareness to specific *chakra centers* (the energy centers of your body), with the intention to 'see' and 'feel' physical and emotional blockages dissolving through focused breath. Pranic work is also about tapping into your physical embodiment to support your spiritual enlightenment; it enables you to fully connect to your inner and outer worlds of consciousness.

As a personal example, when I feel anxious or overwhelmed, I bring my attention skyward and pull breath downward through my crown, consciously tracing my breath as it travels through the center of my brain, throat, heart, and solar plexus, and then lands in the seat of my sacral center's lower belly. While I trace my breath downward through these physical spaces, I visualize myself gathering all heavy energies. I then exhale from my root chakra, releasing these energies into the earth to be transmuted. I also use this downward moving breath to anchor myself during *Yoga asana* (the practice of yogic poses). Through every emotional response that arises throughout my day, with practice, I have learned to automatically invoke my breath. **The breath is always present, every moment.** What a blessing!

27

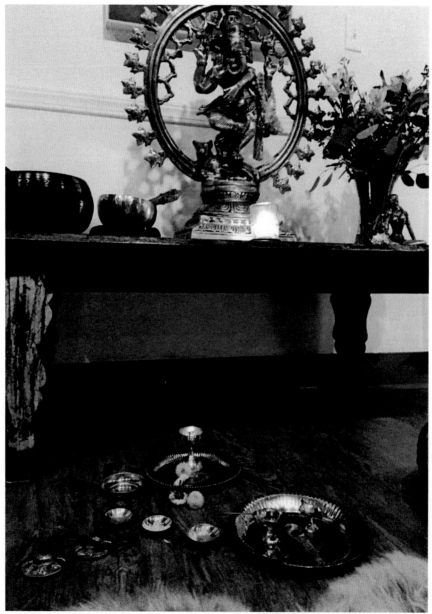

Altar

28

Sacred Space and Altars

The Cultivation of Gratitude and Intention

A path deeper into Yoga is to become aware of the sensation of your physical environment. Here and now, does your space feel peaceful and intentional? How is the light? Is it naturally lit or artificial? Are your lightbulbs LED or soft yellow, bright or dim? Is there a scent? Is it chemical or natural; can fresh air clean the space? Are there any objects in your space that are there out of obligation? Is it clean and intentional? **These first questions have made some students leave my course to never return.**

Being ready to take a deep look into the mirror of your soul while having the courage to examine the cultural soup in which you swim requires great bravery. It requires the willingness to change who you think you are. Sacred Space helps you examine the dimensions in which you hold yourself internally, while also experiencing the external.

The practice of *Sacred Space* honors all faiths, and it is important to incorporate into your home, and in some capacity into your workspace. An *altar* is another term for Sacred Space. Altars can be visualized within meditations and can also be physical expressions. The energy of an altar roots you to the present moment. An altar is also a graceful reflection of your heart, physically and symbolically honoring what you hold precious. Ultimately, an altar is an aspect of gratitude which reminds you of where you've been internally and externally. It's an interconnected link to Spirit.

Taking a few moments in your Sacred Space to connect to divinity at each day's beginning is a beautiful, life-enhancing ritual. This practice is a tool which supports balance of the nervous system, resulting in you feeling grateful; gratitude allows you to be aligned and rooted in all aspects of life. This sacred time can be filled with breathing, prayer, chanting, singing, meditation, and/or crafting your altar (or a new altar) inside and outside your home. Having a space dedicated to spiritual practice supports internal harmony, allowing you to become more receptive to high-frequency energies embodied within the concepts of 'love', 'cherish', 'sacredness', and 'preciousness', which sacred spaces exude.

Even now, ask yourself how you physically feel - and what, if anything, is activated in your body - when you invoke these words:

Love
Cherish
Sacredness
Preciousness

The term 'altar' literally means 'God's Table'. Some traditions and religions have stringent rules regarding altar creation. Altars can be large or small, simple or intricate, and each reflects deep meaning. An altar can be a small empty closet, a corner, or a larger space. It can be a tiny space where you place herbs on the earth, in gratitude. In many traditions, a home altar is in one place and is not used for any other purpose. This dedication to one spot cultivates exquisite energy that will 'supercharge' the space.

Vedic Tradition: The Five Altar Elements

The five elements are often honored in the Yoga Tradition and are explored in Yoga's sister science of *Ayurveda*. The elements are: *space/ether, air, fire, water, and earth.* These five elements (often referred to as *elementals*) are the foundations used in crafting the sacred space of altars.

Elemental symbols are also used in many philosophies, rituals, and ceremonies around the planet. Earth, for example, can be represented by stones, crystals, special rocks, or twigs and sprigs that were picked up on a nature walk. Water is honored with flowers in a vase, with a glass of water that will be enjoyed after a ritual, or a shell from a sea. Fire is seen with a candle flame. Air is honored through incense or candle smoke. Space/ether is honored through physical space, or sound, such as a bell, a singing bowl, or a small musical instrument.

A *Puja* is a form of ritual prayer and reverence. It is a full experience of the senses, which is ultimately an offering of gratitude to be alive in the present moment. All senses are invoked, which ushers in the Pranic energy. Sight, smell, sound, touch, and taste reveal the gift of living in the present moment.

Is the whole picture delicious?

Allow your senses to feast at your home altar.
Does it sound good, feel good, look good, and smell good to you?

1. Space / Sounds Good

How does sound honor your space? Are there unnecessary sounds, like electronics?
Can you hear water, wind, birds, or soothing sacred music?

2. Air / Feels Good

Does the air feel clean with a neutral temperature and good flow?
What is the intention of the space? Does it feel relaxed?
Does the space support quiet sacredness?

3. Fire / Looks Good

Is the space organized and clean?
How is the ambiance? Do colors and light support relaxation in this sacred space?

4. Water / Tastes Good

Enjoy fresh flowers in a vase.
Fruit and tea are often used in rituals and placed on the altar. You may eat the fruit and drink the water afterward or use them as an offering to animals and plants.

5. Earth / Smells Good

Does the air smell good? Is it scented with chemicals or pure oils? Incense or sage?
How often do you open windows to clean the air?

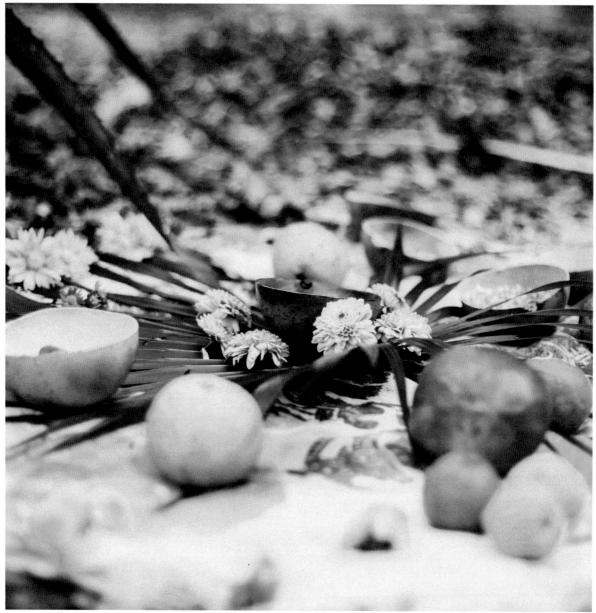

Consciousness Aware of Consciousness

Honoring Interconnection on Your Altar

If you are a poet, you will see clearly that there is a cloud floating in this sheet of paper. Without a cloud, there will be no rain; without rain, the trees cannot grow; and without trees, we cannot make paper. The cloud is essential for the paper to exist. If the cloud is not here, the sheet of paper cannot be here either. So, we can say that the cloud and the paper inter-are. "Interbeing" is a word that is not in the dictionary yet, but if we combine the prefix "inter" with the verb "to be", we have a new verb, inter-be. Without a cloud, we cannot have paper, so we can say that the cloud and the sheet of paper inter-are. If we look into this sheet of paper even more deeply, we can see the sunshine in it. If the sunshine is not there, the forest cannot grow. In fact, nothing can grow. Even we cannot grow without sunshine. And so, we know that the sunshine is also in this sheet of paper. The paper and the sunshine inter-are. And if we continue to look, we can see the logger who cut the tree and brought it to the mill to be transformed into paper. And we see the wheat. We know that the logger cannot exist without his daily bread, and therefore the wheat that became his bread is also in this sheet of paper. And the logger's father and mother are in it too. When we look in this way we see that without all of these things, this sheet of paper cannot exist. ~ Thich Nhat Hanh

Ritual Caretaking

The altar serves as a reminder of divinity in daily life; everything is alive and receptive and from Creator. I recommend that you give yourself permission to become deeply personal and creative in your altar creation. Involve your family! Altars serve as a tool for connection, and children enjoy the task to supply altars with special symbolisms.

Altars must be regularly tended to, as they become a living and breathing organism. And they are naturally in continual motion, so allow the altar to change and evolve by adding and taking away items. Flowers wilt. Incense turns to ash. The constant organic cycle of the altar evokes new energy and perspectives. Altars represent the sweet and precious fleetingness of life. Go with the flow of the altar, but ensure it is fresh and relevant. Altars are mirrors to other aspects of your life.

Be mindful that the thing does not become the Thing, itself.

Not long ago I was in conversation with a man who could not find the 'correct' flowers for his altar, per his guru's instructions. The flowers he needed were not readily available. Though I gave him suggestions for an alternative flower choice, he chose to become panicked, as he was certain his prayer would not be heard if he did not abide by the strictly prescribed ritual, which is traditionally Vedic. However, the desire for unobtainable flowers became the 'Thing' itself. Even if he found the flowers, I believe he still lost the point of it all. I have no doubt that in time he will transform his rigidity into gleeful ease of ritual, abiding in the essence of sweet devotion.

An altar is simply a tool to connect you to your Heart Space through unabashed Intention. The practice of Yoga is recognizing and honoring Divinity within yourself. Altars are tools that invite you to root yourself in peace. They support you in meditation, and in turn, support your understanding of your connection, your adoration of *Bhagavan* (your highest expression of Divine Love). And it's that highest expression of Divine Love that is the essence of *Bhakti Yoga* (the Yoga of Devotion).

Devotion to what?

Devotion to being responsible to Awaken yourself, to muster great courage to be willing to see the Truth of your heart.

Devotion to being courageously vulnerable to change your outer life to live authentically in-line with the Voice of your heart.

Devotion to your ability to change your perspectives of Self and Place. New perspectives that support your embodiment of empathy with all beings. Empathy is the foundation for Compassion, which is the highest aspect of Love. Love leads to Unity. Unity taps you into Bliss that remains ever-present in this wild, Divine Play of Life, which happens to be called *Lila*, which we'll briefly explore later in this book.

My Ever-Transforming Altars

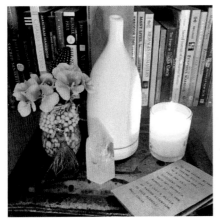 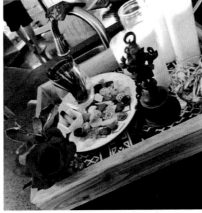 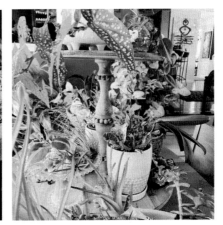

The first image is my altar in my office. I enjoy the physical ritual of lighting candles and working with oils, water, and fire to awaken the space. When this altar is 'alive', I feel more grounded and inspired to research and write. In my relationship with this altar, I close my eyes (to "see" the candle), I smell the healing scents of the essential oil diffuser, and I breathe deeper; my exhales become soothing. I am a lover of poems and wordsmithing and so, on my altar, I have gathered many inspirational poems on special paper that allows me a tactile experience to enjoy what is written. This altar holds space for me to reconnect to my inner muse and makes my office a space I can spend ample time in.

The second image is my altar on my kitchen counter, brimming with tokens full of memory, meaning, and intention-being-manifest. There are shells I've found from beaches around the world; acorns and seeds from beloved forests and fields; sage, incense, and responsibly-sourced palo santo wood. There are the military dog tags of my husband's grandmother, and the perfectly round stone that my grandfather gave me. These treasures rest on a plate that I made in kindergarten. On this altar, I invite the bell of Ganesha to sound, taking me back to when I first heard its radiant *voice* in a tiny, bustling shop in India. And as on all my altars, I have fresh flowers to remind me of the bittersweet preciousness of the moment.

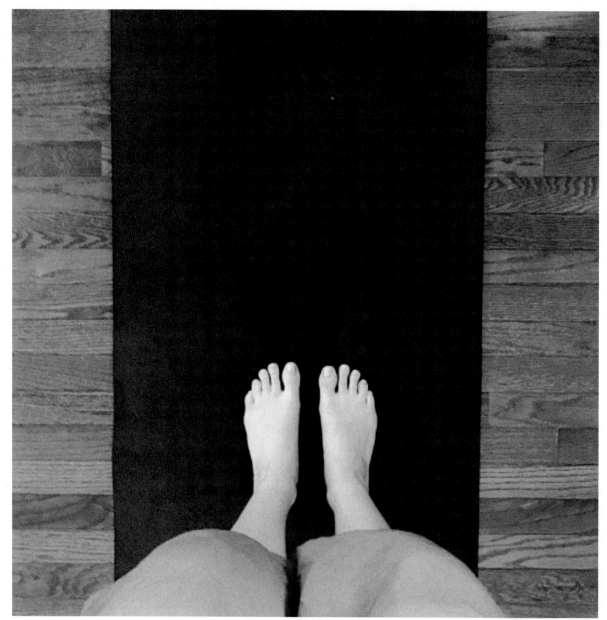

Sacred Altar

36

Every morning, I light the altar candles (even before I grind the beans to make my coffee), which is another ritual filled with my connection to family history and cultural artistry. Not only do I love the warmth of the candle flames, this is my way of saying 'good morning' to my home. It is my physical ritual of being deeply grateful for having a home that I love, which in turn, loves me.

There are more formal altars in my home, used daily as a space to sit and reconnect. I often practice asana and meditation in these spaces. I am reminded to cultivate an authentic, intentional life for myself and hold space for others to be free to live their own journey. These altars hold various personal elements, including: a flute, candles, framed images of inspirations, and many sweet tokens that melt my heart; stones, shells, a pin, a button, a crystal, a feather.

The third image is a peek into my indoor garden, where plants make each room feel sacred. I have over 100 potted plants in my home, and my outdoor flower and herb garden is wild and wonderful in its own right. Inside it feels fresh and alive with life flowing from wall sconces, draping over shelves and spilling over tables. It is especially charming in the winter. And each plant has a personality of its own and unique needs. My relationship to each one is a practice in tending my own internal garden.

Ultimately, to have an altar, you don't need objects and details. This is an image of my Yoga mat; simplicity is *always* my most sacred altar. This is a simple space for me and my deep holistic embodiment and worship of Living.

I sing mantra, pray, and ring bells as I walk around the perimeter of my home's small piece of land. Sometimes I drum, sometimes I hold incense, and often I spread tobacco in the spirit of honoring gratitude and remembrance, calling in protections and blessings. (When I lived in apartments, I would walk around the block, same as I would sacred ground, in full gratitude and blessings for the souls that I shared the special space with.) And always, I connect to the trees, as they are our guardians.

Remember, an altar is simply a tool to connect you to your Heart Space through unabashed Intention. Have your inspirational teachers but know that YOU must be your own Guru. Your true altar is your own Heart. *Blessings on your altar creation!*

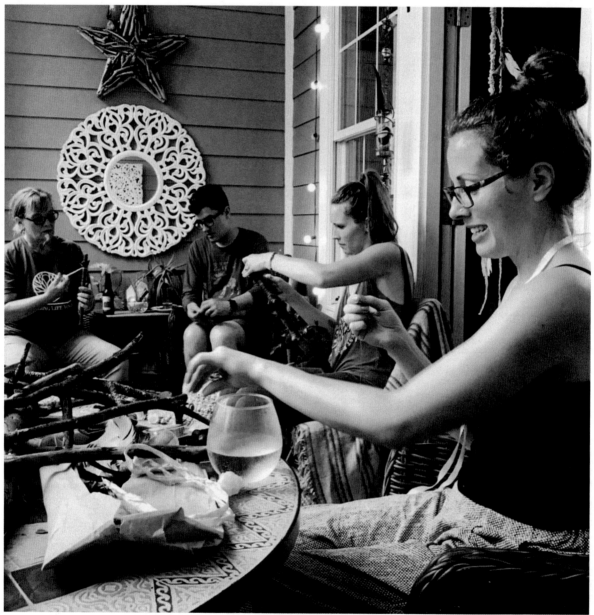

Sacred Space

Sacred Spaces

i am a safe landing for others

i embody

presence
clear of judgement

connection
over competition

support
without expectation

when i hold this space for someone
i send them the message that they matter
just as they are

my heart serves as an invitation
for others to show up + share
their brightest, most authentic light

what a gift i give to the world
when i choose to remain open

~ Danielle Doby, *I Am Her Tribe*

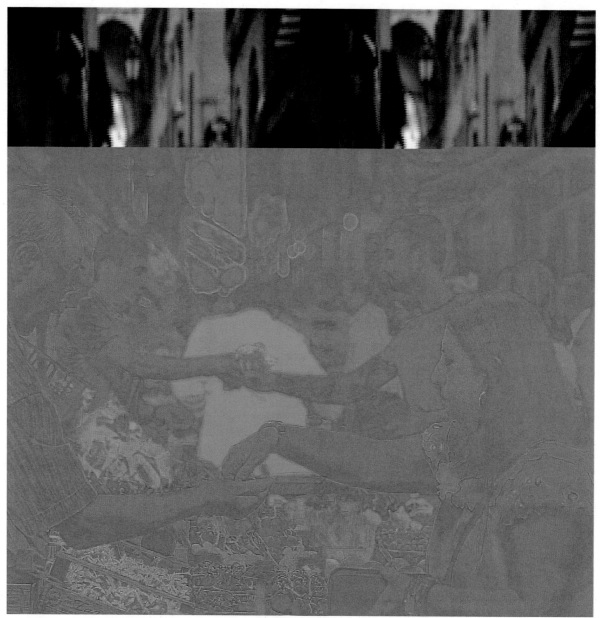

Energy Exchange

Food Relationships and Interconnectedness

Remember that food is the most basic link with the source of life. Be thankful for it, pray over it, honor it. We are not just filling our belly; we are nurturing our mind and spirit as well. Eating with full awareness puts us in harmony with nature - not only with the external world, but also our own inner nature.

~ Carrie Angus

For Whom and When

People are collectively fascinated by the food choice of others. There are personal criticisms and political labels associated with food choice, and people find personal identity by what they put on their plate. Many people assume that yogis are vegetarians, per the *Yoga Sutra's* concept of *Ahimsa*. *Ahimsa* means non-harming and speaks to this assumption. When it comes to food choice, however, you must always consider to whom and when.

Individual body types, ever-changing seasons of people's lives, cultural and religious norms, food availability, among innumerable other factors contribute to the access and the belief systems about food. It is important to note that countless people struggle daily with their body image. Many teens I work with suffer from eating disorders, which I can relate to as I also experienced bulimia. I have often witnessed dangerous food shaming of others from many people who claim they practice Yoga. Also, people may mask eating disorders claiming they eat a yogic diet.

What is a Yogic diet? That is up to you, but I believe it is simply being acutely aware of what is being put in the body. That said, choosing a vegetarian diet is yogic, as the meat industry is one of the planet's leading causes of greenhouse gasses. Not shying away from the facts regarding the raising of animals, separation of babies and their mothers, and inhumane death-procedures a part of factual truths, and truth is Yoga. Knowing the truth about food sources and altering how you always eat is the Practice of Awareness, which may invoke you to change your choices. *Once you know, you know.*

My friend invited me to dinner. "I know you are vegetarian, so I made chicken!" I was initially shocked that my brilliant friend didn't understand what comprised a vegetarian's diet, but I accepted her meal with gratitude. To this day, family and friends make me special meals with meat. When I'm in another country and invited into a student's home for a meal, I never insult their generosity and expression of connection. The energy of gratitude is a balm and blessing for all, regardless of what's on our plates at mealtime.

You will never become spiritually advanced in your food choice. You will never become spiritually advanced by denying yourself joy or occasional splurging. You will never become spiritually advanced by criticizing or shaming others on what they choose for themselves. Ultimately, it is necessary to witness your personal judgments regarding another's plate. I encourage you to honor the needs of your body, and to honor how those needs change.

Creating Space to Eat

You are in a culture of dis-ease regarding time use. (*"If I'm not stressed, I'm not working hard enough." Sound familiar?*) People rush from one event to the next, and for many, the art of food preparation is often reserved to only be received in higher-end restaurants. People eat in a distracted state of mind. Food is swallowed on-the-go in cars, in front of televisions and computer screens, and thawed within minutes in the microwave. We have become disconnected not only from the efforts of those who grew our food, but also from where the food was grown and how it was handled to finally reach you. In this disconnect, we separate ourselves from others.

Greater satisfaction and holistic nourishment can be had by simply holding space with our food. Many people often enjoy the beautiful ritual of prayer before meals, or simply holding hands and breathing deeply together. No matter how the food ritual takes place, the intention blesses the energetic qualities of the food and honors the shared space with others and yourself. Even if you appreciate the colors and textures before you, no matter how simple or for how long, you will more easily be able to recognize the often-complex interconnection that occurred to bring that food to your plate.

Food Trends

Numerous focus groups in the wide-ranging food industry examine endless food combinations. Food trends that develop have their educational place, but they can also be very dangerous. Again, consider the Ayurvedic mantra *for whom and when*.

One of my Yoga-friends has a *high vata dosha* (a concept which will be explored later in the book), expressed as being hyper-busy, prone to hypertension, nervousness, restlessness, and chronic digestive issues, which requires mostly warm and heavier foods to balance and ground holistic energy. This friend attempted to be sustained by juicing for 30-days, ignoring Ayurvedic wisdom. In this short timeframe, her mental awareness and physical body were greatly damaged for months to come. She was in two car accidents, forgot to complete basic daily routines, experienced great confusion with simple tasks, was not functional at her job, lost partial vision, disrupted her digestion, and lost tremendous muscle mass. Her ego was very proud in completing this 30-day juicing challenge, yet she chose not to recognize the damaging after-effects until a year later when she could no longer ignore these results. Recovery is unique to the individual, yet it took her months to feel 'back to normal' after reintroducing proper food into her system, and only then did she question her choice to fast only on cold juice for 30 days.

Choice

Ultimately, we live in an age where many countries are blessed to have access to various food options. In turn, there is growing awareness around ever-changing lifestyle choices and emerging food allergies. Some folks are lactose and gluten sensitive. Vegans are people who consciously choose not to ingest any animal product, including honey, milk, yeast, and eggs. Vegetarians are people who consciously choose not to eat animal flesh, including chicken or fish. Pescatarians are people who have fish as their only meat source. Omnivores are people who choose to eat a variety of meat and dairy, along with a spectrum of grains and vegetables. As an individual, you are often in flux with what feels right for you emotionally and physically, and your food choices reflect that.

NOTE: The chapter *Classical Yoga: Sacred Truths, Sacred Promises* offers a Yoga Meal Awareness Practice that is a loving, enriching way to approach food. Your entire family may enjoy the practice!

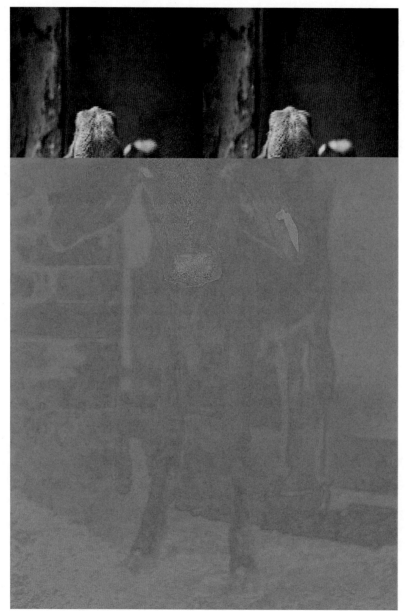

Mirror of My Heart (Rishikesh, India)

Awareness Practice of Presence and Gratitude

Allow food to be a feast for your senses.
This is a meditation to ground you in the moment.

- *Am I distracted from what is before me?*

- *Is my plate created with intention and artistry?*

- *What palate of colors lie before me?*

- *What smells can be individually distinguished and what unified melody is created?*

- *Can I taste the sunshine in this fruit?*

- *Can I feel the energetic health of the soil in which it grew?*

- *Does my food feel that it was loved and honored in its lifetime?*

- *What range of textures unfold as flavors are released in my mouth?*

- *How does this food make me feel emotionally?*

- *Do I feel expanded or constricted when I take this bite?*

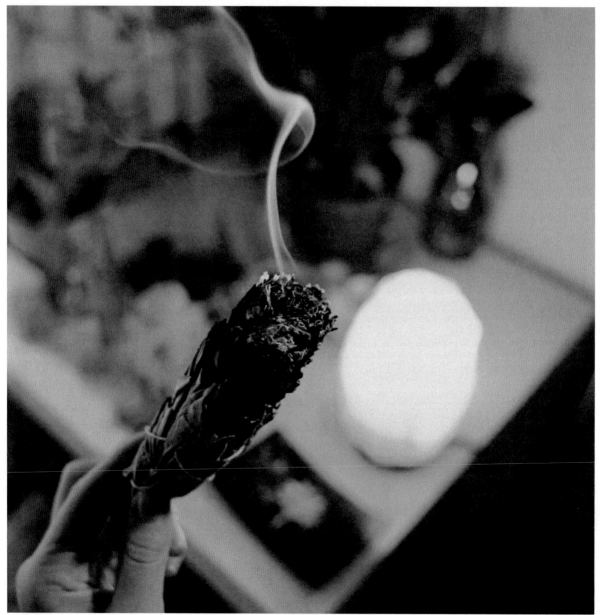

Yoga Off the Mat

Reflection and Discussion

Yoga off the Mat ~ Creating Sacred Space

1) Identify labels in your own life. What label is the most constrictive to yourself and to others? What can you do to dissolve this label?

2) What are benefits of having a sacred space?

3) Many people believe Yoga practitioners are vegetarian. Where does this notion come from? And can you benefit yourself and others by examining your personal relationship and choice to food?

4) **FOR PERSONAL REFLECTION** - Consider the following:

   ❖ Are there rooms or spaces you avoid? Why?

   ❖ If a living area feels neglected, how can you bring beauty and coziness to that space? Consider bringing in plants, art, candles, salt lamps, water features, music, textiles, etc.

   ❖ Does this space energetically change with the seasons?

   ❖ All things wish to be in service. Are there are objects that no longer bring joy or don't have a purpose? Consider donating these objects so another person can find joy and use in them.

   ❖ How often do you clean your space and what intention do you have when you do so? How often do you organize your drawers and cupboards?

   ❖ How do you bring ceremony to bless both the internal and external space of your home?

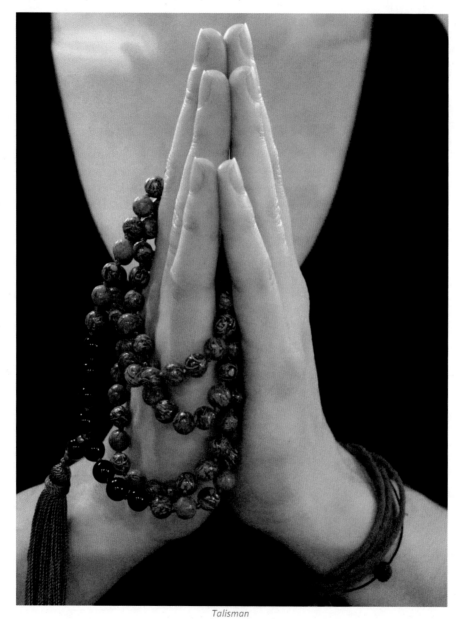

Talisman
(An object marked with some sort of religious or magical powers thought to offer protection and healing to the person in possession of it.)

Chapter 2

Embodiment Tools:

Meditation, Mantra, Mala, Mudra

By this constant intake of spiritual ideas through daily study, gradually there comes about a process of mind-transformation. The old mind is gradually eliminated and a new mind is created within you, a new mind which always thinks spiritually, which always is in a state of awareness.

~ Swami Chidananda Saraswati

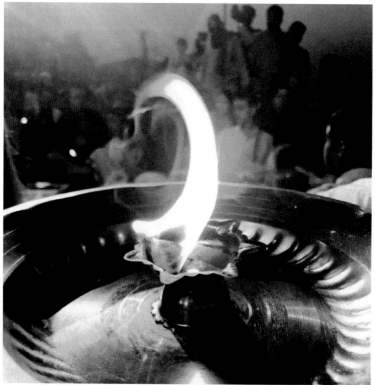

Rishikesh Puja

Chapter 2
Embodiment Tools:

Meditation, Mantra, Mala, Mudra

1. Overview

Chapter 2 introduces embodiment tools: *meditations, mantras, malas,* and *mudras.* By developing an understanding of how to use each tool, the foundation is created for a Yoga practice. Various meditation practices, how to use a yantra, the power of mantras and different Vedic prayers, a mala practice and mudras are discussed.

2. Learning Objectives: I will...

a) Explore various meditation practices
b) Familiarize myself with different traditional mantras
c) Understand meaning behind Vedic prayers
d) Learn about mala and mudra practices to elevate my meditation practice

3. Pre-lecture Assignments

a) Read the chapter and become familiar with the Reflection questions
b) Begin Daily Sadhana - Daily Personal Practice

4. Reflection: *found at the end of the chapter*

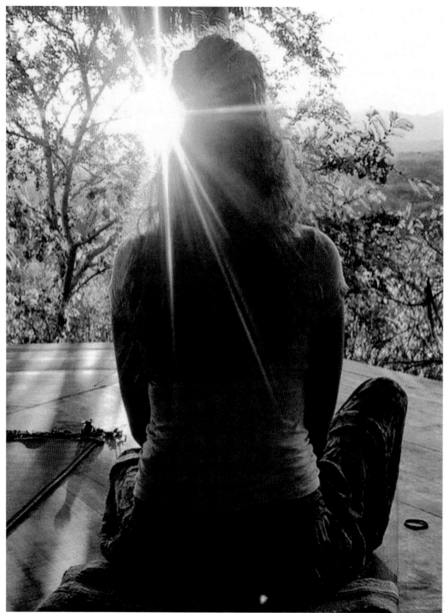

Within, Beyond (Sayulita, Mexico)

Sadhana: Your Dedicated Practice

Do your practice and all is coming. ~ Sri Pattabhi Jois

The practice of Yoga takes discipline, which is called *tapas*. Beginning something new takes tapas-in-action (tapas = dedication), until the mind starts to change. The mind is not going to change automatically, but over time and with dedication, the nature of the mind does change, and you begin to look forward to practicing. This practice is your *sadhana*. Sadhana supports spirit/feeling/interconnection rather than mind/body/ego.

Sadhana is a Sanskrit term meaning a dedicated, disciplined spiritual practice. The practice of Yoga is to keep the mind fixed without desire, attachment, interruption, or expectation of results. Recognizing the fluctuations of the mind and analyzing what causes the undercurrents of these mental waves is a practice within itself. Sadhana is primarily a mental practice that looks like a dedicated asana and meditation practice … for example, the energy put into crafting your own sacred space. It's the dedication of intention-in-action.

Philosophically, connection to the Divine manifests in a mind that holds focus. This is the state of non-doing, called *Nirodhah* meaning cessation or suspension. Here, the still lake of the soul is reflected in the mind, as the mind's waves have stilled to see its own true nature.

All sadhana practices require effort to keep the mind fixed. Because our nature is to allow the mind free reign, and because it requires dedication and concentration to achieve this state of "fixed" consciousness, it could take lifetimes to achieve. On the other hand, it could happen at any moment, even if only for a brief period.

Sadhana offers a path to deep and discerning spiritual development, enhancing all aspects of living, perceptions, and engagements of reality. Being at the heart of the Yoga Tradition, sadhana is a mirror reflecting the integrity and mastery of one's internal thoughts and life experiences. Sadhana amplifies what is aligned and at ease in daily life, as well as highlights what is out of alignment and in dis-ease. The courage to reflect and change is gained through sadhana. But a disciplined, continuous practice of Yoga is key. A teacher of mine once said that when he retires from lecturing about Yoga, he will continue writing about the Yoga tradition - "That will be my sadhana."

An important aspect of sadhana is to question yourself. To experience the dark night of the soul is healthy. It's healthy to have doubts about that which you have not experienced yet; to tear apart and put things back together based on self-exploration and a more stable understanding. If you don't have doubts every so often, you become rigid in your perceptions and beliefs. Ultimately, this rigidity may cause you to become incapable of change, and you may become a fanatic. A fanatic is someone who doesn't want to hear anything that could shake their whole support system.

I've had the honor to see His Holiness the 14th Dalai Lama on four occasions in Washington, D.C. and Indianapolis, Indiana. During one talk, he shared a glimpse into the dark night of his soul. Thick in his dharmic role as the Dalai Lama, he questioned the legitimacy of Buddhism as a whole. He questioned himself and his belief systems. For years, he inquired deep into these recesses and once-blind spots of his atman. This was his Hero's Journey. The Dalai Lama emerged from this dark night more aligned, having moved knowledge-concepts into deep soul-understandings.

Embodiment

While sadhana focuses on the mental body, *embodiment practices* invite you to explore the universe of your physical body. Here, the notion of truth itself can be physically felt within the body, often with the sensations of expansion and contraction. These sensations help you navigate the journey of life. Focusing on, honing, and refining these sensations is also a practice.

Embodiment is honoring the actual *feeling of* what is true for the Self within the physical form and tapping into the wisdom/intuition within the very tissues of the body. Here, the notion of truth itself can be physically felt within the body.

Often, the sensations of *expansion and contraction* are words describing feelings which navigate the journey of life. *Where* you feel these energies moving (or not) in the body can provide important messages. For example, you may feel that your heart is "overflowing", or you may feel a "knot" in the pit of your stomach. These sensations offer the opportunity to lean-in and explore the messages the body is sending, without necessarily being filtered by lenses of the mind. "Why do I feel this way? Have I felt this feeling before? Am I in the energy of *love or fear*? What is the message/truth of this feeling?"

In the self-exploration below, breathe into those expanded/constricted spaces to anchor what is being revealed, consciously or subconsciously.

Ask yourself:

Where do I feel this energy land in my body?
Am I stuck in a story to justify keeping this energy here?

What tools do I have to make the energy flow again?
Am I listening to my heart or my head?

Embodiment practices such as breathing, moving, and meditating can reveal great wisdoms which support an aligned life. Asana, meditation, scriptural study, or *japa*/chanting practices can both balance and enhance your energies. When I teach asana, I often say, "Find eternity in this fleeting moment." Be the one who is breathing. Be the One who is witnessing the breather. Be the breath inside the body. In an asana pose, as in life, all things are fleeting. And it takes dedication and a life-long practice to refine and embody these tools.

Sadhana enhances the relationship of yourself to your Self. Your embodiment practice enhances your spiritual development as well as connects/reconnects you to your body. The purpose of Yoga is to be aware of being aware. Yoga is to be consciously present in the moment. Yoga is how you *show up*.

Sankulpa

A *Sankulpa* is an *intention*. A Sankulpa is the surrender to the present moment by engaging with this universal intention that reflects the nobility of humanity – peace, love, truth, generosity, compassion, kindness, grace, interconnection, among others. These are innate qualities, yet veils of illusion take you from these natural states of being.

The opposite of Sankulpa is *Vikalpa*. Attachment, clinging, fear, and false perception, among others, represent the qualities of Vikalpa. This is the illusion that makes you feel out of control and separate from others. Vikalpa questions truth and intuition and looks outside for answers. This is also responsible for keeping the parasympathetic nervous system in Fight of Flight mode.

Cultivate a relationship with a single Sankulpa with disciplined focus and depth, rather than having various intentions, which can be energetically wide and shallow and ultimately ineffective. If you focus on a single intention for a long time with an open heart, the results will be woven throughout all aspects of your life. A long, uninterrupted time that could be years. Don't become attached to results. In other words, focus on the intention, and the intention will become your reality.

Mantra is a beautiful, powerful tool to use as a Sankulpa. Affirmations are Sankulpas, too.

Approach your Sankulpa with feeling into the intention; feeling as if the intention has already been revealed.

- *What does it physically feel like?*
- *Where do you feel it in your body?*
- *Can you 'stoke' this feeling with breath and mantra?*

The practice of Sankulpa is a tool to recognize and claim your innate, unique potential. Don't lose sight of the actual embodied feeling. Remember, the Seeker and the Sought are the same. You craft your new reality with a Sankulpa.

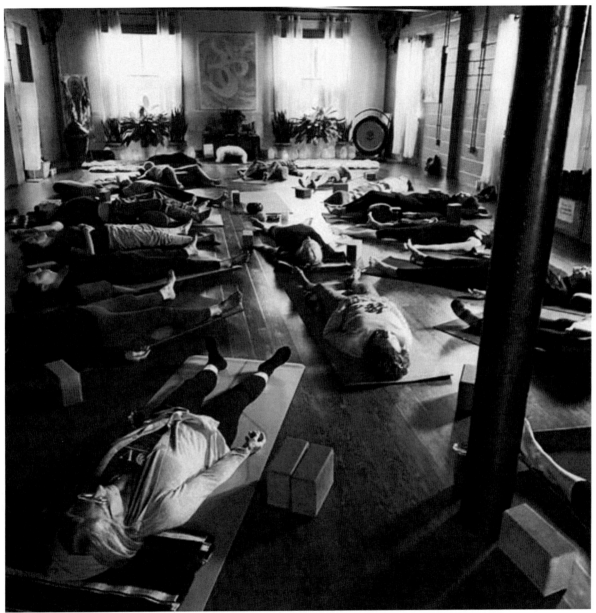

Sadhana

Show Up

**How you show up for the Practice is reflected
in how the Practice shows up for you.**

How do you show up for your art?
How do you show up for your canvas?
How do you show up for your writing?
How do you show up for your instrument?
How do you show up for your honesty?
How do you show up for your relationships?
How do you show up for yourself?

The practice of Yoga frees the mind of desire. Desire is the major undercurrent that gives rise to distracting thought waves. To emphasize this point, 100 of the 700 verses in the *Bhagavad Gita* say to give up desire, which is rooted in *raga* - passion and ignorance. The very nature of desire is always wanting, needing, attaching, grasping.

How is the mind freed from desire? The practice of Yoga is to keep the mind fixed, and thus free from desire. Within a few weeks, the practice of asana can bear the fruit of both physical and mental benefits. When you practice asana, you focus your mind on the body and the breath – on the present moment. The practice of meditation is another, and perhaps the best, means of freeing yourself from desire. For most, developing a meditation practice can take time, perhaps many lifetimes. As you initially begin your practice, know there is nothing mystical or magical about it. It simply takes focused discipline. You must simply begin. And as you continue the practice without interruption, it gets easier, and the results become easier to ascertain.

There is overwhelming data documenting and celebrating the physical and psychological benefits of meditation, including helping you navigate the stresses and anxieties of living in today's often frantic world. This culture demands immediate results, both as a consumer and as a contributor within it. The practice of meditation offers a counter-energy to this cultural pattern. The practice requires patience, dedication, and non-attachment, all of which allow you to focus and explore your internal universe and your connection to Divinity.

The Yoga tradition honors *samsara*, the karmic cycle of life and death of the everlasting atman. As part of this process, you have likely already lived countless lifetimes, and are likely to live many more. To be a human being offers a very special opportunity to clear karmic ties and experience various levels of consciousness. Sadhana allows you to understand that, ultimately, consciousness is simply being conscious of your consciousness. Asana and meditation can help you achieve this understanding. Otherwise, you may have lifetimes of unfulfilled desires and your mind spinning without self-mastery!

How you do one thing is how you do everything. In the Yoga tradition, where the mind is focused at the moment of death dictates how you will be born into your next incarnation. Which means that, with the practice of Yoga, you can better prepare for the moment you leave the Earth (this time around). When Gandhi was assassinated, for example, he looked into the eyes of his assassin while blessing him, chanting a name of god (*Ram)*, as he died. Gandhi's mind was focused and aligned, even amid confusion, a reflection of his life-long practice and heart.

Even if one performs no other rituals or actions,
leaving aside what is commanded
according to one's social estate and stage of life,
the one who dwells within the Heart is a vessel
of enjoyment and liberation, O Goddess of the Heart.

~ 2.50 Kularnava Tantra

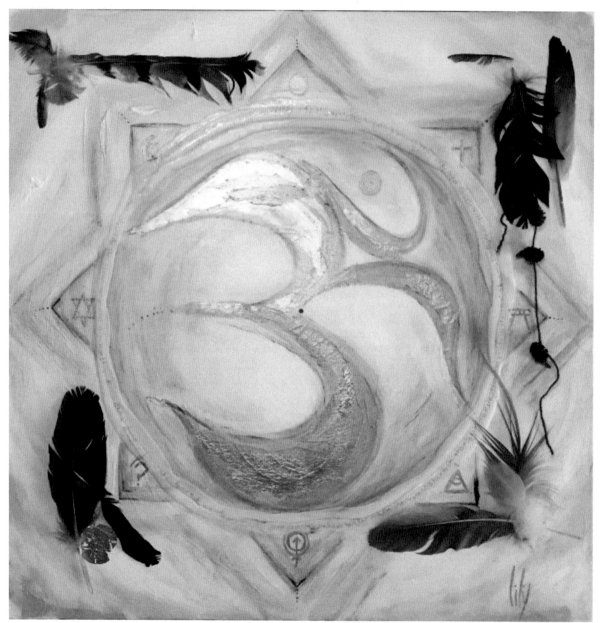

Yantra Om Shanti, painting by Lily Kessler

The Om

Tat Tvam Asi, You are That

"My first night in my apartment in New York City changed my life forever. I laid on my new bed in my new home starting a new life. Having lived in the suburbs, I wasn't use to the continual sounds of the city. I heard my neighbors on all sides, music from the shops on the street, the honking and moving of cars, and it all felt surreal. I began to feel small and out of place. So I used my Yoga tools to realign. As I entered meditation, the mix of sounds around me swelled into the deep and soothing tone of OM. And from that moment on, I learned to allow individual sounds to simply wash over me, yet I could always relish expanding my awareness and drinking in the collection of sounds that symbiotically create the OM. I now profoundly understood that no matter where I go in the world, I am always at home. I am a part of the river of life around me and have fallen madly in love with it all." ~ Justin B.

Everything is energy.

Energy is vibration.

The human body is comprised of compressed energies of light and sound.

The motivating force behind the creation of the Universe (God, Oneness, the Big Bang) resulted in the original sound vibration – the sound of *Om*. Now, the unified collection of all sounds and vibrations within the universe are all part of that transcendent Om. For thousands of years, this powerful, grounding, and aligning tone has enlivened the mind, body, and soul/atman of people within both ancient and modern cultures. It is a tone that enhances all areas of life – it connects you to the present moment and to the universal source of consciousness. Chanting the sacred sound of Om is a foundational practice in the Yoga Tradition.

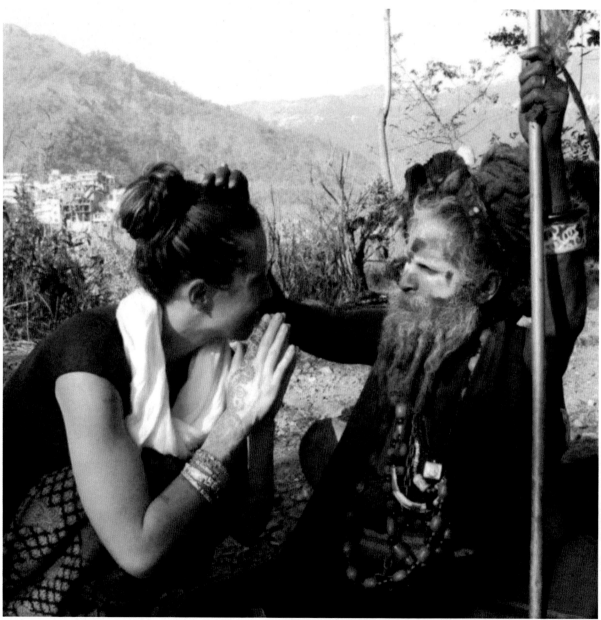

Om is Home

Chandogya Upanishad 1-13,

First Describes Om:

Let us meditate on Om the imperishable, the beginning of prayer.

For as the earth comes from the waters, plants from earth, and man from plants, so man is speech, and speech is Om. Of all speech the essence is the Rig Veda; but Sama is the essence of Rig, and of Sama the essence is OM, the Udgitha.

This is the essence of essences, the highest, the eighth rung, venerated above all that human beings hold holy. Om is the Self of all.

What is rig, what is sama, at the heart of prayer? As rig is speech, so sama is song, and the imperishable Om is the Udgitha. Speech and breath, Sama and Rig, are couples, and the imperishable Om they come together to fulfill each other's desire. For those who, knowing this, meditate on the imperishable Om, all desires are fulfilled. With the word Om we say, "I agree," and fulfill desires. With Om we recite, we give direction, we sing aloud the honor of that Word, the key to the three kinds of knowledge.

Side by side, those who know the Self (and those who know it not) appear to do the same thing; but it is not the same. The act done with knowledge, with inner awareness and faith, grows in power. That, in a word, tells the significance of OM, the indivisible.

~ Chandogya Upanishad

Om As Your Innermost Self

Om is the consciousness that pervades and sustains the entire universe, including your inner most Self. When you chant Om, sink your mind into the mantra of Om without too much thought. Know that Om is not a personal deity but can be associated with one. If you have a strong relationship with a personal deity, you can take the Om and expand it into another mantra including your favorite deity.

The *O* and the *M* have vibrational frequencies that enliven various energetic bandwidths of information that are found within your physical body, your mental body, and your emotional body, opening you to higher perspectives. Chanting Om specifically channels powerful vibrations through the body's holistic systems and is considered medicinal. This nurturing frequency awakens layers of consciousness, as well as activating parts of the body on a cellular level. Chanting stimulates the thinking mind, allowing you to become open to all possibility, where you can more easily flow in the moment with life, aligned and interconnected with all.

Chanting Om means saying YES.

YES to this life, YES to this body, YES to this universe.

Om is about wanting and embracing your life, not someone else's.

O - Reach out

This is the expanded energy field. Toning 'O' resonates with Universal, infinite vibrations. Offer this tone from the solar plexus/belly and imagine yourself casting a net of stars into the cosmos, reaching out with your consciousness as far as it can go in a every direction. Be strong in the spine and soft in the body with eyes closed and gently rolled up to your third eye, heart open, relaxed jaw, relaxed shoulders, relaxed belly, and relaxed hips. The more the system is relaxed, the more sensations can be experienced as the tone courses and emanates throughout the entire body.

With the mind's eye, reach outward into the vast possibility of the universe and gather attributes such as freedom, ease, and courage. Physically *feel* these attributes within the body with the knowingness that they are innately yours to recognize as a part of your wholeness. This refined vibration restructures the energetic shape of the five layers of the body, known as *Koshas*, which we'll explore later. They comprise your energetic, emotional, mental, wisdom, and bliss bodies.

M - Drop in

This is the contracting energy field. Toning 'M' harnesses spherical expansiveness into a single point of consciousness at the upper roof of the mouth. These vibrations stimulate the seat of consciousness in center of the brain – the Pineal gland, the Cave of Brahma, the Third Eye. The 'M' also roots you to the eternal, yet always present, physical moment. When toning 'M' imagine yourself pulling your net of stars, your intentions, back into reality-actualized. It feels nice to experience enlivening vibrations within the upper pallet, teeth, and crown.

AUM

Another Form of Om, of Connecting

Each tone shows up, energetically, as a different shape within the mind and body. The sacred sound of Aum honors the three aspects of existence. Three tones create a unitive, whole, harmonized brain.

Ah - Creation

Expand toward Universal Consciousness; the Unified Field; from the base of the spine to the navel, correlating to the brain stem.

Uu - That Which Pervades

Compresses the Unified Field into a channel; from navel to throat, correlating to the limbic system.

Mm - Transformation

Anchors the Unified Field into an individual expression of consciousness; from throat to crown, correlating to the neocortex.

Naturally incorporate these empowering, healing and grounding tones of Om/Aum into your daily life to experience revelations of your unique, infinite nature and interconnection with all life. The Om supports you in being the steward of your life. It allows your state of mind to move from a defensive *Fight or Flight* mode (associated with the protective personality) to that of high wisdom, larger perspectives, and creative presence.

Vibrations, in all their various forms, are the building blocks of reality. By tapping into these vibrational energies, you can learn to develop a powerful embodiment practice. This embodiment practice is based on awareness of the different states of energy affecting your physical body, emotions, thoughts, etc.

Ask yourself - *Where do I "feel" these energies in my body? What vibration am I emitting? Are there parts of my body that are more activated than others? Am I vibrating in the energy of Love or Fear?*

How you vibrate attracts similar/like vibrations which support both the trajectory of your own life as well as the energetic trajectory of the universe. As a conscious human being, you must be responsible for the course of your energetic trajectory to support the greater good of all beings. Your breath and your chanting of the sacred sound of Om are the greatest tools you have to recalibrate your experience of your present reality.

Tone Om repeatedly, allowing its vibrations to permeate your body, breathe and mind, and allow your levels of consciousness to link with your eternal Self. Tone while driving in the car, while in the shower, while cleaning your home, while gardening, etc. Begin toning when you are feeling out of alignment for any reason, including feeling overwhelmed, angry, sad, or stricken by grief. Also invoke the sacred tone of Om/Aum when you are feeling expanded with the energy of celebration, of honoring, of connection.

Om is a contemplation, yet it constitutes the workings of the physical, mental, emotional, and spiritual realms. Om is the very vibration of life-interconnected, from the microcosm to the macrocosm. Om is the threshold, the door, and the multiverse. Om is empty with everything. You can feel and experience the Unity-Consciousness of Om through the gifts of mantra and meditation.

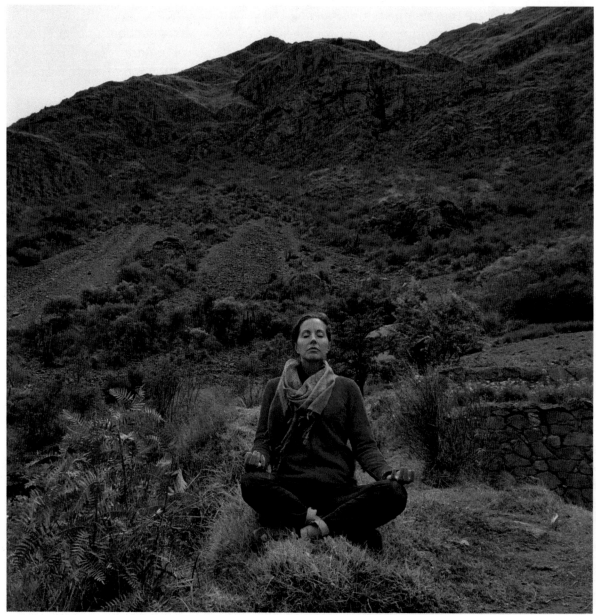

Home From Home

Meditation 101

What is consciousness? This topic is tremendously vast and mysterious, as neuroscientists don't understand the neural basis of consciousness. Ironically, when studying the brain, it is studied from the confines of the brain itself. In the Vedic Tradition in which Yoga was born, philosophers, scientists, and mystics merged insights, discoveries, experiences, and knowledge into realms of possibility beyond what the brain could comprehend. In this, meditation itself is a foundation of the Yoga Tradition.

There are hundreds of meditation techniques comprised of various philosophical backgrounds. The Yoga you are exploring in this book is based on Vedic traditions and is infused with Universal principles.

Meditation can tap you into your essential nature and allow expansion. Just as you don't expect your breathing to stop functioning while meditating, you may not expect that your mind will stop functioning during meditation. Absolutely expect that distracting thoughts and stories will arise during your practice – accept these without judgement. Once you acknowledge the thought and then let go of it, ease arises. Perhaps incorporate your mantra, then simply enjoy the space the meditation allows.

Remember, the human mind is always streaming with thoughts. Personally, I think of sparkling water in a glass. One bubble pops on the surface while more arise, again and again. No surprise! Train your mind to become the Witness of these thoughts and remain curious for what is next without attachment. Your initial focus is to not enter any *story*, and simply feel any emotion as needing to be expressed so it can be released.

Always let arising energies flow while you relax your mind until there is no more *story*. Just the inhale and exhale. Then allow that awareness to relax you into the presence of pure existence. If you touch it, even for a moment, land the feeling into the core of your body.

As with everything in Yoga, there is the concept of Both/And. If your mind and emotions become fixated within a story, you may simply need to be with *what is coming up for you*, without trying to stop it. So allow yourself to drill deep within the story and sit with whatever arises for you.

How to Sit

Feel into your body and let it feel *Good.*

Within traditional meditations there is an important and specific posture that must be engaged. The crown, shoulders, spine, and hips must be aligned.

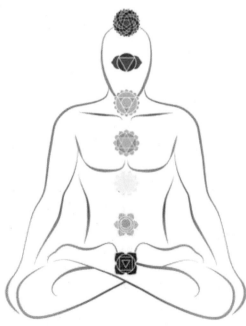

Crown Chakra

Third Eye Chakra

Throat Chakra

Heart Chakra

Solar Plexus Chakra

Sacral Chakra

Root Chakra

Sitting: The WHY At-A-Glance

Alignment of the body allows the chakra system to communicate, and as a result, higher states of consciousness can be had.

From an energetic stand-point, here is a glimpse into the internal communications that the body is comprised of, which the ancient Yogis personally harnessed and then codified. PLEASE NOTE, these topics will be further explored in the book.

The chakras are the gateways to levels of consciousness. The six chakras within/beyond your body are connecting to your crown chakra, which is Interconnection with All. In this, you are linking your Root to the Earth, the Earth to the Crown, which runs along, within, and beyond the spinal system. This is called the Central Channel. The Central Channel is the center of what is called your toroidal field. Every living creature has a toroidal field. This donut-shaped magnetic field of energy dictates your physical health and the very experience of your reality itself.

Your toroidal field is a collection of your pranic energies which are comprised of the quality of your thoughts, the atmosphere of your living situations, the stories you tell yourself, the quality of your food, water, and air, the depth of your understanding of your interconnection with all life, and your relationship with the natural world - just to name a few.

Meditation brings quality and deep, restorative nourishment to each of these aspects. Meditation tunes you in, so to speak.

Meditation is a practice comprised of entering and exiting multitudes of various states of consciousness and experiences.

Sitting: The HOW At-A-Glance

The body is a tool for cosmic transcendence. This is not a New Age concept, but is the oldest examination in human history.

In meditation, you are both relaxed and engaged. The more you 'sit' the more you'll experience how your body strengthens and adjusts to welcome the practice within your daily life. Starting a meditation practice takes both *Sadhana*, disciplined practice, built upon a *Sankulpa*, an intention.

- ❖ **Lift your crown** and **lengthen your spine.** Visualize and feel your Crown over your Root.
- ❖ **Neck muscles slightly *pull-back*,** to balance **head over the shoulders.**
- ❖ **Chin is parallel** to the floor, with a relaxed jaw, and face. Feel lips soften and forehead spread.
- ❖ **Tongue-tip** is resting upwards behind the front teeth. Teeth never touch.
- ❖ A very slight **smile relaxes the body** and allows for deeper breathing.
- ❖ **Shoulders find rest** by lifting them to the ears and rolling them down the back, opening the heart space. Now relax the shoulders while keeping the **heart space broadened.**
- ❖ **Relax arms** with palms in the lap, or **palms resting** facing upward or downward toward knees.
- ❖ Internally lift muscles to **engage the pelvic floor**; this engages the core through the heart space, toning the physical areas of the Central Channel while rooting you to the present moment. Simultaneously, **this enlivens the heart space** and **opens the throat.**
- ❖ Behind closed eyes, **slightly lift the eyes** to the horizon of an imaginary mountain range without straining or crossing the eyes.
- ❖ **Breathe.** Let your belly take up space with each breath, soft, relaxed, and accepting.
- ❖ Behind the **softness of the belly**, feel the **strength of your core** which is always in the continual process of reestablishing physical alignment while you meditate.

Lift your spine. Soften your body. Deep breathe. All is Well.

Meditation 'Sit' Options

For many of these practices, it is traditional to sit in an easy, comfortable pose on a cushion, on the floor, in a cross-legged position. However, sitting for long periods of time, even a short time, is very uncomfortable for many people, including myself. The bodies within Western cultures are not used to squatting. Purposely sitting in physical discomfort with the intention to meditate is not Yoga. Comfort is encouraged.

The Floor

❖ First, consider placing a blanket beneath you to offer additional comfort to ankles and feet.

❖ The focus is to lengthen the spine and relax the legs. Bring height to your hips by sitting on a Zafu meditation cushion (often made of buckwheat), to relieve pressure on your knees, ankles, and spine, and promote proper alignment. A folded blanket, rolled Yoga mat, Yoga block, Yoga bolster, and towel are also great options.

❖ For additional knee support, place folded blankets or pillows underneath them.

❖ Assume proper posture. Consider sitting with your shoulders blades slightly touching a wall.

The Chair

❖ You may also practice meditation in a chair with your feet rooted on the floor, ideally without using back support.

❖ It is important to have your feet flat on the floor. Take off your shoes to connect to the Earth's energy. If your feet don't reach the floor, consider placing a Yoga block under your feet.

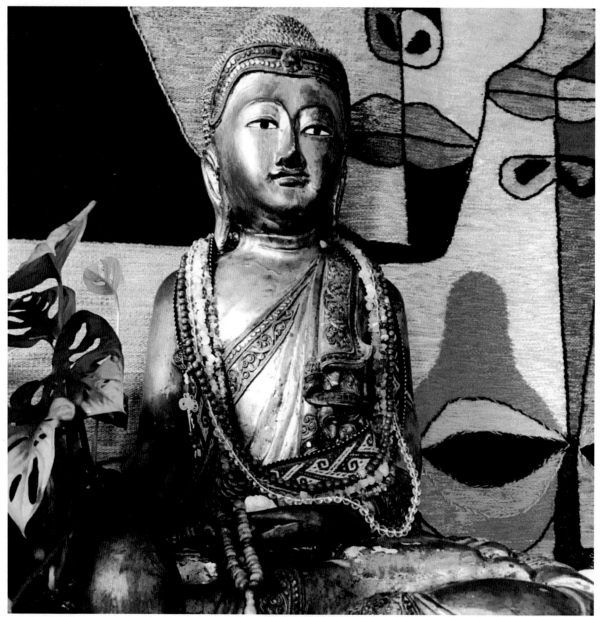

Innate Essence – a home altar

Now Practice the Art of Sitting

- ❖ Considering the suggestions given, sit on a floor cushion, or in a chair.

- ❖ Find comfort with your hands and arms in a position of your choice.

- ❖ Your palms may rest on or near your knees.

- ❖ Palm may face downward for *grounding*, or rest upward for *receptivity*.

- ❖ Sit strong in the spine and soft in the body, slightly tucking your chin to be parallel to the floor to align your crown over your heart and your heart over your hips.

- ❖ Relax your shoulders and elbows.

- ❖ Breathe. Feel breath swell into your body. This *breath of life* is pure prana. It is the source of your life, your energy, and perhaps the very Consciousness of Your Being, *It-Self*.

Other meditations, more appropriately called *concentrated attention* or *reflective awareness activities,* may be practiced while walking, doing dishes, eating, or as part of your other daily activities.

Now that you know how to sit comfortably,
you will be introduced to meditation experiences.

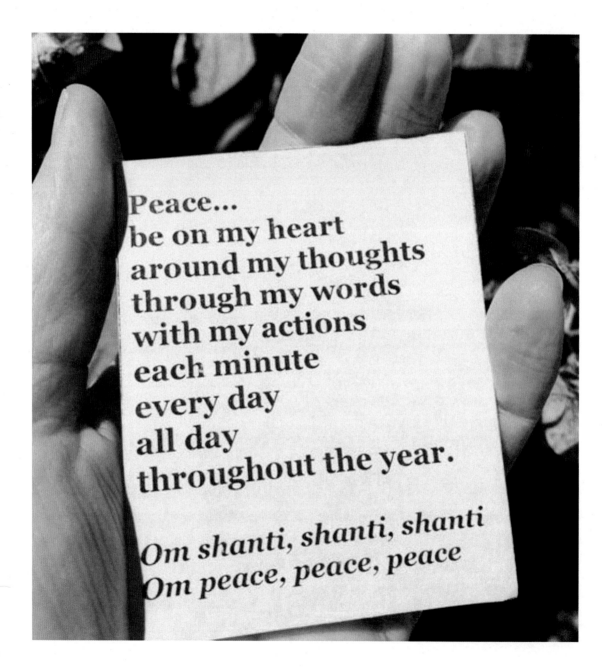

The 3 Categories of Traditional Meditation

Expansive Meditations

(I offer guided Expansive Meditations at the beginning of my classes. Initially, people's energies are scattered from the day's events and to-do lists.) This meditation is the entry point to collect 'parts and pieces' through breath, and is the doorway to deepen meditation further. Allow yourself to embrace your entire internal and external environment. Welcome all sensory perceptions of sound, texture, thought, emotions, smell, etc. The point is to see how these experiences are fleeting and how non-reactive you can be, while harnessing your breath and awareness to the moment.

This meditation strengthens the Witness Self.

Single Focus Meditations

After you settle with Expansive Meditation, focus your attention on one single object. Consider an external object in the form of a yantra, breath, one thought, a body part, a chakra center, a mantra, etc. Flow your attention directly into that chosen form and let all other distractions become silent.

This meditation strengthens the steadiness of attention.

Effortless Being Meditations

Effortless Being is also called Choiceless Awareness. *So Hum* – I am That. *Sat Nam* – Sitting within your *Self*. You begin to dissolve and unwind the thoughts and definitions that keep you constricted. You are simply allowed to Be. Your attention is not focused on anything.

This meditation strengthens the ability to live in the present.

Meditation Practices

Mindfulness Meditation

Intentionally focus on the present moment without judgment and attachment to emotions and thoughts. Breathe in and know you are breathing in and know how it feels to breathe in. Breathe out and know you are breathing out and know how it feels to breathe out. If you enter Story, return to breath awareness. Witness your thoughts coming and going like clouds in the sky. Enjoy Mindful Meditation in your daily activities. Drive without distraction of a cell phone or music. Wash your dishes and *be* with the water, the soap, and the dish. Walk, knowing where you are putting your feet on the earth. Speak with integrity and listen completely.

Zen Meditation (Zazen), Seated Zen or Seated Meditation

With a soft gaze, direct your eyes three feet in front of you. Focus on the in and out movements of your breath, inhaling and exhaling through your nose. Inhale and count to ten, exhale counting to back to zero. If you lose concentration, lovingly focus your attention back to the breath. Remain in the present moment through Effortless Being.

Awareness Fusion

Bring your attention to the moment and to the breath through Expansive Meditation. Simply notice the coming and going of sensations and allow them to dissolve. Then practice Single Focus Meditation and label anything that comes into your field of perception. Label "hearing" rather than *voices*, "feeling" rather than *knee ache*, "smelling" rather than *perfume*. You are objectively observant without subjective attachment, allowing fluid sensations to pass, opening yourself to peace.

Body Scan

Embody *to be here now*. Breathe from beyond your crown and trace the breath downward and out your feet. You can incorporate visualizing and feeling into the chakra centers, or simply with the belly, the heart, and head.

Third Eye Meditation

Gently close your eyes and focus your attention on the "third eye" or the spot between the eyebrows ("*ajna chakra*"). If distracted, bring your attention gently and consistently back to this point. This is a means to silence the mind. With time, the "silent gaps" between thoughts get wider and deeper.

Walking Meditation to Celebrate Living

Go outdoors and stand still, drinking in outer awareness and breath awareness. Notice how you feel in every aspect of your body. Begin a relaxed walking pace, focusing on what is going on physically. Wonder at the intricacies of how your body feels when it moves from left to right, the pressure and balance of the soles of your feet, your arms swaying, your leg placement, the textures of your clothing and the feel of your shoes on your skin … relax and notice that each step is a blessing.

So Hum Meditation to Expand Consciousness

So = Cosmic Consciousness (S/he) / *Hum* = Individual Consciousness (Me). Observe your breath for a few moments. Slowly inhale through your nose as you silently say *So*. Slowly exhale through your nose as you silently say *Hum*. Continue, always returning your attention to the inflow and outflow of breath. Your breath will emulate the sounds of ocean waves.

"Who Am I" Meditation

Inhaling: "Who am I?" Exhaling: "I don't know." Incorporate this meditation during your walking meditation, your Yoga centering, and throughout your day. You can find liberation in softening the walls of your heart and becoming the curious, playful Witness.

Chakra Seed Sound Meditation & Mantra

A *Bija Mantra*, meaning *Seed Mantra*, is a one-syllable sound, holding the full potential of a single vibrational point or *Chakra*. With a closed-eye-gaze resting on your third eye center, inhale and chant LAM, VAM, RAM YAM, HAM, OM. Feel the energy that moves upward through these chakra centers. These bija tones are that of the universal elements. Though the Seven Chakra System has 'assigned' elements for each chakra center, infuse elements where they are needed. As an example, you may need earth/stability in your heart space rather than wind. Chant the elemental mantra of LAM, infusing earth energies here.

LAM - Earth Element: 'Lam' in a rich, deep, earthy tone, feeling your Root
VAM - Water Element: 'Vam' in a watery, rich tone, feeling your Sacral Center
RAM - Fire Element: 'Ram', a name of God, stating it strongly from your Solar Plexus
YAM - Wind/Air Element: 'Yam' like it is a yummy, delicious, savory sound from your Heart
HAM - Space/Ether: say 'Ham' in a guttural breathy voice from your Throat
OM - Third Eye Chakra: 'Om' with your eyes focused, vibrating your Intuitive Center

Mantra Meditation

Focus on a mantra (which could be a syllable, word, or phrase). Know what energy the mantra activates and embody that feeling. The subtle vibrations associated with the repetition of the mantra you choose will also help you enter a deeper state of meditation

80

Candle Gazing

Sit in a darkened room and light a beeswax or soy candle. Move your torso from side to side then find stillness, breathing naturally. Begin to gaze softly below the flame, allowing thoughts to come and go as they will. Focus your breathing paired with a gentle gaze - relaxed, focused, aware. Blink as necessary.

Loving Kindness Meditation (Metta Meditation)

This meditation harnesses energy to support the trajectory of harmony and love for all beings. This work begins within. When you cultivate compassion toward yourself, you can share compassion with others. This increases self and other-acceptance. Generate the physical feeling of kindness and love for yourself, perhaps using a mantra and tapping into empathy. The more you practice this, the more joy you will cultivate. The following progression is advised:

Visualize yourself right where you are, in this very time and space. Observe yourself as you would see a baby for the first time. See yourself in all your ages and stages and bless those to come. Allow yourself to be in awe of your own, unique, human expression of life and all the diverse colors and qualities that make you, *you*. Breathe deep with ease and feel yourself glow with presence and gratitude for being conscious of your consciousness of being alive.

With this same energy of love, bring attention to the following intentions listed below, breathing into them the presence of love, empathy, and compassion (all of which are the energies of Interconnection):

1. *Compassion towards yourself*
2. *Compassion towards a good friend*
3. *Compassion towards a "neutral" person*
4. *Compassion towards a difficult person*
5. *Compassion towards all four of the above equally*
6. *Compassion that incorporates the entire Universe*

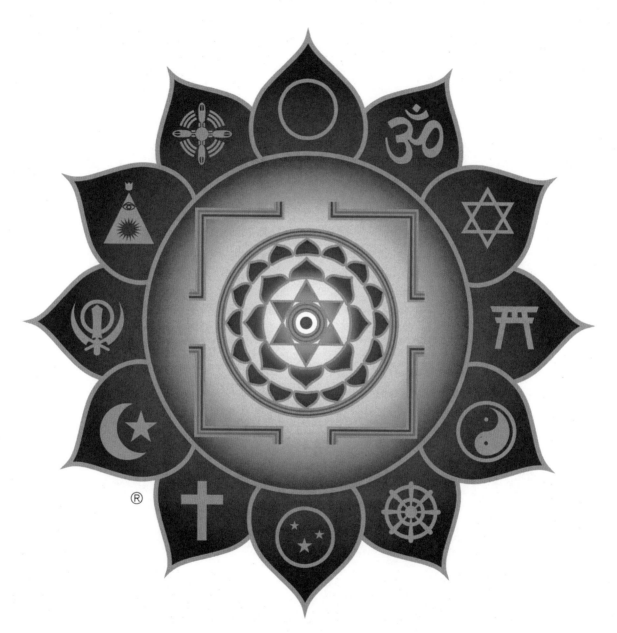

Integral Yoga Yantra

Meditating with a Yantra

There are different types of meditation techniques that support different learning styles. Yantra Meditation is for the practitioner who is more visual, and/or who enjoys eyes open with a soft gaze.

Historically, when mantras were used in meditation, images arose. The same fascinating occurrence applies today, and those images are yantras. Yantras are physical representations of the sacred sound vibration of a mantra. Essentially, a yantra is vibration-in-form. It is said that the first Divine expression was sound. The Bible states, "In the beginning was the Word…"

Ultimately, a yantra is an image of sacred geometry used to support meditation. A Yantra is not defined by a particular tradition or religion. It is Universal. A yantra represents your mind, body, and spirit connection to the cosmos. You can feel the divine qualities of love and peace when meditating in front of a yantra.

In a yantra, Feminine Shakti is represented as a womb in the upside-down triangle. Masculine Shiva is represented as the penis in a point-side-up triangle. The dot, the meditation point, is in the center of the Yantra and is called a *bindu*. This represents merging into the eternal present. A yantra incorporates a drishti, which is a practice that harnesses concentration by focusing a concentrated gaze on the bindu. You breathe into and out of the bindu.

Yantras have an open borders/gates that represent the four directions, how Divinity is vast and infinite, and each gate has a mystical significance depending on the yantra. Different yantras have different deities and mantras associated with gates. Also, the square-shape of the four gateways is said to ground the cosmic energies of mantras and deities into the earthly plane and physical body.

The practice of repeating a mantra while visualizing a yantra is called *Trataka*. Allow a yantra to unfold in the mind without force. During meditation, perhaps a color will reveal itself. Let shapes dance until they merge. Perhaps this will occur, perhaps not. No attachment. If you find a particular yantra that calls itself to you, honor it in a space where you meditate.

The Mantra

A *mantra* is a tool which invokes a syllable, word, or phrase that is often spoken or sung in Sanskrit — the ancient, sacred language of the Vedic tradition. Literally, 'man' means *mind*, and 'tra' means *to free from*. Mantra also means *sound vibration*. Mantra is an especially effective way to activate energy throughout your body and spirit. The more you do it, the deeper your energy body is activated and accessed, moving beyond visualization and the vocal tract.

Sound is always everywhere. Sound can change the course of your life in an instant. Vibration of light reflected from objects allows you to see, whereas the vibration of sound is captured in the tiny hairs of your inner ear, allowing you to hear. Both sight and sound affect the physical and subtle bodies (later explored in *the kosha system*). Mantras work through subtle and physical bodies. The subtle body interpenetrates the physical body. The *subtle body* is an energetic layer of the Self, affiliated with the chakras located along the *sushumna*, or the spine of the subtle body, running from the base of the spine to the third eye center.

The tones of the mantra are often repeated for the purpose of focusing the mind's attention away from repetitive thoughts and habits, clearing the subconscious mind. Doing so alters the neuroplasticity of the mind, as where the mind goes prana flows.

Mantras can be one word or a series of words, chanted in repetition. Mantras are spiritual in nature and are a form of meditation. Each mantra is simple and positive in nature, promoting well-being, manifestation, or transformation. By using a mantra with a *mala*, or *devotional prayer/meditation beads*, the mind can become more controlled, focused, and still. This is beneficial in breaking habitual patterns, reducing stress, and balancing emotions, enlivening consciousness, compassion, and presence.

Mantras harness the power of intentional sound-energy

to create specific energetic responses.

Chaitanya is a term that literally means *one who is conscious*. In terms of mantra, chaitanya relates to when a mantra springs into life and becomes vivid and real – a transformational force. This can happen spontaneously (which is rare but does happen), can happen through steady practice (which is more stable), or can occur through the transmission of one who uses a mantra that is very much alive for them.

Where the mind goes, prana flows.

A mantra may ease you into a meditative state and root your internal energy, so you are in line with and in communication with the perceptively sensitive Universe. The key is the identification of a specific intention you intend to manifest into reality. You may associate a chosen mantra to the form you recognize as God, which is the most practiced type of Indian meditation.

A mantra can be said aloud, it can be whispered, or it can be expressed silently. A combination of all three is fine. The mantra may even disappear when the mind is led deeper and deeper into levels of perception where you may enter the field of pure Consciousness. Many hundreds, if not thousands, of mantras can be invoked. The more familiar a mantra is, the more power it generates, as it becomes a personal tool which can be used with piercing, transformative results. Regardless of the mantra, you must embody the *feeling* of it within your body and welcome it home!

Mantras are like rivers. They allow you to unite with cosmic flow. Mantras are shaped by *purely intentional energy* co-shared by fellow brothers and sisters for thousands of years. When I enter an ancient mantra, I internally and externally feel my connection to Everything. I contribute my own Heart Voice to the current of other Voices. A merging occurs of my energy with the everlasting, timeless connection of others. Ultimately, a mantra is filled with longing and love, gratitude and awareness, humility and a non-dominating, radiant power. Belief moves mountains. You are a LIVING mantra.

It is noble to be called to deepen your practice, but there is a fine line of attachment. Do the practice for the sake of the practice without expectation of the fruits of your actions.

Bringer and Removal of Obstacles ~ Ganesha Mantra

Om Gam Ganapataye Namaha

I see possibility within every obstacle, which strengthens my spirit and opens my heart. I bow to Ganesha for giving me the obstacles I need and reminding me of my ability to overcome them.

Unifying and Grounding

OM

In the beginning was the Word and the Word was God (Om).
The Sacred Sound that connects us. Our Source.
Our Truth. Our Vibrational Essence.
Everything begins and ends with Om. Indescribable.

Peace for All

Lokah Samastah Sukhino Bhavantu

May all beings everywhere be happy and free
May the thoughts, words, and actions of my own life
Contribute in some way to that happiness and to that freedom for all
Om, Shanti (peace in spirit), Shanti (peace in mind), Shanti (peace in body)

The Great Redemption

Oṁ Namaḥ Śivāya

I bow to the knowingness of my ultimate Divinity
I breathe into to my Essential, Authentic Self as I am the Oneness in All

Protection ~ Durga Mantra

Om Dum Durgayei Namaha

I embody Divine power, protection, and abundance. My light always shines bright.

Healing

Om Shree Dhanvantre

May I abide in the strength of my Divine Nature. May I slow down and breathe. May I understand that all is well and is in the service of my Highest Good.

Love and Devotion ~ Hanuman Mantra

Om Shri Hanumate Namaha

I invoke unbound love, giving strength and success to my devotional activities which reveals the power of my soul to triumph over adversities, revealing my highest realizations.

Spirit of Enlightenment

Om Mani Padme Hum

Generosity, Ethics, Patience, Perseverance, Concentration, Wisdom

Inner Peace

Om Shanti Om

Peace … be on my heart, around my thoughts, through my words, with my actions each minute, every day, all day, throughout the year.

Maha Manta (Great Mantra) of Adoration

**hare kṛiṣhṇa hare kṛiṣhṇa kṛiṣhṇa kṛiṣhṇa hare hare
hare rāma hare rāma rāma rāma hare hare**
I focus my mind on purifying my consciousness; absorbing consciousness with Divinity.

Honoring the Guru of my Heart

**Guru Brahma, Guru Vishnu, Guru Devo Maheshwara,
Guru Sakshat Param Brahma, Tasmai Shri Gurave Namah**
I invoke the Creator, the Preserver, the Destroyer. All life experiences are a guru. May I be strong enough to remove ignorance and blindness. I am my Ultimate Guru.

Transformation

Sa Ta Na Ma
Sa - Existence, *Ta* - Life, *Na* - Death, *Ma* - Rebirth
This mantra supports emotional balance, habit-breaking, and memory support.

Universal Mantra

So Hum
I Am That I Am
Inhale with 'So, 'and exhale with 'Hum'.

Abundance

Om Shreem Maha Lakshmiyei Namaha
The universe is full of abundance, and abundance is mine to receive within my non-dominating heart. I call upon the energy of Lakshmi, the Goddess of Wealth, Good Fortune and Happiness. May I receive abundance in holistic wealth, health, and joy to all I encounter.

Sanctuary

Om Namo Narayana
I bow to the Interconnectedness of all beings.
May all living entities rest in the sanctuary of my healing presence.

Joy and Bliss

Om Radha Krishnaya Namaha
Om, I bow to the Love manifested in Krishna and Radha, and I hear the Divine Calling in the beat of my heart. God (Krishna & masculine) calls the Soul (Radha & feminine) and the Soul calls God. The Seeker and the Sought are the same. Everything I need is here.

I Am Thou

Ra Ma Da Sa, Sa Say So Hung
God is within me.
Ra - Sun / *Ma* - moon / *Da* - earth / *Sa* - infinity / *Say* - the personal embodiment of Sa
So - personal senses merging with Sa / *Hung* - Reality Vibrating

89

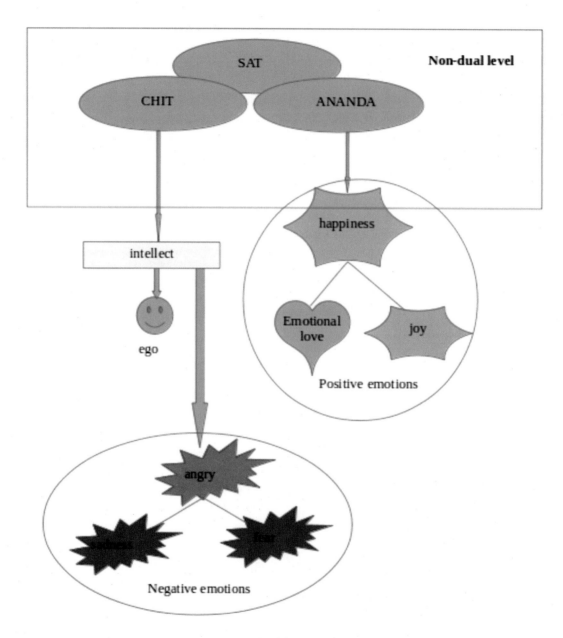

Sat Chit Ananda

The Self-Realization That ALL is Divine

Sat means Existence. Inside Existence is Consciousness. Inside Existence is Bliss.

You being alive in this *here-and-now* moment delights the Universe, as you are loved without condition. Your existence is and always has been everlasting. You embody such wonderful uniqueness as your absolute Truth! God comes in all forms, and you are no exception. You represent the essence of absolute Love, as you are a Child of the Stars, Divine and perfect no matter the situation. There are many paths that open the endless doors of the heart, and all are holy.

Chit means Consciousness. Inside Consciousness is Existence. Inside Consciousness is Bliss.

Our Practice is to live from the wisdom of the heart, not the protective personality of the head. Your life's journey is to understand the depths of your wonderful Existence. You can experience your atman's (soul/seer) vastness and emotional integrity with your inner eye. With your outer eyes, you can see your interconnection to all life forms. Your heart comprehends that it beats as one with Existence. Namaste is a word that represents Consciousness. Namaste must be born from the sacred inner temple of interconnection and shared by speaking with locked eyes with others, without condition.

Ananda means Bliss. Inside Bliss is Existence. Inside Bliss is Consciousness.

Our natural state is Love. The Consciousness of being alive is innately wrapped in the freedom to experience unbound joy and happiness. Bliss is everlasting and pure. Bliss promises the ability to live as Heaven is on Earth. May your thoughts be born from Bliss, which grace your words. May your actions contribute to compassion. When veils of conditional love are lifted, may all beings rest in the Bliss Consciousness that their Existence is perfect, here and now.

Vedic Prayers

Mother of the Vedas and all Mantras ~ Gayatri Mantra

**Oṁ bhūr bhuvaḥ svaḥ
tát savitúr váreṇ(i)yaṃ
bhárgo devásya dhīmahi
dhíyo yó naḥ pracodáyāt**

We meditate on the glory of Divinity
Who has created the Universe, worthy of adoration
Who is the embodiment of Knowledge and Light
Who is the remover of ignorance, enlightening our hearts

Prayer for Awakening ~ Asato Ma Sadgamaya

**asato mā sadgamaya
tamasomā jyotir gamaya
mrityormāamritam gamaya
Oṁ śhānti śhānti śhānti**

*Lead me from ignorance to Truth
Lead me from darkness to Light
Lead me from death to Immortality
Om, peace, peace, peace*

92

Song for the Heart ~ Twameva Mata Prayer

Twameva mata cha pita twameva
Twameva bandhush cha sakha twameva
Twameva vidya drvinam twameva
Twameva sarvam mama deva deva

You are my Nourishing Mother & Illuminating Father
You are my Family & Eternal Friend
You are my Divine Knowledge & Liberation (Wealth)
You are my Everything

Embracing Holistic Liberation ~ Maha Mrityunjaya

Om tryambakam yajāmahe
sugandhim pushti-vardhanam
urvārukam-iva bandhanā
mṛtyormukṣīya māmṛtāat

I bow to my Divinity, my expression and communion with life.
My intellect, emotions, body, and Divine Spirit are One.
I am illuminated in the radiance of my own Light.

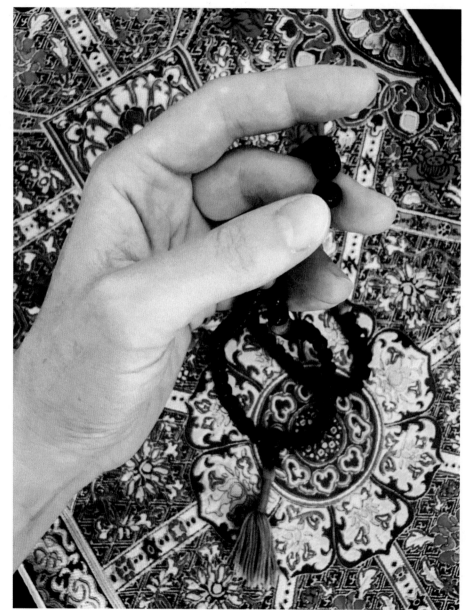

Rosewood Mala

Japa Practice: The Mantra and Mala

A *Japamala*, or *mala*, is a simple, effective meditation tool, which can help to focus the mind, reduce stress, and enhance wisdom, patience, and health. Mala meditation is an ancient technique, adopted across the planet in many cultures and religions. The mala is believed to be the inspiration for rosary beads, and the mala is a tool in a *japa practice* (chanting mantra), which may include *mudras*. Japa chants the *Name*. The gross form penetrates the subtle form, then you can go even subtler still.

For example, what if you concentrate on Om? In the beginning, it is just a sound. The more intensely and devotionally you chant – *and there must be embodied devotion* – then the Om can manifest into the form of God/Ishvara/Bhagavan, or whatever name speaks to you. If you have a vision of God, the japa practice can merge you with God.

Fix the mind on the mantra and keep its meaning in mind. When you chant the mantra, it is with a loving feeling. *God is in the name.* You go into the beloved name through the tools of your mind and heart. This takes dedication and focus. So, get up early, which is *tapas* (dedication), take a shower, get on your mat, get your mala out, and surrender the mind, devotionally.

Japa meditation is not only a meditation style, but it is a lifelong, devotional practice of chanting a sacred sound/mantra, often paired with the use of a mala.

A mala is a prayer strand of 108 beads (or its derivatives, such as 27 or 54 beads) traditionally strung together on silk thread with one larger bead, called the Guru bead, from which hangs a tassel. Why 108? This auspicious number represents the names of God, among other representations. According to the Vedic Tradition, the physical and subtle bodies contain 108 channels of energy, the *nadis*. Saying a mantra 108 times sends energy into each of those channels. These nadis lead into the *Anahata chakra*, the heart gate. Chanting a mantra 108 times fills your nadis with balanced vibration supporting holistic alignment.

Japa Meditation Benefits

❖ Improves focus and concentration in all areas of life.

❖ With focus, the mind is calmed, reducing stress.

❖ The physical heart is fortified, as blood pressure and heart rates decrease.

❖ Negative thoughts decrease while general mood elevates.

❖ Positive emotions are cultivated and last longer in all areas of life.

❖ *Commitment / Tapas / Effort* within a practice increases prana in all areas of life.

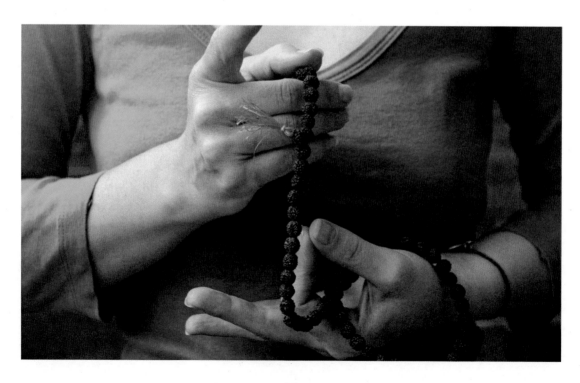

HOW to Practice Japa Meditation

- ❖ Find a comfortable seat with eyes closed. Sit tall in the spine and soft in the body, aligning your chakra centers. Let your chin be parallel to the floor, shoulders and arms relaxed.

- ❖ Ensure your mala does not touch the floor. Some traditions state that you should not use your index finger while engaged with your mala, as it represents the ego.

- ❖ With your right hand, hold the 109th bead - the larger Guru bead - between your thumb and middle finger. Tune into your mantra; the feeling it evokes. The Guru holds all the prayers that are ever said on your mala, hence its sacredness.

- ❖ With the mala resting over the middle finger, starting with the bead to the right of the Guru bead, use your thumb to pull each bead toward your heart as you say a mantra or seed sound. Ensure you touch each bead when you say your mantra, either out loud, in a whisper, or silently.

- ❖ Do not cross over the guru bead. If you wish to chant more than 108 times, when you reach the Guru on your 108th bead, turn the mala and continue your mantra and count, starting again from the last 108th bead.

- ❖ As you chant, be mindful of your breath and spinal alignment, but focus on the mantra blooming in your mind and body. Notice the natural fluxuations of the mind-stuff, and let it transform without judgement.

- ❖ After chanting 108 times, you may find yourself ready to release both the mantra and mala and enter the meditation that it inspired. Remember, don't get hung up on rules. When the thing becomes *the thing* itself, the point is lost.

Japa and Different Traditions

Japa Meditation is used in Hinduism, Buddhism, Jainism, Sikhism, Shinto, and other traditions. Other forms of prayer beads are similar, such as the rosary, which the West is familiar with.

The term "Mala" means a garland of flowers, just as the term "Rosary" means a garden of roses, for in all traditions a bead upon which one prays is also an image of the world-flower. In the East, the World-Flower is the Lotus. In the West, it is the Rose.

According to various traditions, there are many ways of understanding your relationship to Divinity. There is also a difference in how people chant Japa; there is a difference in what their goals are; there is a difference in their orientations. All are possible.

I urge you to think carefully what you want the focus of your japa practice to be. Simplistically, do you seek your *atman* - your inner most Self - to experience pure consciousness? Or do you seek a blissful relationship and absorption into Bhagavan as Other?

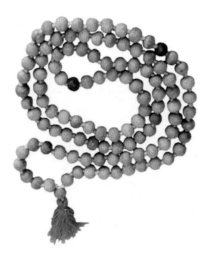

Combining Mantra and Meditation

Choose a Mantra

- ❖ Be clear in your intention/purpose. Choose a mantra that is specific to supporting your intention.
- ❖ Internally feel into where this mantra lands in your body.
- ❖ What chakra area is this?
- ❖ What does that area represent?

Practice

- ❖ Set your practice at a specific time of day that you can dedicate yourself to. It is recommended you practice in the morning (upon rising) and before bed. From a mystical, yogic perspective, it is a potent time to practice in the *ambrosia hours* of sunrise and sunset, when the veils between dimensions are thinnest.
- ❖ Practice without interruption or expectations for certain results. It may take years.
- ❖ Set a specific place where you will be comfortable to practice. You are creating sacred space.

Length

- ❖ At first, try to practice twice daily, while additionally enjoying small mindfulness breaks throughout the day; enjoy anywhere from 1 to 21-minute pauses (or anything in between) to tune into yourself. The more you pause and collect yourself, the more you naturally infuse the practice within your day.
- ❖ The repetition of mantra can be as often as possible over a specific amount of time, but keep in mind that 40 days: changes energy, 90 days: confirms new energy, 120 days: new energy is embodied, 1000 days: mastery of new energy

Ganesha Mudra
(To Overcome all Obstacles)

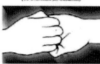

Kubera Mudra
(For Achieving Your Goals)

Pushan Mudra
(For ...)

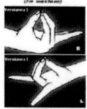

Bronchial Mudra

Asthma Mudra

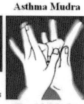

Prithivi Mudra
Earth Mudra
(For energy deficit in the root chakra)

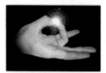

Prana Mudra
Life Mudra

Linga Mudra
Upright Mudra
Practice the Mudra for Frequent Cold,
Congested Chest and Incurable Infections

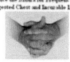

Apana Mudra
Energy Mudra
For Urinary and Liver Strenghtening
Cleanses & purifies the body

Shankh Mudra
Shell Mudra

Surabhi Mudra
Core Mudra

Shunya Mudra
Heaven (Akasha) Mudra

Apan Vayu Mudra
Mrit Sanjivini Mudra
Lifesaver: first aid for
heart attacks

Suchi Mudra
For chronic Constipation

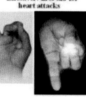

Detoxification Mudra

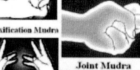

Mushti Mudra

Mahasirs Mudra
Large head mudra

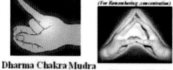

Hakini Mudra
(For Remembering ;concentration)

**Supreme Wisdom
Mudra**
fist of ... six
wisdom ... element
mudra

Karuna Mudra
(compassion)

Joint Mudra

Dharma Chakra Mudra

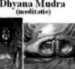

Dhyana Mudra
(meditatie)

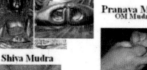

Pranava Mudra
OM Mudra

Anjali Mudra
(salut and veneration)

Abhaya Mudra
Shiva Hand;("fear not")

Kwan Yin

Shiva Mudra

Varada Mudra
Implinirea dorinte,
juraminte

Jnana Mudra

Vitarka Mudra
(dezvaluire;daruire;predare;invatare)

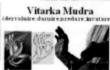

Lotus Mudra

Artist Unknown

Mudras

The origin of the mudra is unknown, yet throughout time, mudras have historically been a part of spiritual traditions around the world through prayer rituals, meditations, and chanting.

The body is a sacred temple, and mudras can unlock the temple doors to connect to Divinity. The term *mudra* means 'seals.' Practicing Mudra Yoga is a meditative practice that evokes your deepest self to immerge, inviting sensation, clarity, and healing to be experienced. In Sanskrit, *mudra* means symbolic gesture, seal, symbol, or posture. Mudras are used to stimulate and lock in energies that affect specific feelings or states of being. They are created through intention, pranayama, meditation, even asana, and are powerful enough to awaken the five levels of the *koshas* (the energy bodies comprising awareness).

*Thumb ~ Fire * Index ~ Air * Middle ~ Ether*

*Ring ~ Earth * Little ~ Water*

Mudras are mostly engaged in through the hands and fingers. Each finger represents and accesses one of the five elements. Fingers link the brain to energy centers due to their networks of nerve endings and nadis (*Streams of Prana*, explored later). When engaged in mudra, one must exert a small amount of pressure to tap into the nadis to harness emotional energies and harmonize them throughout the body.

Common mudras are explored on the following pages.

Guyan Mudra and Active Guyan Mudra

GUAN MUDRA ~ Tip of the thumb touches the tip of the index finger, *stimulating knowledge ability.* The index finger is symbolized by Jupiter, and the thumb represents the ego.

ACTIVE GUAN MUDRA ~ The first joint of the index finger is bent under the first joint of the thumb, *invoking knowledge and universal wisdom.*

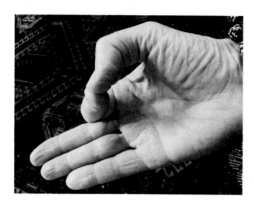 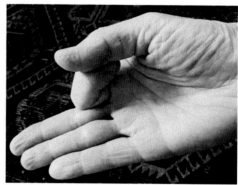

Shuni Mudra

Tip of the middle finger (symbolized by Saturn) touches the tip of the thumb, *invoking patience.*

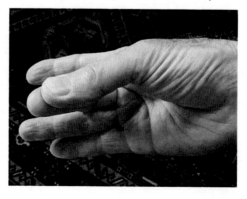

Jupiter Mudra

With the two index fingers together, the power of Jupiter, or good luck and expansion, is activated. Together, they focus your energy to break *through barriers*.

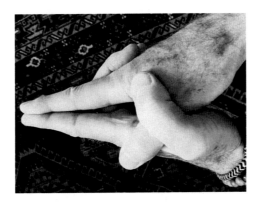

Surya or Ravi Mudra

Tip of the ring finger (symbolized by Uranus or the Sun) touches the tip of the thumb, *invoking energy, health, and intuition.*

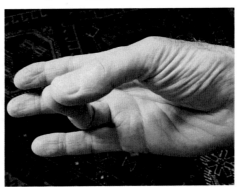

Buddhi Mudra

Tip of the little finger (symbolized by Mercury) touches tip of the thumb
for clear and intuitive communication.

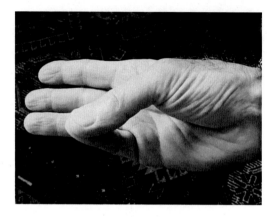

Buddha Mudra

The right-hand rests on the left for men, left on right for women, palms up,
thumbs touching each other to *invoke being with what is, and receptivity.*

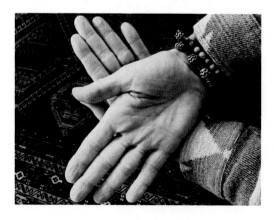

Venus Lock Mudra

Interlace the fingers with the left little finger on the bottom, with the right index finger on top for men and the left for women. The Venus mounds at the base of the thumbs are pressed together, *channeling sensuality, sexuality, and glandular balance, helping to focus and concentrate.*

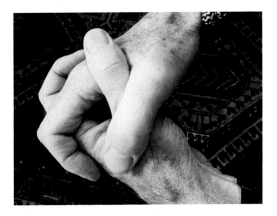

Bear Grip Mudra

The left palm faces out from the body with the thumb down, the right palm faces the body, thumb up, fingers curled and hooked together to *stimulate the heart and intensify concentration.*

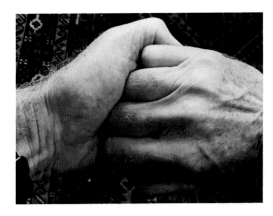

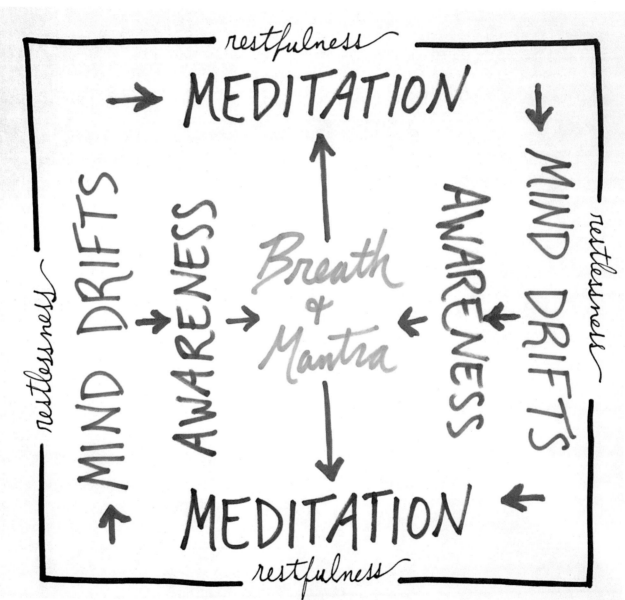

Stages of Meditation

"I Can't Meditate"

When meditation is mastered, the mind is unwavering, like the flame of a lamp in a windless place. ~ Bhagavad Gita

The human mind needs an anchor point to land consciousness. Consider using your precious pranic energy to be a ghost to the past or a ghost to the future; in a story of what was, what could be; not living in the present moment. These *in-between states of presence* is the place where many people reside nearly permanently, especially in this age of device addiction and social media. This is also the realm where fear and anxiety are born. Yet meditation is the bridge uniting you with your Essential Nature.

Importantly, know this … while you meditate, your mind will wander again and again and again. This is human nature, and even the most seasoned of meditators experiences this mental spin. Noticing that you are not in the present moment and then harnessing the mind back into a meditative state is THE practice of Yoga and meditation.

Mantra is a tool to anchor the mind. Understand what your mantra means and feel into the meaning with every fiber of your body. This is a powerful way to invoke a new reality. I will speak more of this in Bhakti Yoga.

Simply know that everyone can meditate. Just be prepared to witness the spinning of the mind, and by using the breath, pull yourself out of the mind and back into the body. The more you show up to the practice of meditation, the more the practice shows up for you.

With practice, you will cultivate a sense of feeling at home within yourself.

This is called Alignment. And Alignment is a holistic energy that expands.

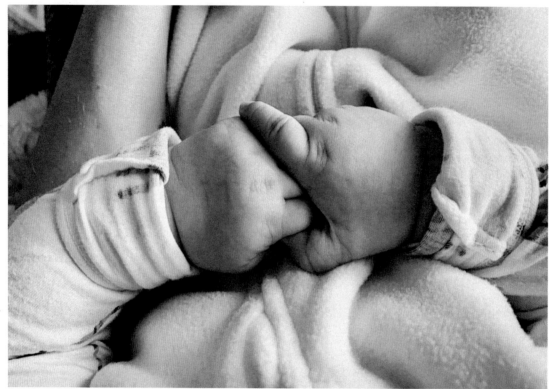

Henry's Mudras

The first thing my family noticed about my nephew
Henry - the only baby born into our immediate family - was his hands.
Since the day he was born, his large, elegant hands have fluttered
with emotion and communication, naturally invoking mudras.

108

Reflection and Practice

Embodiment Tools: Meditation, Mantra, Mala, Mudra

Begin your Meditation Sadhana.

- ❖ Meditation paired with mantra creates great personal change.
- ❖ Choose a specific meditation technique or mantra - and perhaps a mala for a full Japa Practice - that feels right for you, for a minimum of <u>21 minutes a day for 42 days</u> to infuse the vibration into your personal frequency. Having a dedicated time of day to practice is ideal.

Why 21 minutes?

- ❖ A 21-minute meditation routine can lower your pulse rate and improve concentration.
- ❖ You may enjoy increased feelings of stillness.

Why 42 days?

- ❖ Practicing for 21 days can change your habits; old mental images dissolve while new ones form.
- ❖ 21 days can rewire your brain, allowing your brain to work with higher perspectives and with more mental ease.
- ❖ 42 days of practice allows this new habit - and its effects - to take root.
- ❖ After 42 days, chose another meditation technique or mantra, and perhaps use a different mala, if you choose.

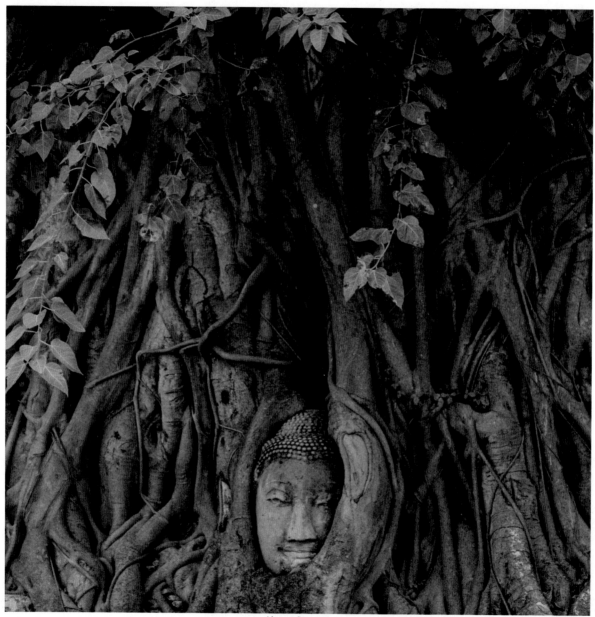

Always Present

Chapter 3

The Roots of Yoga: Potential of Self

Historical Timeline

PRECLASSICAL YOGA ERA

INDUS-SARASVATI AGE: 6500-4500 BCE
- SANATANA DHARMA: "ETERNAL LAW"
- INDUS RIVER VALLEY & SEALS

VEDIC AGE: 4500-2500 BCE
- CONSCIOUSNESS EXPLORED
- VIBRATION OF INTENTION & CAUSATION
- CAUSE & EFFECT: MANTRA & KARMA

SAMKHYA YOGA: 8000-100 BCE
- REALITY EXPLORED: PRAKRITI/PURUSHA
- BODY'S CONSTITUTION: DOSHAS
- AYURVEDA

UPANISHADIC AGE: 2000-1500 BCE
- NON-DUALISM OF ATMAN/BRAHMAN
- DISTILLATION OF VEDAS
- MEDITATION

BHAKTI YOGA: 1000-500 BCE
- ADORATION
- HINDU EPICS / UNIVERSAL INSIGHTS
- 3 BRANCHES OF YOGA

BUDDHISM: C. 500 BCE-PRESENT
- INDIVIDUALITY / MONASTIC TRADITION
- MIDDLE WAY
- FOUR NOBLE TRUTHS / EIGHT-FOLD PATH

CLASSICAL YOGA ERA

CLASSICAL YOGA: 75 BCE-100 CE
- THE YOGA SUTRA'S OF PATANJALI
- EIGHT-LIMBED PATH
- HARNESSING THE MIND

ESOTERIC AGE

TANTRA: 600-1300 CE
- 6 + 1 CHAKRA SYSTEM
- WESTERN NOTION OF EMBODIMENT
- SUBTLE BODY (NADIS, CHAKRAS, ETC.)

HATHA YOGA: C. 1300-1400 CE
- MIND V. BODY
- HATHA YOGA PRADIPIKA
- ASANA / BREATH / BANDHAS / MUDRAS

RISE OF MODERN YOGA

SWAMI VIVEKANANDA: 1872-1950
- INFLUENCED RISE OF MODERN YOGA
- INTRODUCED YOGA TO THE WEST

SRI T. KRISHNAMACHARYA: 1891-1989
- YOGA'S EXPANSION
- FATHER OF MODERN YOGA
- MODERN CONTRIBUTORS

Chapter 3

The Roots of Yoga: Potential of Self

1. Overview of Lecture

Chapter 3 explores the ancient roots of Yoga in relation to the Vedic (Indus-Sarasvati) Age. The timeline of the Story of Yoga is reviewed. In relation to the Vedas, vibrational energy and the power of Sanskrit are discussed.

2. Learning Objectives: I will...

a) Recognize the advanced civilization from which the Vedas and Yoga was born
b) Analyze my use of vibrational intention in thought and language

3. Pre-lecture Assignments

a) Read the chapter and become familiar with the Reflection questions
b) Read *The Four Agreements* by Don Miguel Ruiz
c) Recommended Film: *Heal - Change Your Mind, Change Your Body, Change Your Life*
d) Daily Sadhana - Daily Personal Practice

4. Reflection: *found at the end of the chapter*

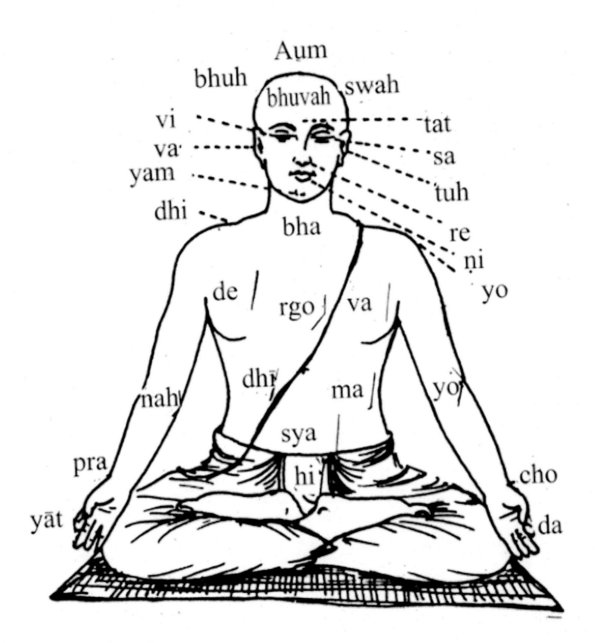

114

Gayatri Mantra

Oṁ bhūr bhuvaḥ svaḥ
the material world   the physical world   the celestial world

tát savitúr váreṇ(i)yaṃ
the Supreme Being   the source   to be worshipped

bhárgo devásya dhīmahi
the Divine Light   its sacred truth   we deeply meditate

dhíyo yó naḥ pracodáyāt
the Intellect   which   to us   may Light be endowed

The Gayatri is a mantra known as the Mother of the Vedas, or *Vedasara*, The Essence of the Vedas. It is a prayer to the Transcendent Divine - The Self. This auspicious and ancient Sanskrit mantra first appears in the Rig Veda with the intention of illuminating the intellect, inspiring wisdom, and offers protection. is a sacred mantra invoking physical, emotional, and mental healing. The Gayatri Mantra purifies karmas and opens doors to possibility.

❖ **The image shows how Sanskrit tones of the Gayatri Mantra *light up*, or activate, different parts of the body. Each part of the body has energetic, psychological, and elemental qualities. Knowing these qualities and discerning them supports self-understanding.**

The Roots of Yoga

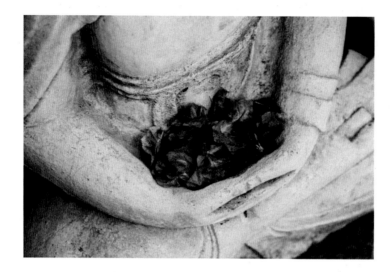

The roots of Yoga are traditionally traced back to the area known as the Indian subcontinent. The journey begins in the Indus-Sarasvati Valley, located in what is now Pakistan, and travels south to a land previously known as Bharata. Less than 200 years ago, England gave the name 'India' to the land previously known as Bharata and gave the name 'Hindu' to label an otherwise religiously diverse group of people in this geographic region. *Bharata* means both 'nourished' and 'the land that loves knowledge'.

Sanatana Dharma was the spiritual essence of the people of Bharata. Sanatana Dharma posits as truth that there is an eternal order to the world. This eternal order merges duality – yin and yang, vertical and horizontal, masculine and feminine energies – to create balance, or sattva. But this eternal order does not belong to any particular group of people, time, or place. It is universal.

The practice of Yoga, which is sometimes referred to as a "living fossil", embodies Sanatana Dharma as the foundational element of the human story. *Truth is one, paths are many.*

Indus-Sarasvati (the Harappan Civilization)

Early evidence of the Yoga tradition can be found in the once flourishing Indus-Sarasvati Civilization of the Indus River Valley, located in modern-day Pakistan. The largest cosmopolitan cities of this time have been identified as Mohenjo-Daro, in the south, and Harappa, 350 miles to the north. Together, they comprise some of the world's largest civilizations of antiquity. The people were called *Aryans*, meaning Noble Ones.

Mohenjo-Daro, home to over five million people, is thought to be the oldest known civilization in the world, dating beyond 9000-3000 BCE. The word *Mohenjo-Daro* translates to 'The Mounds of the Dead'.

Archeological remains of this immense and advanced Neolithic civilization were discovered in 1921. Thus far, approximately 60 of 2,500 known sites have been excavated. These excavations continue to bring to light the advanced and elaborate nature of city planning that pre-dates Roman advances and covers an area larger than Sumer, Assyria, and Egypt, combined.

The sheer size of Mohenjo-Daro is estimated to be 500 acres, suggesting a high level of planning. The city was divided into two parts - the Citadel and the lower city. The Citadel supported public baths and could hold approximately 5000 citizens within its two large assembly halls. However, there are no obvious palaces, temples, or monuments. Moreover, there is no evidence of a king or queen, or a place of central government.

This city was very organized, built in a very specific, focused way. Water was a priority, so planned developments, aqueducts, and wells (for city and individual use) were numerous. The city's heart held a central marketplace with a large central well, and smaller wells were found throughout the city. Over 700 wells were present, which was unheard of in other civilizations at the time. Individual houses obtained water from these smaller wells, although many homes had their own well, which was a profound advancement. Many individual homes found within the city also had a water-proofed bathing room with drainage. One building was found to have an underground furnace that fed a hypocaust, which is a hollow space under a floor into which hot air is used to heat a room or heat bath water. Excavations also revealed a water-tight pool called the Great Bath. Perched on top of a mound of earth and secured with baked brick, this building is considered the closest structure to a temple found in the city. Wastewater was channeled to covered drains that lined the streets. Cleanliness was a central way of life, based on the belief that the river would clean both your body and atman-consciousness, and that the body was a temple.

The Indus-Sarasvati Civilization gave birth to many scientific, technological, and artistic advances, including navigation, astronomy, the number system, and the seven classical notes of music. The Indus-Sarasvati Civilization followed and practiced *Ayurveda*, the Science of Life, and also gave rise to many other advances in medicine (such as cesarean sections and cataract surgeries). Important as well, the Indian spiritual tradition is a scriptural tradition with ample documentation. India was a very literate culture and produced more books than any other pre-modern civilization.

Catastrophic climate and tectonic events dried up the culture's life-giving Sarasvati River around 1900 BCE. In 60 of the known 2,500 sties, archeologists have found massive amounts of radiation. There are some scientists who believe this civilization may have created an atomic bomb that went vastly awry. Within two generations, the Aryans endured a forced but peaceful mass migration to the Ganga River Valley, bringing with them the Rig Veda, the text believed to be the origin of Yoga, and other early scriptures.

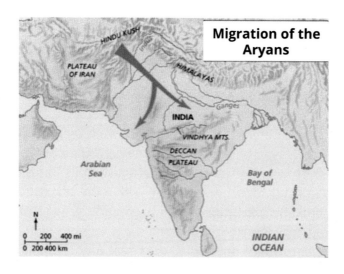

118

Yogic Evidence

Yoga historians rarely agree about dates regarding events within the Yoga Lineage. However, what is generally noted as the first artistic evidence of Yoga are the Indus-Sarasvati soapstone and terracotta seals. These seals depict plants, animals, and mythological figures that are reminiscent of shamanism, Goddess worship, and today's Hindu deities.

Among these early seals are those containing images of a human form, perhaps in meditation. As seen below, one of these seals is believed to contain the first images of Shiva, a representation of the first yogi called Adiyogi. Another seal contains an image of Pashupati, Lord and Protector of Animals.

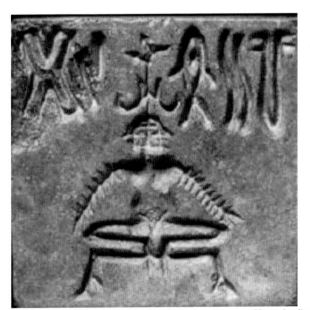 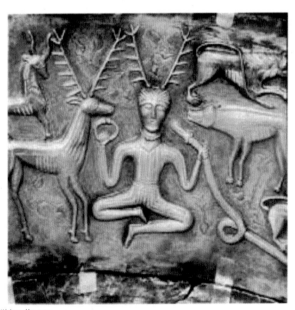

Photo Credits: Wikipedia.org

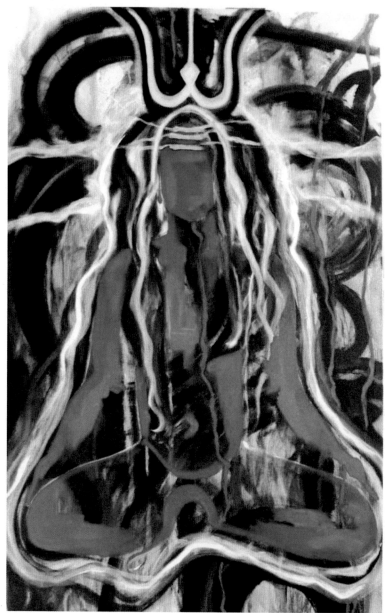

Adiyogi, painting by Lily Kessler

The Adiyogi ~ The First Yogi

The name *Shiva* means 'That Which is Not'

In the Vedic Tradition, Shiva is known as the Adiyogi, the first yogi and the first guru. Shiva is the supreme example of how one can lead a life from the place of the one created to that of also being the Creator. In yogic lore, Shiva attained the ecstasy of enlightenment by dissolving the distinction of his boundaries between Created and Creator. If you have known a moment of ecstasy in your life, those moments happen only when the notion of who you thought you were expanded into the awareness of being the one who is also the creator of the expansion.

Yoga is not defined by a particular exercise, pose, or technique. Yoga is the Science of Creation and explores how to take this piece of creation – that is you – to its ultimate possibility. Yoga is your relationship with your Source.

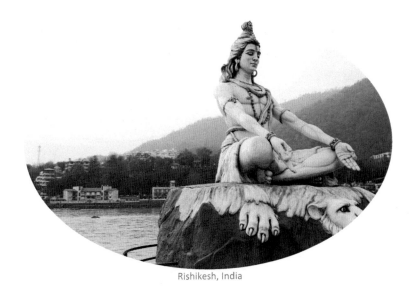

Rishikesh, India

121

The Sanskrit Alphabet

अ	आ	इ	ई	उ	ऊ
a	ā	i	ī	u	ū

ए	ऐ	ओ	औ
e	ai	o	au

ऋ	ॠ	ऌ	अं	अः
ṛ	ṝ	ḷ	aṅ/añ/an/aṃ	aḥ

क	ख	ग	घ	ङ	Guttural
ka	kha	ga	gha	ṅa	
च	छ	ज	झ	ञ	Palatal
ca	cha	ja	jha	ña	
ट	ठ	ड	ढ	ण	Cerebral
ṭa	ṭha	ḍa	ḍha	ṇa	
त	थ	द	ध	न	Dental
ta	tha	da	dha	na	
प	फ	ब	भ	म	Labial
pa	pha	ba	bha	ma	

य	र	ल	व
ya	ra	la	va

श	ष	स	ह	क्ष	ज्ञ
śa	ṣa	sa	ha	kṣa	jña

122

Sanskrit as a Matrix

The Microcosm and the Macrocosm of the Universe

The word *matrix* means a system that can birth various expressions of itself. The Latin root of matrix means 'mother'. But it also means 'a carefully balanced system that can produce countless iterations of itself'. *Matrika* in Sanskrit is an affectionate term for Divine Mother, and it directly references the Sanskrit alphabet. Some traditions consider the alphabet itself a deity. The mantra of this alphabet is mapped onto the subtle body within you.

Why is this significant?

In linguistic mysticism, the 50 phonemes of the Sanskrit alphabet also stand for the 50 principles of reality that make up the entire universe. When you are experiencing the phonemes of the Sanskrit alphabet in you, through mantra, you are also affirming to yourself that all fundamental principles, the building blocks of reality, are in you. Everything is in you. *The Seeker and the Sought are One*.

Your energy body is conceived of as a microcosm and the macrocosm, particularly in every form of Tantric Yoga. In other words, the pattern of the whole universe is within you, and you are a microcosm of the whole. This is important because the teaching is not stating you are a part of God, or you are a part of the whole. *You are the whole!* Everything is within you because this is the nature of a self-similar universe, which is also called a *fractal*.

The same patterns are iterating on all scales in this self-similar universe. So that means that anything any human being has ever experienced is possible for you to experience. There is nothing unavailable to you, if you are patient enough, because the potentiality for every experience exists within each one of us. It must be this way, just as each cell of the physical body has DNA for the whole body. As a 'cell' of the universe, you contain the pattern of the whole. That is the significance of the Sanskrit alphabet. It's the primordial sounds of the universe, recorded and codified.

Sanskrit and the Vedas

May the good belong to all the people in the world.
May the rulers go by the path of justice.
May the best of men and their course always prove to be a blessing.
May all the world rejoice in happiness.
May rain come in time and plentifulness be on earth.
May this world be free from suffering and the noble ones be free from fear.

~ Vedic Literature

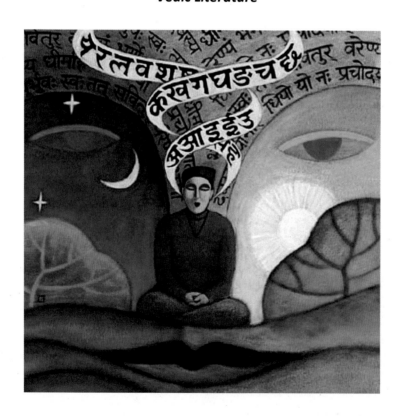

Yogic wisdom has developed through Śruti (or *Shruti*) and Smriti. *Śruti* is that which is heard, and *Smriti* is that which is remembered. The *rishis* (the sages), who experienced Śruti directly, downloaded wisdom through the ether of their consciousness, creating what is the *Vedas*.

The word *Veda* means 'knowledge' or 'essence of truth'. This enormous prehistorical collection of 20,000 verses is broken down into four books: the Rig (Rg) Veda, the Sama Veda, the Yajur Veda and the Atharva Veda. The Vedas inquire into the microcosm and the macrocosm of Humanity. They inquire into the question of what it means to be human. *What is the ultimate principle of this vast universe and how does it relate to my own being? What is the soul?* The Vedas became a source of information on everything from when to plant crops, when to marry, rituals for birth and death, the deities, and beyond. They encompassed information regarding the energies of love and fear, and how to balance nature and natures' effect within one's body.

The Vedas are considered the earliest philosophical and religious manuscripts in the world. They are considered *Aparurushey*, meaning the Vedas were divinely gifted to humans by the Divine or cosmic Star Nations. The historian and philosopher Adi Shankara stated: "The Vedas were never created or destroyed. They merely get illuminated and de-illuminated but remain in Ishwar (Divinity)." The Vedas remain a living entity of how-to live in harmony within yourself and within the world; same/same. The Vedas are a guide for understanding that humans are spiritual beings in a spiritual body having a spiritually human experience.

A foundational Vedic tenet is that there is a spark within you that is matched by a cosmic, luminous Source. Ultimately, the Truth has always been here. Truth is Universal and available to all because it resides within every cell of your being, within every life form. Through vibration, intention, and reverberation, you transform flesh and bone into a godlike entity, and a godlike entity into flesh and bone. You are the same energy as the Divinity but on a different level of operation and awareness. Through this vibrational technology, you can manifest and express these different levels of Divinity.

Originally, the Vedas were preserved by oral tradition, passed from father to son, and learned through mathematical precision to ensure they were not corrupted. Some scholars believe the Vedas led to the formation of the current major world religions and philosophies. Sections of the Vedas became the foundational layer of Hinduism, while other sections do not have a religious context. Many of these contribute to Indian philosophies, including the philosophies that comprise your understanding of Yoga. Although all four Vedic books have spiritual wisdom within them, the *Rig Veda*, meaning 'Praise Knowledge', is the primary book from which current yogic traditions are derived.

Moving from the oral tradition, the Vedas were written in Sanskritam, or Sanskrit. *Shabdarashi* is a term describing Sanskrit as the mass of sounds. Sanskrit is considered the most ancient and richest of all languages of the world: The Language of God and Bright Beings; the Hanging Gardens; Mother of all Indo-European languages. Sanskrit is seen as the sacred language of God. The Aryans believed Sanskrit was Śruti, written in the ether by the collective unconscious, and it was Divinely revealed to the most esteemed members of society, the Rishis. The Rishis, the Seers, intuited Sanskrit, 'finding' and embodying the language through their inner eye while in a state of meditation. Sanskrit was a language only for the priestly cast, not laypeople. Today, the Sanskrit language remains known only/primarily to scholars.

Sanskrit has dominion over reality. *Sanskrit*, which literally means 'well-made', comprises reality's building bricks and is a language of shaping experience using precise sounds. These sounds are energies that vibrate due to tongue placement in the mouth, which activates the brain, sinuses, and subtle body. When speaking Sanskrit, one internally feels these energies in specific places. For example, *sharanam* means 'sanctuary'. When repeated, the essence of a sanctuary - peace, healing, safety - will tap the chanter into the actual state of *sharanam* where it's energy can be moved into reality as a blessing for another or manifest in the chanter's own life experience.

All matter is made of small particles that vibrate. Wherever there is a vibration, there is a sound. Sanskrit is a 'found' language that expresses this vibration through human voice. Sanskrit embodies and manifests the actual essence of an object or quality. The power of speech - *vac* - is harnessed through the chanting of mantras. The whole of existence is sound vibration and sounds open dimensions. Every sound is a mantra and is honored as a key to existence. When spoken, or more appropriately, uttered with a sense of pure intention at the proper moment, the mantra manifests as an extension of one's energy. Where the mind goes, *prana* (life force) flows.

126

The Vedas primarily contain sacred mantras and instructions for correctly performing Vedic rituals. These rituals honor the universal order of life, or *rta*. Rta predictably manipulates the universe through cause-and-effect relationships, ultimately invoking karma.

The following includes a sampling of the scope of the Vedas: *knowledge of the seasons; actions of the sun, moon, planets, atomic energy, solar energy; the process of death, birth, life; worship and Yogic Philosophie; agriculture; knowledge of politics, administration, architecture, business; rules about men, women, children, marriage; Brahmacharya (energy control); education; and clothing.* All knowledge from the sprouting of a seed to the knowledge of God is found in the Vedas.

"MAY THE GOOD BELONG
TO ALL THE PEOPLE IN THE WORLD.
MAY THE RULERS GO BY THE PATH OF JUSTICE.
MAY THE BEST OF MEN AND THEIR SOURCE
ALWAYS PROVE TO BE A BLESSING.
MAY ALL THE WORLD REJOICE IN HAPPINESS.
MAY RAIN COME IN TIME
AND PLENTIFULNESS BE ON EARTH.
MAY THIS WORLD BE FREE FROM SUFFERING,
AND THE NOBLE ONES BE FREE FROM FEAR".

– FROM THE VEDIC LITERATURE

In early Vedic civilization, women held important roles in Vedic rituals, and caste was a fluid system where one could change professions and, thus, change caste. By the end of the Vedic civilization, the status of women declined, and the caste system had solidified into a highly rigid, hierarchical system in which one was born into a particular caste with no mobility to change professions or caste. The Vedic priest, who held the highest caste, held the power in society as they were the only ones who could perform the Vedic rituals, a service for which they eventually heavily charged. Toward the end of the Vedic Age, societal unrest increased. People became disillusioned with the increasingly corrupt Vedic ritual system. Furthermore, people yearned for a deep and personal spiritual experience instead of having a priest perform the ritual on his/her behalf. Ascetic tradition increased. The stage was set for a spiritual revolution.

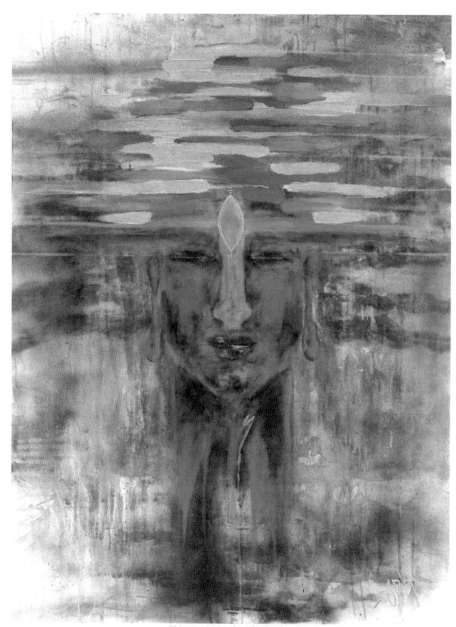

Shiva, painting by Lily Kessler

Essence of the Vedas ~ Cause and Effect

Mantric Causation of Rta and Vac

Sound is the Building Block of the Universe.
Sound is energy, intention/mantra, manifestation.
Where the mind goes, prana flows.

The key concepts of the Vedas are based on *Rta* and *Vac*. Both terms have similar meanings and require awareness and responsibility. *Rta* means 'sound has power to create change'. *Vac* means 'speech has power'.

Sound is considered alive, and in Sanskrit, *the name of a thing* is *the sound of the thing itself*. There is an order to the universe, which can be manipulated through proper rituals and mantras by specially trained priests.

The Vedas reveal a very deep understanding of sound. Sound is honored as a key to existence, and mantra is a device to change or alter existence. When sounds are uttered with the right sense of intensity, at the right moment in life, new things unfold.

Don Miguel Ruiz, author of *The Four Agreements* says, "Be impeccable with your word. Speak with integrity. Say only what you mean. Avoid using the world to speak against yourself or to gossip about others. Use the power of your word in the direction of truth and love."

Glimpses into the four Vedic books are briefly shared in the coming pages.

129

Rig (Rg) Veda

Book of Mantra and Knowledge of God

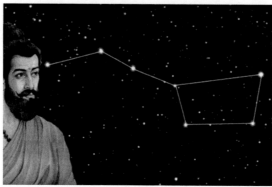

Photo Credit: Google Images

The Big Dipper has another name! It is named The Saptarishi's, which honor the Seven Sages, who spread various forms of Yoga around the world. The seven Yoga's are: Bhakti/Devotion, Karma/Action, Raja/Mind, Jnana/Knowledge, Mantra/Primordial Sound, Tantra/Energies, Hatha/Balanced Gross and Subtle Body.

❖ All Vedic Philosophy flows from the *Rig Veda*, Knowledge of the Almighty. It is one of the oldest Indo-European language texts containing poetic hymns and chants.

❖ Contains several mythological and poetical accounts of the origin of the world, with hymns praising the forms of Divinity and ancient prayers for life, prosperity, etc.

❖ Contains a series of prescriptions that help people overcome ailments: Ayurveda, *the Science of Life*, as well as the concept of Rta, which posits there is order to the universe which can be manipulated through proper rituals and mantras by specially trained priest.

Yajur Veda

Book of Ritual and Karma

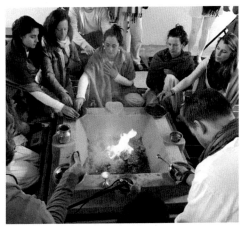

Lingering After Ceremony

❖ A manual on how priests are to perform mantras and sacrifices, providing guidelines and context for ceremonies to honor Divine Guidance in daily living.

❖ Focuses on mantras used during fire ceremonies to honor God.

❖ In the heart of Yoga, you internally replicate this ceremony through *Tapas*, your internal dedication. Tapas is seen through the element fire. When you make offerings to fire, you recognize what you have in life, and the offerings are a balance of *give and take*. This balance is called *sattva*.

❖ Every moment, the five elements of ether, air, fire, water, and earth are sustaining and nourishing the body, and you pay reverence to that. When you value your body and the body of loved ones, should you not value the ingredients which make this body?

Sama Veda

Book of Song and Worship

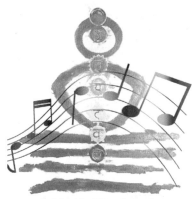

Invisible World by Lily Kessler

❖ Liturgical (public worship) collection of melodies and divine hymns are set to music. Musical renditions of the essence of the Rig Vega are sung by priests.

❖ The breath prosody (rhythm) needed to sing these metrical hymns forms the basis of pranayama.

❖ Same chants as those mantras in the Rig Veda, but at times, the recitation of hymns was re-arranged to suit their intended hymn.

❖ Sound energy was being thoroughly studied in how it affected the human mind and body, which codified Chakra tones: *LAM, VAM, RAM, YAM, HAM, OM, silence.* Correlated to the chakra tones, the seven classical notes of music (sa, re, ga, ma, pa, dha, ne, sa) were solidified.

❖ Through vibration and intention - through reverberation - you transform flesh and bone into a godlike entity. You are the same energy as Divinity but in different levels of operation. Through this sound technology, you can manifest and express these different levels.

Atharva Veda

Book of Medicines and Ishvara

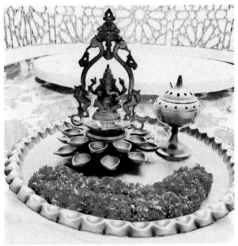

Ritual

❖ Also known as The Veda of Magical Formulas, and Knowledge of Philosophy & Rituals, containing hymns, mantras, spells, astrology, and prayers.

❖ Focusing on prolonging life, healing illnesses within the body and mind, finding love, and explores the concepts of good and evil.

❖ Incantations for material gain, protection from evil, disease, illness, natural disasters, etc.

❖ Provides a platform for the practical implementation of the wisdom enshrined in the Rig Veda, so human society can easily benefit from Divine Knowledge.

❖ Considered to be an early reference that inspired Yoga, Tantra, and breath techniques.

133

The Wheel of Karma

Cause and Effect

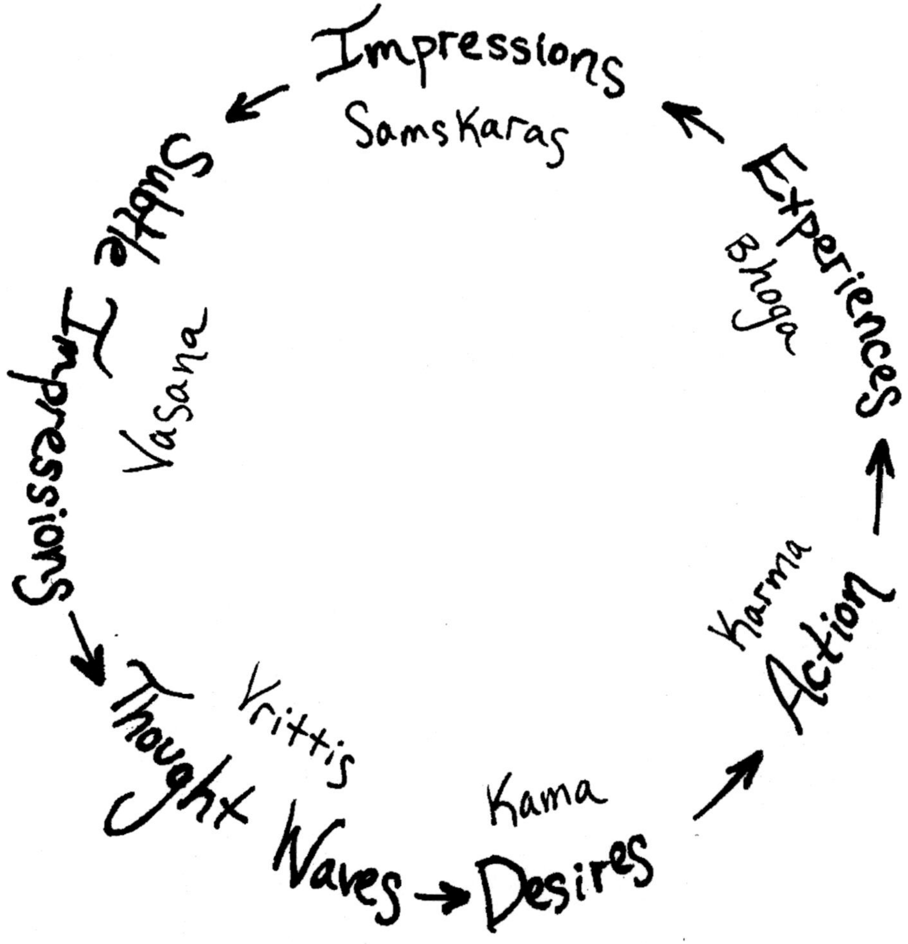

Impressions
Samskaras

Experiences
Bhoga

Subtle Impressions

Vasana

Action
Karma

Thought Waves

Vrittis

Desires
Kama

The mind is the cause of your bondage and the cause of your liberation. You have a mind and get to use it however you wish to use it. Whatever the mind chooses creates effects that you will experience.

The concept of multiple lives is not a New Age idea. This is deep spirituality based on humanity's oldest tenets of religion and philosophy.

The Vedic Tradition is based on the concept that the atman is everlasting. Atman and Brahman are one in the same. Transmigration, rebirth, reincarnation, and other terms harkening to the atman's eternal nature are major, historical concepts and the foundations of this tradition. Basically, it is a reminder that each atman is evolving, and there are lessons to learn in each life experience.

Mental impressions are ties that bind the atman to the Earth plane. Yoga offers the opportunity to explore more refined dimensions, higher realms where you are no longer subject to the cycle of birth and rebirth, or *samsara*.

A *vritti* is a Sanskrit word meaning 'a mental thought wave'. A *samskara* is a mental and psychological impression created from conscious and subconscious thoughts and actions; from experiences of past lifetimes and current experiences, which are rooted in both pleasure and pain. Samskaras and *vasanas* (meaning "wishes" or "desires") are born from the ego's protective personality, which conditions future responses that limit potential based on fear-patterns. They are the source of impulses and dispositions, misidentifying the atman as separate from Source, which is the cause of suffering.

Suffering exists because of misidentification and misunderstanding. Explored later, the five roots of misunderstanding are called *kleshas*. These false identifications create mental impressions (*samskaras*) from experiences that form fear and desires, which then condition future behavior and responses. This creates the cycle of life, death, and rebirth (*samsara*). Samskara imprints are accumulated lifetime to lifetime and passed on to future life experiences, influencing karma.

Think of a samskara as a scratch on a record. *Why do I always attract this sort of relationship/person/situation?* But rather than focusing on the fear and negativity, you can use these experiences as opportunities to "fill in the gaps" and evolve beyond them. Stumbling blocks can be powerful steppingstones. So let nothing be shunned, ignored, or shamed, as what you resist persists. Samskaras dissolve when fear is leaned into; when boundaries are made; when people-pleasing ceases; and, when alignment of your inner world matches and mirrors your outer world.

Here is what that looked like for me:

I avoided going to the *shala* (another name for a yoga studio) day after day because I didn't want to see a friend who would most certainly be waiting for me there. She had a key to the space, was an incredible support for the studio, and was well-liked in the community. The problem was she demanded my energy in a way that I couldn't give her. I couldn't go to the studio to meditate, practice, or clean in silence, because she always seemed to show up, and I could never be alone to relish my creation. For years, my mind justified the good she was doing for the studio, even as my heart became oppressed, and so, I avoided attending. My friend became more and more jealous, and she began to feel dangerous to me. I decided to close the studio.

I soon recognized I had made a drastically desperate decision. I was setting myself up for self-sabotage, based on being a people-pleaser. I was simply scared to share my truth, and because of this, I gave away my personal power. And with this rattling recognition, I was finally moved to stand for what I needed. My old and detrimental decision-patterns of trying to never 'cause waves' had led me to always wear masks that hid my inner pleadings. This was my default samskara programing - until it wasn't. I leaned into my fear by having an open conversation to establish boundaries. *Bravery and vulnerability are often needed to embrace a samskara.*

However, I also saw myself as a hypocrite. I taught self-care, the bravery of truth, boundary-making, and embodiment principles daily. But where was my authenticity? Where was the power behind my teachings? Was I a sham?

Guilt began to creep into my heart.

It's important to recognize that nothing in life is truly linear. We heal our samskaras layer by layer, consciously and subconsciously. To transform my guilt, I reflected on past experiences and celebrated my growth as a person. We are always moving from an unknowingness to an awareness and knowing, an understanding of things, which is a main reason why I teach. And that act of teaching also holds me accountable in honesty to my Self. Honesty must begin within. Truth must begin within. Bravery must begin within.

When I shared my truth - what I needed - with her, the remnants of our strained relationship died in a matter of moments. Despite her colorfully violent reaction, I remained aligned, still, and grounded from the inside out. I was aware that my old self would have given in and apologized, yet now I was able to remain solid in my truth, and this truth was shared out of respect for us both.

When in the *eye of a storm*, this type of new rootedness becomes an upleveled feeling of alignment. A samskara/vasana begins the path to greater healing or is completely liberated.

No matter what, I know I can't serve a friendship, or any role, out of obligation, and I broke my pattern of being a people pleaser by expressing myself honestly with as much grace as I could muster. Though a bit of drama erupted with the community, due to her exit, it was a relief-filled blessing, as 'negative' energy was replaced by authentic energy. To remain rooted, I kept breathing into *the feeling* I was embodying, and I was able to maintain that feeling of being inwardly aligned. I was her teacher as much as she was mine, and I am so grateful for the experience. Each person who enters your life is a blessing for greater growth, and I now welcome a plethora of teachers to come.

Samskaras are where your greatest gifts and potential lie. They may seem like unsurmountable obstacles, pits, or voids. But when you open the door of fear, you realize there is nothing to fear on the other side. There is simply non-dominating self-empowerment. When you stand aligned, the world has no choice but to rise with you.

When you are addicted to something, there is a driving force, and where does the driving force come from? A desire. If the desire is not fulfilled, you keep trying to re-create it. When you can't recreate it, the drive becomes deeper. It's as if it becomes a groove in your brain, like a record continuously spinning, stuck in a rut in the vinyl. It takes great focus to alter that pattern. Mantra and prayer are fantastic tools to get to the other side of any rut.

The Cycle

Thought waves lead to the forming of desires, which lead to taking actions to fulfill the desire. In turn, actions lead to experiences and impressions of those experiences, forming subconscious perceptions of reality and beliefs. These beliefs rise to become their own thought waves, and the cycle continues.

Yoga is awareness of these conscious processes and offers you the courage to explore the subconscious. *"Why do I think the way I think?"* Remember, labels and tribal belief systems form both conscious and subconscious behavior. Questioning everything and the willingness to break out of cycles is the practice of Yoga.

Desire and Attachment

Desire and attachment are inherent in the human condition, until they are not. If you have a desire of wanting a relationship, for example, that unfulfilled desire may grow stronger and stronger. Based on that desire, you may engage in action to "find" someone who can fulfill your need. If you don't get what you want when you want it, though, thoughts questioning your worthiness can arise. Or you may get angry because your desires are not being met. If you do find a relationship, however, it can be a good experience or an unpleasant one. Either way, impressions will be created that are either pleasant or painful, or perhaps even both. With fulfillment of desire comes attachment. You have now achieved your goal, and you believe you need to keep, or maintain, what you have or else you will suffer from loss. The cycle repeats itself, not necessarily focused on relationships, but on all your desires and attachments.

Impressions

Using the same example as above, assume you have achieved the relationship you desire. But also assume there is an injury in the relationship that leaves a very bad impression. As a result, you may become reluctant to enter into another relationship (no matter how badly you might desire it) because your subconscious (in the form of a subtle impression) has been affected. In the extreme, you may even fully resist the very thought of another relationship.

The mind is a container. It's not anything unto itself. So, what does it contain? Everything that enters the mind creates a samskara, which sits in the mind. In other words, it's samskaras that come from the outside, and whatever comes from the outside becomes your mind. These are imprints. Imprints are things that you allow to be fed though your senses. They leave their imprints, and your consciousness then flows through these imprints and into the world. People are subject to chasing desires, illusions, and other cravings/desires/*ragas*, which are born from their memories.

Samskaras and Impressions

Karma is samskara. Everything you do, every thought you have, and every word you speak, creates the seeds of your vasanas, or desires. It is from the seeds of your desires that your samskaras grow.

Ultimately, Samskaras are your life experiences, and these experiences navigate your future; your labels, judgments, and choices are all colored by your samskaras. Some samskaras come from past experiences, but most are newly created in this lifetime. Samskara can be both personal and ancestral. Certain samskaras may be based on family or lineage. Unfulfilled desires and the samskara they create may go deep to the bottom of your psyche, and the impressions they create may not manifest for lifetimes. These impressions can be so deep they become like the sediment that lies at the bottom of an ocean.

Even pleasant impressions can create samskaras. Because of attachment to pleasurable experiences, you may fear their absence or loss. When you recount a happy memory and bring that memory into the present moment, for example, you may shed tears of unhappiness because the events associated with the memory are not happening at this moment. Samskara is created.

All impressions and the samskara they generate, whether deep or superficial, provide opportunities for learning and healing. Angelic beings may choose to come into the most difficult situations, which provide the greatest opportunity for learning and healing. These beings may choose to engage in extreme hardships in order to address, and eventually resolve, their samskara and develop the strength to handle the fullness of life. Through this process, they come to realize that a single lifetime is but a blip in the eternity of time. They realize that you can choose what you do along the Wheel of Karma again, and again.

Karma is not fate. Your fate is created by your thoughts and your actions. But you are newly creating your fate right now, in every moment of your life. Even quantum theories posit that your future selves are supporting your spiritual development, now.

Vasanas

The mind is filled with past life memory impressions, which are vasanas. (Samskaras is a word that tends to be used for imprints from this lifetime, though it can also be past life imprints.) Vasanas are samskaras from past lives. They are deep-level and most often are subconscious. The mind is filled with past life vasanas.

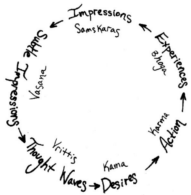

Wheel of Karma

This diagram of the Wheel of Karma is from the guru of Rama Jyoti Vernon, a beloved teacher of mine. Understanding the Wheel of Karma can help prevent future pain if you recognize it in this life. In other words, you can stop at the thought wave, which is the purpose of meditation. A mantra, or *japa*, may stop the thought waves, create an inspirational aspect of the thought wave, or it can stop desires. You can look at it and turn it back in on itself. Or you may take the action, and as you do, watch yourself as a Witness, which is your Inner Witness, looking at and discerning a situation in different ways so it doesn't grow deep roots in your psyche. And once you have experienced it, you can use Yoga asana, psychotherapy, or various models of philosophy to address how you allow the samskara in your life this time around.

The ancient Yogis and modern sages believe that your last thought determines your next birth. *Where the mind goes, prana flows.* Whatever thoughts you think throughout life become the composition of your next thought. I deeply consider this in my everyday life. Therefore, I try to stop the vasana somewhere on that 'wheel' before my imperceptions gets too deep, which may influence one of my next incarnations.

You incarnate according to the specific gravity of the atman/soul. How much *gravity* are you creating in these moments in your lifetime? How many samskaras are you working out from your past? Samskaras and vasanas are held in the cellular memory of your body!

Mantra

Mantras may be a sacred message, text, charm, spell, or other words of wisdom, and can help you craft your reality, both consciously and subconsciously. Mantra is important because it helps to erase impressions within your brain. *Japa* is a one-word repetition, a seed sound, which is a part of mantra. When you engage in japa throughout the day, it can help lessen the impact of the 6,000 thoughts that pass through the human mind on any given day, the vast majority of which tend to be negative or repetitive. Replacing those thoughts with thoughts of the Divine will free you from negativity and allow you to achieve a state of serenity or even bliss. That is Karma Yoga, too.

When you establish a relationship with a particular mantra, you feel how the mantra can shift the shape of energy in your body. The mantra becomes you.

I included various, traditional Sanskrit mantras at the beginning of the book. Out of thousands, or perhaps even millions of mantras, I chose the few I did because I have a personal and beloved relationship with each one of them. Each mantra has shaped me. I have used them for embodiment meditations and for other reasons, for every aspect of my life.

I also use mantras that are in English. *Om, Today, Love, And Now, Us, Cherish, Peace, Truth, Rise, Be, Present, Precious, Aware, Trust*, and many more are in my mantra toolbox. I introduce mantra through these relatable, high-frequency words to my university students. Many people begin here, like I have done with you, yet end up gravitating to the development of their own personal relationships with Sanskrit mantras. Others find great satisfaction with words from their own religious traditions. No matter which avenue you choose, when you show up for the mantra, the mantra shows up for you.

What you think you become. What you feel you attract. What you imagine, you create.

So again, what does your mantra invoke? Where does its energy land in your body? Does it then activate and vibrate your whole system?

Mantras lighten the load of mental thoughts. After a lifetime of practicing a mantra, that mantra comes in your last moment, your last breath, your last thought. Your life's Practice is what allows the mantra to come in during your last breath. In the Vedic tradition, on the moment of death whatever you think that is what you become. You leave your body and your soul enters that on which your mind is centered. Consider the energies of Love or the energies of Fear.

8.5-8.8 in the Bhagavad Gita, Krishna speaks to Arjuna.

(5) Those who remember me at the time of death will come to me. Do not doubt this. (6) Whatever occupies the mind at the time of death determines the destination of the dying; always they will tend toward that state of being. (7) Therefore remember me at all times and persist on. With your heart and mind intent of me, you will surely come to me. (8) When you make your mind one-pointed through regular practice of meditation, you will find the supreme glory of the Lord.

Tree of Cause and Effect

FREE WILL
Creation of new impressions

BRANCHES
Result of past actions
that lead to impressions

SEEDS
Creation of
new impressions,
& some take root
into new karma →

TRUNK
Birth, Life Span, Parents,
Family, Body, Mind, Values

LAYERS OF IMPRESSIONS

SUBTLE IMPRESSIONS

LATENT EFFECTS IN SUBCONSCIOUS
Unconscious: positive/negative

DEEP IMPRESSIONS
From past experiences

Another Look: Dissolving Vasanas for Liberation

There's no way out but through.

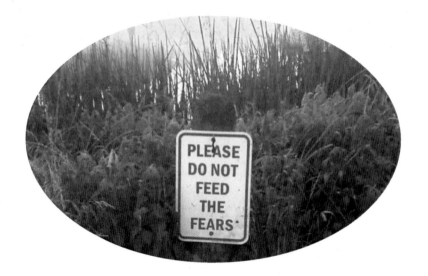

Yoga is discovering equanimity, seeing beyond fear and labels into new understandings. As noted previously, there are multiple levels of samskaras and vasanas. Some are dissolved at the time of death, but the deeper vasanas are carried from lifetime to lifetime until they are healed. Some theories postulate that this is an explanation as to why people have intense and traumatic emotional reactions that seem disproportionate to a situation. Past-life samskaras are said to explain phobias that don't stem from this-life experiences. But even intense fears can be dissolved, little by little, by cultivating the ability to simply allow them to pass through you.

Yoga is an umbrella-term for many traditions and philosophies that strive to understand the levels of consciousness and aspects of the soul. Recognizing when your emotions arise, where they are felt in your body are the first steps toward inward explorations that may lead to healing and dissolving vasanas.

1) Open the body

Engage in Yoga asana to open stagnant energy within the body, releasing emotions.

2) Open the emotional core

Meditate, meditate, meditate. Be willing to see what needs to be seen and feel what needs to be felt.

3) Self-Reflection

This is critical self-inquiry through careful inspection. Look your emotions *in the eye* with honesty. This requires truth, bravery, humility, and cultivation. A teacher or spiritual therapist may be a support to illuminate your *blind spots*.

4) Embrace experiences

When samskaras are triggered, the universe is supporting your path to liberation (*though it often doesn't feel like it at the time!*). When the emotion/desire is arising (fear, aversion, pain, craving, etc.), remain fully present. Notice the emotion and breathe, allowing it to pass through you. Importantly, resist judgement, as this not only dissolves samskaras, but prevents samskaric seeds from germinating. When you let new experiences and emotions pass through you, without clinging to them or resisting them, no samskara is deposited.

On a personal note, I recommend that you do not speculate much about your past lives. This is not necessary in cultures that embrace rebirth. The ego often paints the past with new stories, and you do not need to reengage with painful experiences to heal them. An asana and meditation practice will, in and of itself, eventually resolve all samskara. And this will happen at a rate determined solely by the clarity of your intention, the rigor and honesty of your self-inquiry, and the dedication to your holistic practice.

The Sound of Truth

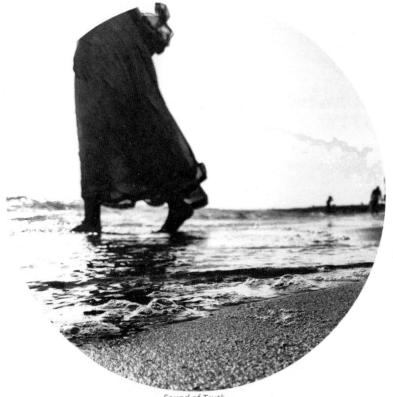

Sound of Truth

There was once a yogi well-versed in mantra. She focused her energy on one particular mantra, which provided her great insight into the other realms of Yoga. Though her humility was far from perfect, she enjoyed years of successful teaching. The yogi felt very confident that she had very little to learn from others, however, she heard of a famous sage who lived nearby as a hermit. Her curiosity could not pass up the opportunity to visit this allusive individual.

The sage lived alone on a small lake island. The yogi hired a boatman to take her for a visit. Upon her arrival, she was met with warmth, and they both shared tea. The yogi was very respectful to the elder woman, and together, they shared their spiritual experiences.

The sage did not have a teacher, nor any spiritual practice, except for one mantra. The yogi was so pleased to hear that the sage used the same mantra she did! She asked the sage to speak the mantra, but when she did so, the yogi was horrified.

"I'm sorry to say this," the yogi said, "but you are not speaking the manta appropriately. You may have wasted your life because you have not been saying it correctly this whole time."

"Oh my, that is a pity," the sage replied. "How should I say it?"

The yogi taught the elder sage the correct way in which to chant the mantra. Together, they practiced it, again and again. The elder was truly grateful to the yogi and asked to be left alone on her island so she could practice the mantra right away to make up for lost time.

The yogi was being rowed back across the lake, her eyes fixed on her destination. She was feeling very accomplished as a teacher, as well as sad at the fate of the hermit elder. *She is so fortunate that I came along. In her remaining years, at least, she will have a little time to practice before she dies.*

Just then, the boatman froze, looking quite shocked. The yogi turned to see the sage standing on the water next to the boat, respectfully waiting for her attention.

"I'm sorry to bother you," the sage said. "Can you please repeat the proper pronunciation of the mantra, as I've already forgotten it?"

The yogi stammered the mantra, and the old woman greatly thanked her. She then walked gracefully on the water back to her island, repeating the mantra carefully and deliberately, over and over again.

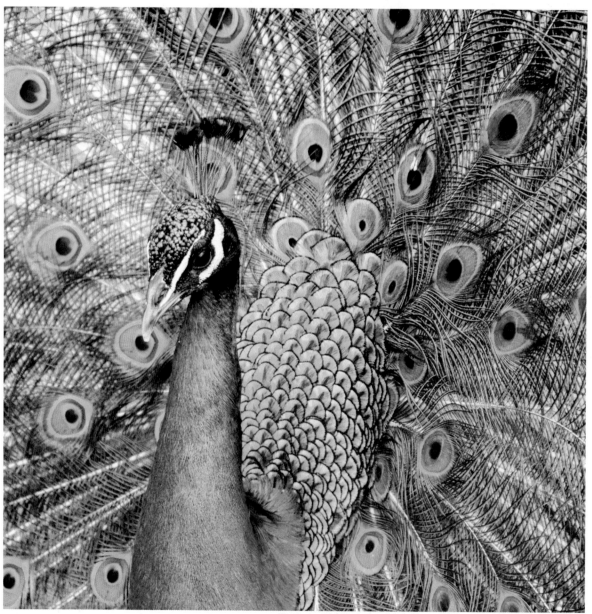

Mayūra

148

Reflection

The Roots of Yoga: Potential of Self

1) Describe the essence of Sanskrit.

2) What is the first historical evidence of Yoga?

3) What are the Vedas and why are they important?

4) A major concept in the Vedas addresses *The Power of Intention / The Power of Vibration*. What are your thoughts, if any, on the interconnection between intention and vibration?

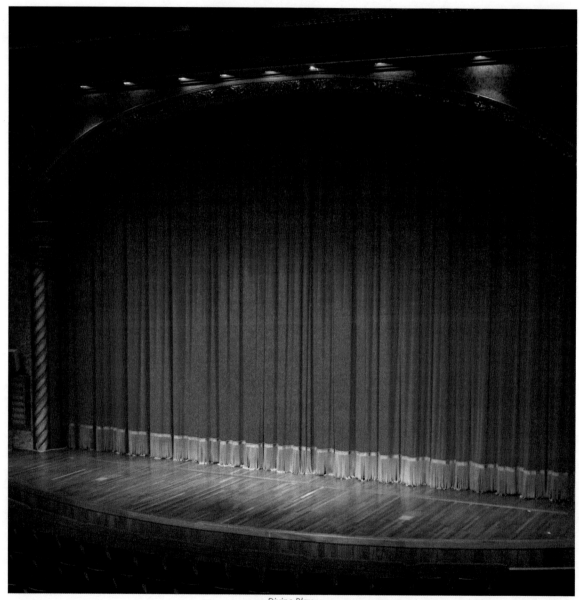

Divine Play

150

Chapter 4

The World is a Samkhya Stage: Perception, Reality, and Ayurveda 101

Historical Timeline

PRECLASSICAL YOGA ERA

INDUS-SARASVATI AGE: 6500-4500 BCE
- SANATANA DHARMA: "ETERNAL LAW"
- INDUS RIVER VALLEY & SEALS

VEDIC AGE: 4500-2500 BCE
- CONSCIOUSNESS EXPLORED
- VIBRATION OF INTENTION & CAUSATION
- CAUSE & EFFECT: MANTRA & KARMA

SAMKHYA YOGA: 8000-100 BCE
- REALITY EXPLORED: PRAKRITI/PURUSHA
- BODY'S CONSTITUTION: DOSHAS
- AYURVEDA

UPANISHADIC AGE: 2000-1500 BCE
- NON-DUALISM OF ATMAN/BRAHMAN
- DISTILLATION OF VEDAS
- MEDITATION

BHAKTI YOGA: 1000-500 BCE
- ADORATION
- HINDU EPICS / UNIVERSAL INSIGHTS
- 3 BRANCHES OF YOGA

BUDDHISM: C. 500 BCE-PRESENT
- INDIVIDUALITY / MONASTIC TRADITION
- MIDDLE WAY
- FOUR NOBLE TRUTHS / EIGHT-FOLD PATH

CLASSICAL YOGA ERA

CLASSICAL YOGA: 75 BCE-100 CE
- THE YOGA SUTRA'S OF PATANJALI
- EIGHT-LIMBED PATH
- HARNESSING THE MIND

ESOTERIC AGE

TANTRA: 600-1300 CE
- 6 + 1 CHAKRA SYSTEM
- WESTERN NOTION OF EMBODIMENT
- SUBTLE BODY (NADIS, CHAKRAS, ETC.)

HATHA YOGA: C. 1300-1400 CE
- MIND V. BODY
- HATHA YOGA PRADIPIKA
- ASANA / BREATH / BANDHAS / MUDRAS

RISE OF MODERN YOGA

SWAMI VIVEKANANDA: 1872-1950
- INFLUENCED RISE OF MODERN YOGA
- INTRODUCED YOGA TO THE WEST

SRI T. KRISHNAMACHARYA: 1891-1989
- YOGA'S EXPANSION
- FATHER OF MODERN YOGA
- MODERN CONTRIBUTORS

Chapter 4
The World is a Samkhya Stage

1. Overview of Lecture

Chapter 4 introduces key concepts in Samkhya Philosophy: *Purusha* and *Prakriti*. *Purusha* is Consciousness and Truth. *Prakriti* is unconscious material existence, always changing, and is mistakenly understood as Truth. Analyze how these concepts play out in everyday life, and how they influence the construction of experience and perception. Included in this chapter is an overview of Ayurveda, the Knowledge of Life. Doshas (the physical body's constitution) is examined as to how it affects how reality is perceived.

2. Learning Objectives: I will...

a) Understand that my Witness Self is also known as Purusha
b) Examine how Prakriti has influenced qualities of *the three gunas* – the attributes of creation
c) Identify my primary and secondary dosha
d) Explore how to balance my dosha through the concept of Ayurveda and awareness

3. Pre-lecture Assignments

a) Read this chapter and become familiar with the Reflection questions
b) Read *The Power of Now* by Eckhart Tolle
c) Daily Sadhana - Daily Personal Practice

4. Reflection: *found at the end of the chapter*

Lila, the Divine Play of Life

All the world's a stage, and all the men and women merely players: they have their exits and their entrances; and one man in his time, plays many parts. ~ William Shakespeare

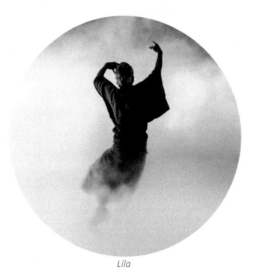

Lila

William Shakespeare said, "Life is but a dream, within a dream." *Lila* is a Sanskrit term describing life and all reality, not as a dream, but as a divine play. Lila is the stage upon which life unfolds. The definition of Self and place in the universe is explored through Lila. Labels and judgements are explored through Lila. Life lessons are learned through Lila. Lila describes all reality, which manifests on earthly, cosmic, and interdimensional realities.

Lila is the 'play of life' on the stage representing reality. In the Vedic tradition, Lila is the nature of Shakti, feminine energy, representing the most powerful form of energy in the universe. *The Bhagavad Gita* states, "Act for action's sake but do not be attached to the fruits of your actions." This means to live deeply involved, but to trust that all things will unfold with divine timing; all things unfold perfectly.

Brahman is Supreme Existence and Absolute Reality. *Brahman* is also the stage of your personal life experience on which Lila unfolds. *Brahman* represents the absolute aspect of perfectionism and possibility. Energies comprising reality, as it is known, are formed from Brahman. These energetic forms are categorized as good or bad, familiar or unfamiliar. This is a dualistic point of view. In striving to make an irrational world rational, stories are created, as are defining labels of self, place, and other. The more life is lived through this limited scope of labels, however, the less freedom can be experienced.

When experiencing an event on a horizonal, earthly reality, labels arise. This is due to *Maya*, an ever-changing magical illusion which conceals the true character of spiritual reality. Maya is the curtain, the veil, that establishes the boundaries between the seen world and the invisible world. Seeing beyond the veil, therefore *seeing within Maya*, is looking behind the actor's mask, looking behind the curtain, dismantling any story of self-limitation, including victimhood. Seeing within Maya pierces illusion, so that freedom and holistic interconnection can be experienced.

Reality can be experienced in a non-dualistic manner by recognizing the nature of Lila and each role within the Divine Play in which every person and life form is participating. Labels, patterns, and perceptions create the illusion of the play you are participating in. By living only within the illusion, you limit your perspective of reality; it becomes a dualistic story – a story of me/other, me/Divine. Once you recognize this, you can step out of the play and experience life in a non-dualistic, non-limiting way.

To be more authentically in control of your life, cease labeling *who* and *what*. Think of these energies of reality as simply being *heavy* or *light*, and both qualities are of great service to existence. Lila explores these energies as three modes of nature, which are *the Gunas*, which will be explored later in this book.

All qualities co-exist in harmony. Harmony demands a dance of birth, preservation, and destruction. The role of a conscious human being is to widen their inner and outer vision to see Brahman, Divinity, in all aspects of life, known and unknown. Everything that is encountered in life is the unfolding of a divine play, where all roads lead to Bliss. Bliss opens when the emotional, mental, and physical vision becomes expanded wide enough. Lila offers that all experiences are done for your betterment, including heartbreak, yet your heart must be open to receive the gift. It can take time and high perspective to see it, but once you do, healing takes place. But this work is done in the realm of Lila, as the soul expands.

155

Samkhya Philosophy of Creation

The purpose of Samkhya is about liberating the human soul.

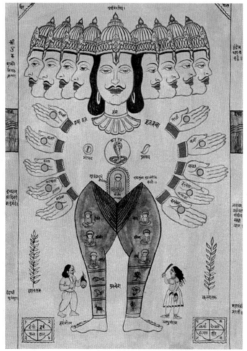

Cosmic Man

Sam- means to bring together with experiential discrimination, and *-khya* means to enumerate. *Samkhya Yoga* is a Vedic philosophy that has no identifiable date of origin yet is considered the oldest known school of philosophy. However, the roots of Samkhya philosophy are thought to be older than the Rig Veda; beyond 8000 BCE. Samkhya lays a massive foundation for spiritual and religious traditions. Samkhya philosophy is also the basis for Ayurveda, the Knowledge of Life.

Breaking it Down: Dualism and Non-dualism

Samkhya Yoga is a dualistic system and is often referred to as a Metaphysical Dualism. Metaphysics is a branch of philosophy that looks at the nature of reality; what is *there*? Is it energy in a being, substance, nature? *What is reality?*

Mono is a prefix that means one, only, single.

The term *monism* means a reality made of one thing. In other words, everything that appears is an expression of the same fundamental stuff; everything is One.

Examples of monism are *Idealism* (reality is an expression of ideas), and *Advaita Vedanta* from the Indian Tradition. In the Advaita Vedanta tradition, everything is ultimately an expression of Brahman. Brahman is eternal and singular, and there is only one *thing*, and that is the Absolute Consciousness of Brahman. The goal of Yoga practice is to merge with that Absolute. Everything starts from Purusha's consciousness, and everything is Brahman. Every difference/form/thought is an illusion, yet truly Brahman.

Dual means consisting of two parts, elements, or aspects.

Dualistic examples include the *Saiva Siddhanta System*, where God is always the leader and the soul is always led. From the Christian Orthodox perspective, there, too, is no merging with God. However, the poetry of Christian mystics describes a merging, and every tradition has its own esoteric form of the experience of monism. There always remains point of view through personal tendencies.

Non-duality is <u>not</u> saying there is only one thing, but <u>it is saying</u> there are not two things. This is an important, yet subtle, distinction. The non-dual is what is experienced in meditation.

Non-duality is an attempt to articulate a state of consciousness that has been experienced in the context of meditation, where the experience is that *difference is non-separate from itself*; there is no separation between what appears as multiple. You navigate through the world of Prakriti as you would in a connective state; an extension of the world that is experienced in larger perspective states of consciousness. In Kashmir Shaivism, Shiva and Shakti are never separated because they are consciousness and energy. Both are needed for the other to exist.

The intention, or *Sankulpa*, of Samkhya is to liberate oneself from suffering; to find a mode of existence that transcends the ordinary structure of human experience. Here, there is recognition of the fact that there is suffering in your inner world. The question is, *how do you get out of the cycle of suffering?*

Suffering is based on the entanglement of Purusha in Prakriti. Classical Samkhya and Classical Yoga are both traditions based on dualism. They are about dis-union, not union. The goal of Yoga is dis-union. Disunion of what? The disunion of Purusha from Prakriti.

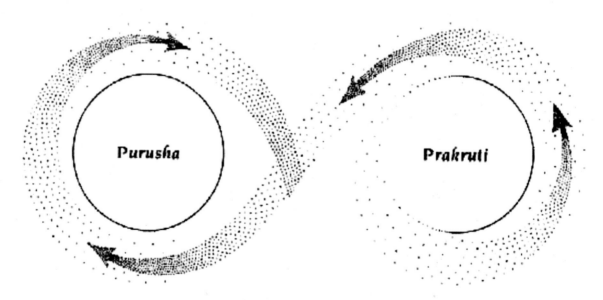

Metaphysics in Samkhya Philosophy

Purusha and Prakriti, Gunas and Doshas

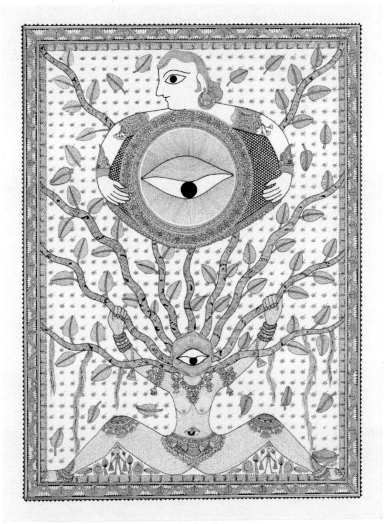

Photo Credit: Google Images

Samkhya Dualism of Purusha and Prakriti

I recognize there is something observing everything that is happening. I can acknowledge that Witness, unperturbed, despite the changeableness of what is being perceived. There is a fact of consciousness, and there is fact of the world that I'm witnessing. I am conscious of my consciousness.

Purusha

Purusha is the Witness; the Fact of Consciousness. Purusha is pure existence, passive, unbiased, content-less Consciousness, likened to the Spectator of Life. Purusha is the father-force, pure potential. Purusha is unmanifested, formless, the absolute Reality; Ishvara, beyond attributes, beyond cause and effect, beyond space and time. Purusha is pure Existence. Purusha is referred to as the *Cosmic Man*, in the early Rig Vedas.

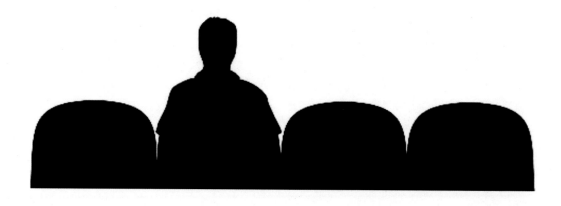

Prakriti

Prakriti is the Witnessed; the Content of Consciousness; Substance. Prakriti is extended from material reality to the subtlest aspects of psychology; both physical and psychological. If it can be witnessed, it is a part of Prakriti. Prakriti is the creative force of action, likened to the Interpretive Dancer of Life. Prakriti is the mother-force, ever-changing, manifestation of Purusha's potential. Prakriti is matter composed by three forces which are the building blocks of reality; elemental combinations called *the gunas – rajas, tamas, and sattva*. All experiences and perspectives are guna-driven, driven by the qualities of your nature. Prakriti offers you all obstacles necessary for your liberation. Equanimity gained through action and love are key.

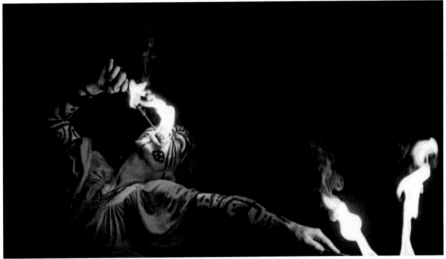

Dancer

Purusha appears as what it is not.
Prakriti appears as what it is not.
Only by appearing as what it is not
can Purusha be what it is.

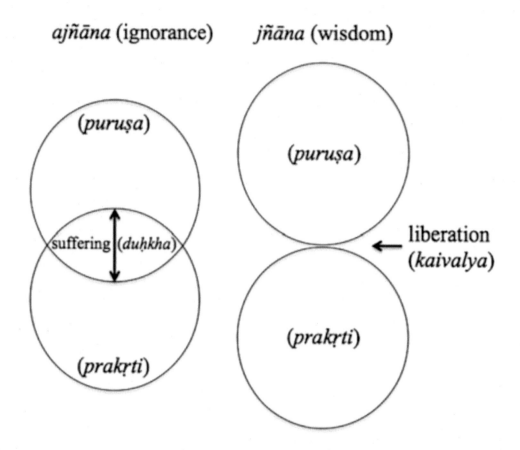

Sāṃkhya, Fig. 2 Ignorance (*ajñāna*) and knowledge (*jñāna*)

Samkhya explores different levels of consciousness, which define the universe based on the existence of two states of reality - *Purusha* and *Prakriti* (also spelled/spoken *Prakruti*). All substance is Prakriti, and Purusha is the pure witnessing present (the witnessing of all substance), the fact of consciousness into the world. Prakriti is translated crudely as matter or nature, or material or physical. All of cognition and all the material world are a part of Prakriti. Purusha is the pure, witnessing presence of consciousness.

Just as fire is different from the sparks that ignite it and the smoke that billows from it, the body is connected to the Purusha, yet is not the Purusha. Purusha is the true Self that every individual lifeform has, and it is a very complex concept with diverse meanings. It is the all-pervasive Universal Principle. Purusha is unchanging, pure potential, non-perceivable, it encompasses the principles of nature. Purusha is the Self, the universal thinker behind thoughts, the seer behind sight, the knower behind words. Purusha, is always the witness to the play of life, the play of consciousness, which is *Lila*.

While Purusha represents pure potential, Prakriti is the manifesting force giving rise to physical form and the creative force behind actions. Prakriti is manifested from the unmanifested, primordial condition. Prakriti is the undifferentiated plentitude of reality; the undifferenced *Ocean of Being* before it manifests into differentiation.

Purusha can't be experienced in the knowledge of the Prakriti realm. You are in Prakriti, using body/mind tools, such as a language to express and infer the existence of something that can only be experienced from or in Prakriti.

The universe, described by Samkhya, is one created by the interaction of Purusha and Prakriti, resulting in various permutations and combinations of enumerated elements like senses, feelings, activity, and mindfulness/thoughts. During a state of imbalance, Purusha remains in bondage, due to its false identification of self with *chitta* (mind-thoughts). The end of this imbalance or bondage is referred to as liberation, or *moksha*.

Because of the differences and proportions of the three gunas, each individual person is interacting with their own play of consciousness based on their own 'gunic mix' of what is happening in the *buddhi*, the intellect.

The Three Gunas

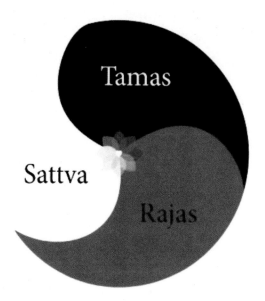

Each person is born into, according to the Laws of Karma, a particular constitution. Prakriti assumes qualities from a combination of the five elements – earth, water, fire, air, and ether – that exist both in nature and in every being. Specific combinations of these elements constitute the three energetic forces called the *gunas*. The gunas are the attributes of creation and the building blocks of reality itself.

Guna means strand. The three gunas are *rajas, tamas, and sattva*. *Rajas* is dynamic movement and activity. It is the vital life force of the body and moves the organic and inorganic universal materials of the other two gunas. *Tamas* is static, inertia. Though tamas is not active, it is pure potential which needs action to manifest. *Sattva* is pure balanced essence, and like tamas, needs rajas to manifest creative potential.

Dosha and Guna Relationships

Every living being is born with specific tendencies and constitutions formed through a unique combination of the five elements and their properties that comprise the three gunas. All beings embody all three gunas. (Combinations of the three gunas, which we'll discuss later in this chapter, give rise to *the three doshas* – the combination of elemental forces affecting physical, mental, emotional, and spiritual existence. The doshas contain all five elements in nature, but each dosha is predominantly composed of two elements.) The gunas thus help explain the characteristics and tendencies of a person on both a physical and psychological level. What you see as reality, influenced by labels and stories, is really a series of perceptions distilled through the lenses of the gunas. Your dominant guna, or combination of gunas, will define how you experience reality at any given point in time.

The fabric of your existence is thus woven by the strands of the gunas, which cause you to see the world through various veils of contrast and diversity, limiting your ability to connect with your higher Self. For this reason, the gunas are sometimes described as "the ropes that bind the soul to the world." In other words, these ropes bind you to a reality that separate you from the state of Oneness. Realization that life is Lila, comprised of Prakriti, and Purusha is separate from Prakriti, is a gateway to achieving the bliss-state of liberation. When the mind is stilled and the gunas are in the balance of sattva, truth is revealed.

Here is a visual for the cycle of suffering, Samsara (Rebirth), and Moksha (Liberation).

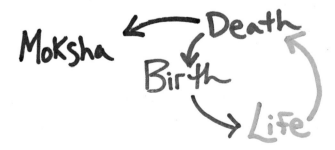

The goal of Samkhya philosophy is to experience the liberating knowledge that Purusha is separate from Prakriti. This knowledge leads to *moksha*, another word for liberation.

Suffering exists because people misidentify themselves as only Prakriti. This false identification creates mental impressions (*samskaras/karma*) from experiences that form fear and desires, therefore conditioning future behaviors and responses. This creates the cycle of rebirth (*samsara*).

Reality, as you experience it, is not the truth because it consists of ever-changing perceptions and mental impressions that are influenced by the gunas. Through Prakriti, you experience the influence of the gunas as everything, gross and subtle. The gunas affect your thoughts, resulting in actions, and, thus, germination of the *bija*, Sanskrit for the seed of potential. This is the moment in which you manifest your reality.

By training the mind and recognizing how you are being influenced by your gunas, you have the ability to pierce the veils of Prakriti and recognize the Purusha-Self. As you move into this Purusha state, you experience a reality of greater freedom and, eventually, full liberation, or moksha. As your practice develops, you can move in and out of these states, tasting these levels of consciousness.

According to Samkhya philosophy and the central principle of Yoga, the goal is to return to a state of Purusha consciousness. You can achieve moksha by stilling the fluctuations of the mind.

The Bhagavad Gita states, "In the still mind, in the depths of meditation, the Self reveals itself. Beholding the Self by means of the Self, an aspirant knows the joy and peace of complete fulfillment." (6.20)

The Yoga Sutras states," Then the Seer (Self/*Drashta*, referring to Purusha) abides in One's own nature." (1.3)

Samkhya Summary on Suffering and Moksha

❖ The nature of Prakriti is made from the three gunas. Whatever is produced will change, die, decay, and is not the Self.

❖ Prakriti falsely identifies with feelings of misery from rajas and tamas, forgetting its capacity to see beyond the veil of false identification.

❖ Purusha needs Prakriti to distinguish itself from Prakriti, so it can realize its true nature. The activity of Prakriti must be guided by Purusha's intelligence.

❖ By understanding this, you will become liberated in your lifetime. Upon physical death, you achieve Moksha, never to be reborn in a human form unless by choice.

❖ People who choose to return are known as *siddhas* and *bodhisattvas*, and can be seen in the forms of Krishna, Jesus, Buddha, among many, many others. They teach from an authentic-life experience rooted in universal integrity.

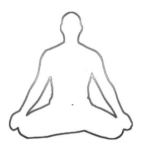

Originally, self-realization through Samkhya philosophy was learned under the guidance of an enlightened guru, a *Jivanmukta*, who drew from their personal experiences. The teacher/student (*guru/shishya*) relationship was the fundamental means by which knowledge was transferred and obtained.

Samkhya's 25 Tattvas

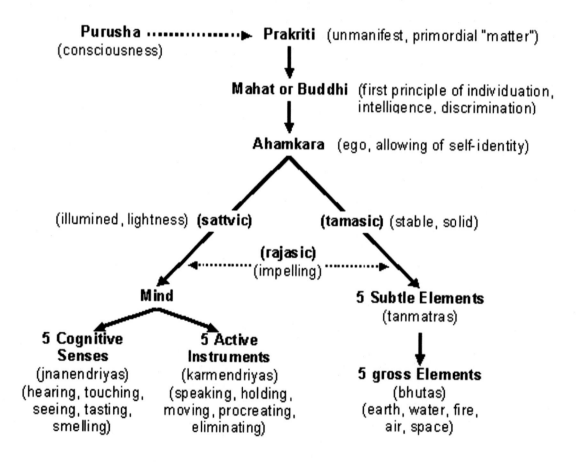

Purusha ·····························▶ **Prakriti** (unmanifest, primordial "matter")
(consciousness)

Mahat or Buddhi (first principle of individuation,
intelligence, discrimination)

Ahamkara (ego, allowing of self-identity)

(illumined, lightness) **(sattvic)**   **(tamasic)** (stable, solid)

(rajasic)
(impelling)

Mind   **5 Subtle Elements**
(tanmatras)

**5 Cognitive   5 Active
Senses   Instruments**
(jnanendriyas)   (karmendriyas)   **5 gross Elements**
(hearing, touching, (speaking, holding,   (bhutas)
seeing, tasting,   moving, procreating,   (earth, water, fire,
smelling)   eliminating)   air, space)

In a nutshell...

Samkhya is a philosophical school based on a systematic enumeration and rational interpretation of the world. There are *25 tattvas* (elements or true principles), and 24 levels of Prakriti that influence its distinction and separateness from Purusha. Its ultimate objective is liberation.

1. **Unmanifested Purusha** - Soul, pure, contentless consciousness

2. **Prakriti** - unmanifested energy, primordial materiality

3. **Buddhi/mahat** - intellect, the pre-egoic awareness space

4. **Ahamkara** - Ego, I-ness, existence of self

5. **Manas** - perceptual mind, emotions

6 – 10. **Buddhindriya**- Five sense organs: hearing, touching, seeing, tasting, smelling

11 – 15. **Karmendriyas** - Five motor organs: speaking, grasping, walking, excreting, procreating

16 – 20. **Tanmatras** - Five subtle elements: sound, touch, form, taste, smell

21 – 25. **Mahabutas** - Five gross elements: space, air, fire, water, earth

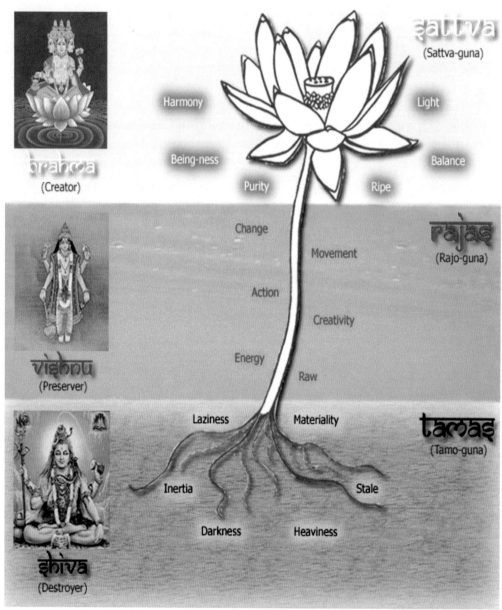

Photo Credit: Google Images

Prakrti and the Three Gunas

Expression of Energy, the Building Blocks of Reality

Prakriti is a Sanskrit word which means "original or primary substance; the natural form or condition of anything." The pure energetic source of *Purusha* (masculine/potential) gives rise to *Prakriti* (female/manifestation). Everything you think (cognitively, morally, psychologically), everything you feel (emotionally), and everything you experience (through your senses and the material/physical world) is Prakriti.

Prakriti is characterized by the three gunas. *Guna* literally means strand, as in weaving the tapestry of the universe. Each of the three gunas has an innate quality of its own. The combined balance of the gunas is the basis of all observed reality. Gunas are always in flux between being balanced and imbalanced, which results in life experiences of harmony or friction. These expressions and strands of energy are transformed and manifested in the world that is experienced through cause-and-effect relationships.

The gunas are the building blocks of the universe and reality itself, both the tangible and intangible. The three gunas (as mentioned previously) are *tamas, rajas,* and *sattva*. Understanding the nature of each guna will support a deeper recognition and communion with the manifesting source of Purusha. The gunas are how you understand the human organism (the microcosm) and the world (the macrocosm). The psychological reflects the physical.

Tamas - inertia, inactivity, ignorance, apathy, dullness. This energy is slow and grounding and necessary for rest. When overabundant, you feel dull, depressed, lethargic, heavy; and it is difficult to feel physically and mentally enlivened. Tamas-overabundance hides awareness and hinders self-inquiry, and in this state, your personal fears interpret your daily experiences.

Rajas - passion, motion, activity, energy, desire, fire of life, ego. The generating force that keeps things moving. This energy is extroverted, its passion, and it's needed for motivation. When overabundant, however, you feel fidgety, anxious, moody, agitated, or bored. Rajas-overabundance hides awareness, hinders self-inquiry. Your behavior might be called manic, and your desire interprets your daily experiences.

Sattva - harmony, purity, creative, luminous, serenity, balance of Rajas and Tamas. This energy is grounded, calm, and aware. It is a balance of Tamas and Rajas, which allows your spiritual expression to move outward into your physical self. Sattva is liberation through holistic balance. This groundedness is accomplished through breath work, a Yoga practice, what you eat, how you interact with the world, the music you listen to, how you appreciate your home, how you appreciate and approach all beings, and how you receive all things you encounter. Your outer world reflects your inner world. A sattvic state is more conductive to greater alignment, it's more open to the nature of *Samadhi*; it's the Bliss State.

> *sattvaṃ laghu prakāśakam* - Sattva is buoyant and shining
> *iṣṭam upaṣṭambhakaṃ calaṃ ca rajaḥ* - Rajas is stimulating and moving
> *guru varaṇakam eva tamaḥ* - tamas is heavy and enveloping
> *pradīpavac cā'rthato vṛttiḥ* - They function for the sake of the Puruṣa like a lamp
> ~ *From The Samkhyakarika, the earliest text of the Samkhya School of Indian Philosophy*

When unbalanced, one guna manifests and dominates the other two gunas, resulting in a particular lens of perception. The gunas are aspects of how you perceive your unique relationship to reality, offering a training ground for you to explore your mental and emotional walls, which are linked to your body's physical expressions and limitations, and your thoughts, words, actions, and ultimately, your daily life experiences. You will experience your physical reality in a different way from another person. Your manifested Prakriti is a result of the moods and dispositions of your pre-egoic awareness space.

The goal is to experience reality in a sattvic way. The more you become sattvic, the more you can burn through samskaras to reach the liberation of living in the present moment, which is the purpose of the practice and is the essence of meditation. Meditation is a practice to be conscious of your consciousness, and to live fully in the now, to be more *sattvic*. This energy focus dissolves the density of samskaras.

TAMAS	SATTVA	RAJAS
Darkness, Moon	Balance, Ambrosia Hour (sunrise/sunset)	Light, Solar
inertia, inactivity and materiality	harmony, peace, joy, intelligence	energy, action, change, dynamic movement
Needed to: Sit still, listen, sleep, be with what is	**Needed to:** Make liberation possible, *Moksha*	**Needed to:** Rise from bed, daily living, clarity, motivation to alter, attraction
When out of balance: Dull, depressed, repressed, neglectful, denied, ignorance, underactive	**Always Balanced**	**When out of balance:** Chaotic, manic, obsessive, addicted, greed, selfish lust, overactive, longing, attachment/binding to work
Avoid: Oversleeping, over eating, inactivity, passivity, yin yoga	**EMBRACE:** Activities and environments that promote inner joy, self-accountability, yogic lifestyle	**Avoid:** Over-exercising, obsessive work / long work hours, loud music, excessive thinking, over consumption in general, only practicing hot, energizing yoga
Foods to avoid: Heavy meats, microwaved food, chemically treated, processed, refined	**Foods to EMBRACE:** Fresh fruits and vegetables growing above ground, whole grains, legumes, living water	**Foods to avoid:** Wine, fried foods, spicy foods, stimulants

*We can't talk about our own health without understanding our place
in our environment, because in order to fulfill our potential we have to live
in the context of our surroundings. We have to know our place in
the ecosystem of which we are a part, and this means living 'consciously':
being aware of nature and how it affects us and how we, in turn, affect nature.*

~ Sebastian Pole

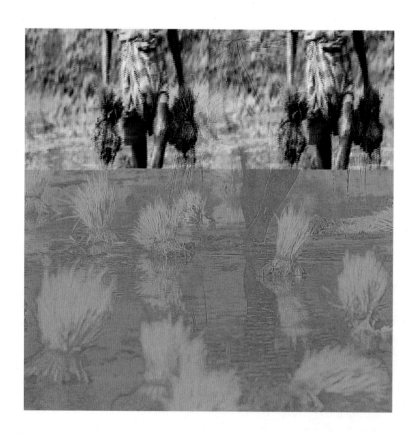

Without insight and practice, the mind's psychological qualities are unstable. The predominant guna of the mind acts as a lens that determines the perceptions and perspectives you form of your reality.

Too Much Tamas Too Much Past	SATTVA PRESENCE	Too Much Rajas Too Much Future
guilt	harmony	unease
regret	lightness	anxiety
resentment	joy	tension
grievances	peace	stress
sadness	freedom	worry
bitterness	balance	fear
depression	clarity	agitation
apathy	openness	desire
ignorance	intelligence	egotism

Ayurveda 101: A Brief Introduction

*One who is established in Self, who has balanced dosha (primary life force),
balanced agni (digestive fire), properly formed dhatus (tissues),
proper elimination of malas (waste), well-functioning bodily processes,
and who's mind, soul, and senses are full of bliss is called a healthy person.*

~ Sushruti Samhita 15.38

Ayurveda and Yoga are sister sciences. *Ayurveda* is premised on the understanding that the macrocosm of the universe mirrors the microcosm of the universe within the human body. It explores the concept of "for whom and when" and applies that concept as the approach to deciding what is best for a specific individual. Ayurveda also explores how external, natural cycles and seasons can affect one's internal system balance, therefore influencing how one perceives and experiences reality.

Ayurveda comes from *ayuh* meaning life or longevity, and *veda* means 'study of.' *Ayurveda* is known as the Science/Study of Life. The most accurate term expressing Ayurveda is *Knowledge of Life*. It is one of the world's oldest sciences; a system which uses the principles of nature and the five elements (air, water, fire, earth, and ether) to help maintain health by balancing the mind, body, and spirit. Ayurveda exceeds 6,000 years of history and has contributed to the foundation of the healthcare system. This system protects health and eliminates diseases and body dysfunctions based on an individualized approach.

Ayurveda is about creating balanced, embodied conditions of the physical form, which therefore affects mental forms. These conditions are the necessary foundations which support the processes of deep meditative insight and self-realization. Ayurveda is about cultivating a sattvic state and has to do with the decisions you make at the level of your own lifestyle in order to live in that state.

If one system in the body is in disharmony, all systems will not function properly. Illness and the ability to heal is based on how well prana flows in the subtle body, the physical systems of the body. Understanding why and how prana moves is key to optimal, holistic health. Ayurveda looks at the whole picture of the person – from lifestyle and belief systems to the sounds of the voice, to posture, gait, gestures, stance, and more.

There is an overidentification with the forms of suffering. For example, "I am my depression. I am my anxiety." Ayurveda is coupled with the understanding that *you are not your disease (dis-ease)* or any of the conditions of your embodiment.

The root of suffering is *avidya*, ignorance. Ignorance is manifested through misidentifications with various tattvas. *Tattvas* are various levels of individuality, personality, and truth. Here, you overidentify with your identified states of affliction, and you have difficulty leaving them because you know them so well. There is something scarier about leaving the condition you know and identify with than moving into a more sattvic kind of condition accompanied by an experience of self that is alien to what you have considered yourself to be.

The practice of becoming more sattvic is partly a practice of disidentifying yourself from everything you've come to think of as you – your forms of suffering and your forms of joys. That doesn't mean that you are beyond or above emotional states. Rather, you don't become so identified with any of them or the labels you give them. You don't identify yourself with moments of joy, because when joy leaves, you won't be in a position of profound suffering because you wanted that joy to stay there.

You have happy periods in your life, which you want to cling to it, and when life turns bitter, then you have not cultivated the flexibility to be able to hold space for that shifting character of the gunas. The gunas, as you know, are always in a state of permutation. There is constant transmutation, and a mixing of the gunas, that is different at every stage of your life, and that change will not stop until your final liberation. The gesture of attachment is one that tries to make permanent what is impermanent.

Ayurveda works with the five elements that make up all that exists in the universe – earth, water, fire, air, and ether (space). Each element has a unique mind and body constitution, and when they're combined, they make your Ayurvedic fingerprint, called a *dosha*.

A *dosha* represents a constitutional body type, referred to as *Prakriti* - essential nature. **Doshas are made by combinations of the universal elements, which are comprised of the gunas' qualities.** The three doshas in the Ayurvedic system are *Vata, Pitta,* and *Kapha*. Each dosha has varied amounts of each element.

Understanding and balancing your main dosha is where your inner work lies.

Your dosha(s) affects your physical and emotional characteristics. Identifying what dosha(s) rules your system allows you better insight into your behaviors and allows you to make choices to obtain sattva (balance). Understanding your dosha will nurture and balance your holistic intelligence so you may make clear and grounded choices to support your wellbeing. This enables you to stand in your Authentic Self. Doshas facilitate the mind's dialogue with the body. Imbalance of the doshas disrupts the mind-body physiology, causing dis-ease. Disease. Once the doshas are restored to balance, the body and mind enjoy ease.

IMPORTANT: What is your Dosha?

The coming pages will examine the concept of Doshas.
Before you move on, determine your main dosha by taking a quick online dosha quiz.
Simply Google, 'Dosha Quiz' and many good options will pop up.

❖ *Remember that you embody all doshas. When taking the test, allow your initial 'gut' response help you determine what your main dosha is.*

The 5 Elements of the Universe and Body

Ether (space): all encompassing, pure potentiality, light, subtle and clear
Air: movement, change, light, mobile, clear, rough, and dry.
Fire: transformation, hot, direct, assimilation, digestion, metabolism, sharp, fluid, penetrating
Water: cohesion, protection, taste, heavy, wet, lubricating, cool, soft
Earth: solid structure, form, grounded, stable, thick, dense, solid, hard, heavy, stable

	Space / Ether	Air	Fire	Water	Earth
Sense	Sound Hear	Touch Feel	Sight See	Taste Taste	Fragrance Smell
Organ	Ears	Skin	Eyes	Tongue	Nose
Motor	Vocal Chords	Hands	Legs	Reproductive Organs	Excretory Organs
Chakra	5th Throat Vishuddha	4th Heart Anahata	3rd Solar Plexus Manipura	2nd Sacral Svadhisthana	1st Root Muladhara
Bija/Seed Sound	HAM	YAM	RAM	VAM	LAM

Guna and Dosha Relationship

Your experience with the Gunas are directly related to your dosha, your body's constitution.

The gunas can be balanced by understanding your dosha (your body/mind constitutions), paired with your willingness to explore new perspectives on daily living and the choices you make.

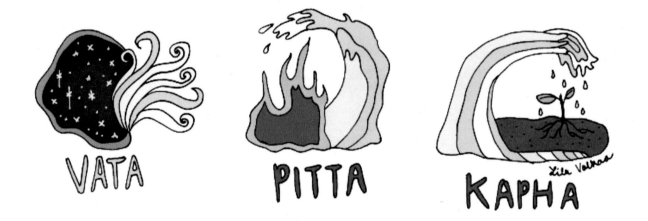

In Ayurveda, like attracts like, which causes imbalance, while opposites heal.

Recall that Prakriti consists of the three gunas: rajas, tamas, and sattva. Rajas has more dynamic fire qualities, while tamas has heavier earth qualities. Sattva is a balance of the elements of space, air, fire, water, and earth. Understanding the doshas in relationship with the gunas, one can better navigate day-to-day emotions and choices.

The three doshas incorporate the primary elements. Vata is ether and air, kapha is water and earth, and pitta is fire and water. All three doshas exist and interact within the constitution of all creatures, and the relative effect of each dosha may change from time to time. In general, though, you are influenced by a primary dosha that has specific dominance resulting from the combination of a specific set of elements. Like the gunas, like attracts like, and you tend to engage in activities, or be attracted to things, that "align" with your dominant dosha. But, while this "alignment" may feel natural at the time, you may find that you need more of the "opposite" to help balance a dosha that is out of alignment.

Each dosha is influenced by the gunas. Though guna and dosha comparisons are not cleanly 'cut and dry', in general, they are as follows: vata has more movement qualities and is prone to rajas; pitta's fire qualities are also prone to rajas; and kapha has earth qualities and is more prone to tamas.

In Ayurveda, one's perception of reality is based on how balanced these qualities ~ representing space, air, fire, water, and earth ~ are within the body's systems. Sometimes, the combination of these influences can create an overabundance of an element(s). This overabundance, in turn, can alter how one experiences and perceives reality. Agitation, anxiety, depression, and lethargy, for example, are symptoms of being unaligned. These symptoms could result if there is an overabundance of tamasic influence on a person with a dominant kapha constitution. Similarly, too much air may cause anxiety if you are vata, and too much fire may cause irritation if you are pitta. Although you may be attracted to your "likes", you have heard that too much of a "good thing" can just be too much!

On the other hand, opposites can heal. So, when you are feeling flighty and unable to concentrate, you may want to engage in some grounding behavior to help balance your system. Understanding when you are out of balance, and thus out of alignment, allows you to use learned tools and take the measures needed to regain sattva (balance). In other words, when an imbalance is perceived, consider what qualities are associated with the imbalance and look for what opposing qualities can be brought in for balance (lifestyle, diet, thought patterns, Yoga, etc.).

Each dosha also has an associated time of day, a lunar cycle, and season associated with it. For example, autumn and early winter are vata seasons, which are dry, light, and cold. Both late winter and early spring are considered kapha seasons, which are wet, heavy, and cool. Summer is the pitta season, being liquid and hot.

It is energetically beneficial for Yoga teachers to craft appropriate classes that are in-line with the season, which will then support the balance of all doshas. However, if a dosha is out-of-balance, regardless of the time of year, remember opposites heal. For example, the pitta dosha may gravitate toward a hot Yoga class after a demanding day at work. But if there is an overabundance of pitta, a slow, soothing class may be a more appropriate way to cool the internal fire, rather than continue a day of stress with more action and competition transferred to the mat. Likewise, the kapha dosha may gravitate toward a cooling Yin Yoga class. But an energizing Yoga class that raises the heartbeat, builds muscle, and invokes sweat will also balance the thicker qualities that are innately kapha. Vata dosha may be drawn to fast-paced, flexibility-inducing classes. However, a slow, warm, grounding, and strengthening class will soothe and ground this spinning energy.

The following pages will support a larger look into how the doshas are played out in daily life.

Interesting to Note:

- Doshas change throughout life. Younger people are more Pitta, as this is a season of exploration, learning, and asking, "Why". As one become older, Vata naturally increases.

- Kapha, pronounced in Southern India is *kapp-a*, as there is no -f sound in Sanskrit. Kapha, pronounced in Northern India is often *kaff-a*, per rules of the English language, as this language and phonetic standards were influenced by English rule.

Tendencies of the Three Doshas

VATA Ether & Air	KAPHA Water & Earth	PITTA Fire & Water
Wind Movement & change	Earth Structure & fluidity	Transformation & digestion
Vata Qualities: Light, Dry, Cool, Rough, Irregular, Mobile/Quick, Subtle	**Kapha Qualities:** Cold, Wet, Heavy, Slow, Solid, Soft, Cold, Oily, Smooth, Dense, Stable, Sticky/Slimy	**Pitta Qualities:** Oily, Sharp, Hot, Light, Spreading, Liquid, Fermenting, Churning Mind
Vata tends to overextend/leak energy in many life-areas resulting in adrenal fatigue. Are often are physically hypermobile and muscularly tense.	Kapha tends to need motivation in some life-areas if energetically sluggish. Are often physically hypermobile and need additional core strength.	Pitta tends to hyper-focus and overextend/push energy in many life-areas, energetically overheating causing stress. Are often physically competitive and strain the body.
Found in: Joints, hollow organs, bone cavities, colon, thighs, ears, nervous system	**Found in:** Cells and forms of muscle, fat, bone, and sinew	**Found in:** Blood, oil, and acidic secretions, small intestine, stomach, eyes
Controls: All body movements and thought movement	**Controls:** Body structure and strength in muscles, tendons, bones, and cells	**Controls:** Digestion, metabolism, energy production
Physical Characteristics: Thin, light frame, arthritis, agile, energetic bursts, fatigue, dry skin and hair, cold hands and feet, light sleep, hypertension, sensitive digestion.	**Physical Characteristics:** Strong body and stamina, large features (eyes, lips, breasts), radiant skin and hair, regular sleep, regular digestion.	**Physical Characteristics:** Medium size and weight, fiery nature in body and mind, warm temperature, thinning hair or baldness, regular digestion, regular sleep, strong sex drive and appetite, lustrous complexion.

Prone to weight loss, constipation, weakness, skin conditions, dryness, hyperactivity, anxiety, arthritis.	**Prone to** sinus conditions, congestion, excess weight, excess sleep, fluid retention, allergies, asthma, diabetes.	**Prone to** rashes, ulcers, hypertension, acne, indigestion.
Emotional Characteristics: Energetic, creative, social, flexible.	**Emotional Characteristics:** Grounded, calm, thoughtful, loving, routine-oriented, patient, supportive.	**Emotional Characteristics:** Good concentration, intellect, precise, direct.
Prone to restlessness, scattered mind, confusion, anxiousness, insomnia.	**Prone to** be stubborn and depressed.	**Prone to** be busy, hyper-tension, anger, over-stressed, controlling.
Balance With: Pitta & Kapha doshas. Heavy, Warm, Nourishing, Dense (embodied), Stable, Smooth, Soft	**Balance With:** Pitta & Vata doshas. Light, Hot, Dry, Penetrating, Fluid, Hard, Mobile, Subtle, Clear	**Balance With:** Vata & Kapha doshas. Dry, Cool, Dull, Soft, Slow, Smooth, Dense (earthy, grounded)
Tools for Balance: Slow down, meditate, eat regular, cooked and grounding meals, prolong sleep, walk barefoot.	**Tools for Balance:** Stay active with daily routines, awaken early, exercise, cleanse sinuses.	**Tool for Balances:** Go slower. Eat regularly, rest regularly, enjoy nature, surround with cool colors, enjoy coolness and calming exercises.
Avoid cold in and on the body.	**Avoid** cold, damp, and stagnation.	**Avoid** heat and agitating exercise.
Nutritional Guidelines: Heavy & warm. Must include warm cooked sweet, sour, and salty tastes for building, nourishing, and grounding. Eat amply. Incorporate oils, heavy fruits, nuts, cooked vegetables, dairy, spices. **Limit** beans and raw vegetables.	**Nutritional Guidelines:** Lighten & warm. Must include light, dry, and cooling foods. Incorporate spices, beans, vegetables, clear teas, lighter fruits, soups. **Limit** sweets, red meat, salt, oils, wheat, oats, dairy.	**Nutritional Guidelines:** Sooth & cool. Must include cooling foods to calm the mind and body. Incorporate dairy, oils, sweet fruits, most vegetables, soothing herbs, most grains. **Limit** sour fruit, spicy herbs, spicy vegetables.

Harmonious Cycles of Days, Weeks, Seasons

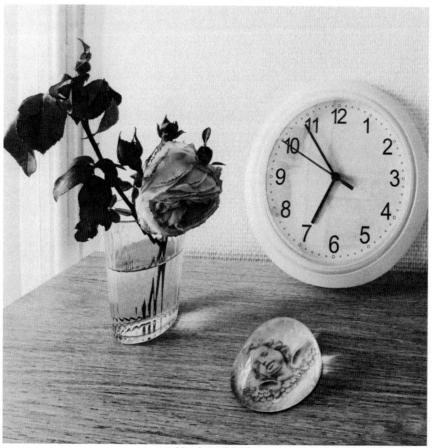

Dinacharya Rituals

186

Dinacharya

Your Daily Self-Care Ayurvedic Routine

Ayurveda's 3 Pillars of Health are:

Ahar: **Nourishing diet & proper digestion (food and emotions, and physical and mental digestion)**
Nidra: **Nourishing rest**
Brahmacharya: **Healthy relationships (proper sex) with others & healthy relationship with self**

Perceiving the circadian rhythms of nature and aligning with these rhythms support the health of the mind, body, and spirit. This new, fast-paced, technology-filled 'norm' that has reigned in the past few decades is not in rhythm with the ancient natural world. The sensitive human system is bombarded by artificial light and sound, the ceaseless demands of social media and communication, as well as other technological and chemical distractions. The effects of these stresses are linked to the overwhelming disconnect humans have with nature.

The night sky is no longer dark. The migration patterns of animals have been destroyed for multitudes of species, and new generations of people have never seen the stars and are unable to comprehend the vastness of the universe and the holy balance of interconnection between life forms. This disconnect from the natural environment has limited the imagination and mystery for so many people. Ultimately, this disconnect has caused depression and stresses in unprecedented forms.

Practicing *Dinacharya* is a profound practice to remain balanced in a world that seems imbalanced. *Dinacharya* is an ancient Ayurvedic way of life that supports the natural state of the human system. A moderate lifestyle with routines of work, play, and rest, and a diet rich in natural foods, are the largest contributors to holistic health. **In the following pages are the basics of Dinacharya. Experiment to see what feels right for your body type.**

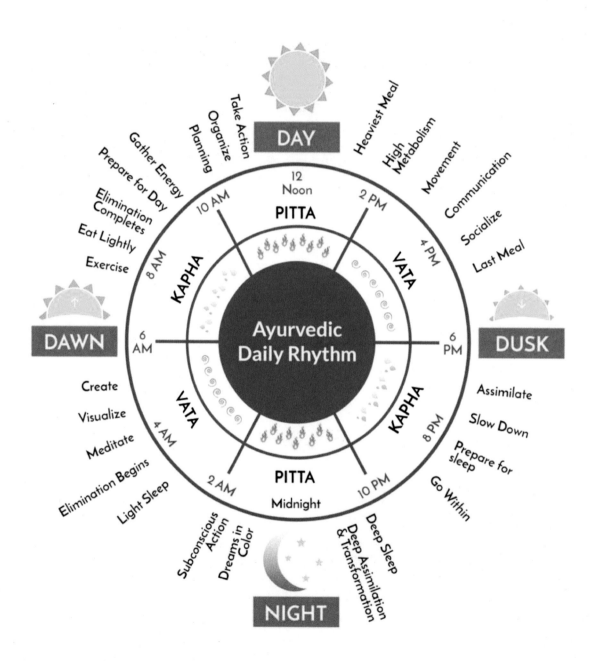

24-Hour Dinacharya Cycle

A pillar of Ayurveda is Brahmacharya, which is living in alignment with nature's rhythms. When in flow, rather than in force, life has ease and harmony, so it is important to honor the elements and how they relate to daily, monthly, and seasonal cycles, including the larger cycles of the sun, moon, and planets. This knowledge gives additional insight on how to balance the holistic system.

2am-6am: Vata elements rule
- ❖ The Ambrosia Hour where the veil between dimensions is thin
- ❖ Connect with meditation and pranayama

6am-10am: Kapha elements rule
- ❖ Cleanse
- ❖ Practice asana and complete physical chores/errands

10am-2pm: Pitta elements rule
- ❖ Eat the largest meal of the day
- ❖ Enjoy mental tasks in this flow of momentum

2pm-6pm: Vata elements rule
- ❖ Enjoy creative tasks to not get lethargic
- ❖ Include a planned break such as a pranayama meditation, nap, or nature walk

6pm-10pm: Kapha elements rule
- ❖ Soothing heart connection and grounding of the body and mind
- ❖ Eat 2-3 hours before bed, turn off electronics to support the nervous system

10pm-2am: Pitta elements rule
- ❖ Sleep
- ❖ Rest, digest, restore, heal

Dinacharya Day At-A-Glance

Morning

- ❖ Wake early to see the sunrise (Kapha wake at 5am, Pitta wake at 5:30am, Vata wake at 6am)
- ❖ Invoke gratitude and intention for the day-yet-unwritten
- ❖ Drink a large glass of room temperature water
- ❖ Mouth-Care: gently brush teeth with natural cleansers
    - o Scrape the tongue back to front
    - o Oil Pull swish (sesame oil=spring, winter, autumn / coconut oil=summer)
- ❖ Body-Care: awaken by washing the face and eyes (use pure rosewater)
    - o Abhyanga (oil self-massage) optional
    - o Oil the nose with nasya / skip if congested
- ❖ Evacuate bowels
- ❖ 30 minutes of exercise: a brisk walk, Yoga, breath work, 5-10 minutes of meditation
- ❖ Bathing/Showering
    - o Abhyanga (self-massage oil into skin, and feel all parts of the body) in shower
    - o Protect your skin by using warmed water, not hot
- ❖ Breakfast 7-8am: eat a hearty meal to satiate you to lunch
    - o Limited amounts of lukewarm water or hot tea is encouraged; too much liquid may cause bloat; cold liquid slows digestion

Afternoon

- ❖ Lunch, 11-1pm: the largest meal of the day
- ❖ Drinking limited amounts of lukewarm water or hot tea is encouraged
- ❖ Take a walk outside after eating
- ❖ Re-energize throughout the day with water and moments of rest through breathwork
- ❖ After completing work/study, meditate for 10-15 minutes to clear the mind and heart

Evening

- ❖ Dinner 5-7pm: the lightest meal of the day
- ❖ Drinking limited lukewarm water or hot tea is encouraged
- ❖ No caffeine after 4pm to ensure better sleep
- ❖ No alcohol after 6pm to ensure better sleep
- ❖ Unwind and reflect on a short walk
- ❖ Socialize and connect with others without electronics
- ❖ Mouth/Body-Care with a light shower/bath with abhyanga (self-massage with oil)
- ❖ Read a light-hearted book to rest the mind
- ❖ Oil the nose with nasya (if feeling dry)
- ❖ Sleep in a fully dark room without electronics
- ❖ Invoke gratitude for the day. When your head hits the pillow, it is a celebration!

Weekly Schedule and the Planets

Monday	Moon White/Silver	Tune into the cooling, grounding, nourishing motherly energies of the moon. This is a good day to be extra gentle with yourself to better connect to all beings.
Tuesday	Mars Red	Tune into the energy of Mars, which is courage and inner strength. Harness your non-dominating willpower, as today is a day to complete tasks.
Wednesday	Mercury Green	This is a day to polish your brilliance by relishing new ideas and seek new knowledge to expand the heart. This is a good day for communication and attention to detail.
Thursday	Jupiter Yellow/Orange	This is the day to honor the inner Guru, enjoy the bliss of nature, and expand perspectives. This is the day to do things that require strength internally and externally.
Friday	Venus Pink/Purple	Beauty is the focus of the day, so enjoy the diversity in the arts and find ways to delight the senses. Relish in self-care and enjoy deep connection with loved ones.
Saturday	Saturn Blue/Black	This is a day of quiet and contemplation, reflecting on the inner workings of the mind and heart. Journaling is recommended, and enjoy gentle yogic practices.
Sunday	Sun Orange/Gold	The mantra of the day is *Namaste*. This is the day for present connection with loved ones. Also, enjoy nature and safely tune into the healing rays of sunlight.

Doshas and the Moon Cycles

NEW MOON	WAXING MOON	FULL MOON	WANING MOON
Vata	Vata / Kapha	Kapha	Pitta
Focus on: Inner Exploration, dedication, finding deep clarity of an intention, slow down, enjoy ample rest so you may further shine.	**Focus on:** Vata energies rule for one week followed by Kapha. Manifestation / germination of the New Moon seed and is a good time to start new projects.	**Focus on:** This is a highly energized time for celebrating life, working with community, and entering a space of gratitude for all things.	**Focus on:** This is a time to catch the osmic momentum and to complete projects.
Lunar Yoga: Yoga Nidra, floor practices, Yin, Restorative	**Lunar Yoga:** Backbends and heart openers	**Lunar Yoga:** Dynamic asana, Warrior Poses	**Lunar Yoga:** Folds and inversions, meditation

❖ The next page includes suggested asanas, mediations, and breath to support each dosha.

Balancing Your Dosha with Yogasana

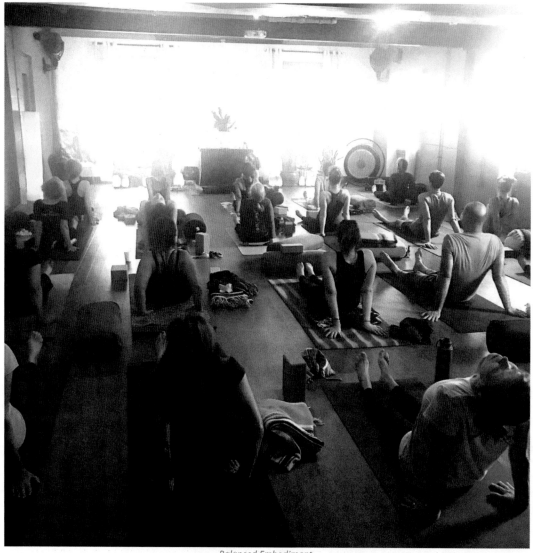

Balanced Embodiment

VATA	KAPHA	PITTA
Autumn / Early Winter	Late Winter / Spring	Late Spring / Summer Early Autumn
Ground & Heat Afternoon for Vata Yoga Class	**Move & Strengthen** Morning for Kapha Yoga Class	**Slow & Cool** Evening for Pitta Yoga Class
Vata Yogasana: A warmed yoga room with a calming practice. Include grounding, long-held floor poses paired with lengthened pranayama with focus on the exhale. Needs joint mobilization poses to lubricate the joints.	**Kapha Yogasana:** A warmed yoga room with a heat-based, strengthening flow balanced with a faster paced and energizing practice. Be playful in poses. Needs accountability, dynamic movement to increase sweat heart rate.	**Pita Yogasana:** In a soft-lit, slightly warmed room let go of competition and make an intention to disconnect from stress by focusing on the present. Moderate dynamic poses, with cooling, longer-held floor poses. Ample time for a long Savasana, slow breathing, meditation, and chanting.
Poses: Ample floor poses, slow-paced Sun Salutations, cat/cow, cobra, throat and heart-opening poses, arm binds to loosen shoulders, inversions, reclined knee to chest, plow, forward fold, restorative poses	**Poses:** Sun Salutation, dynamic standing poses, Warrior Poses, abdominal work, balancing poses, heart openers, inversions, stretch spine in all directions, neck mobilizations, less time laying on the floor	**Poses:** Moderately dynamic poses, eart and shoulder openers, playful poses that invoke joy, twists to wring out heat, back-bends. Avoid too many inversions and arm balances.
Meditation: Yoga Nidra, visualizing sinking roots into Earth, forest bathe, sun bathe (with precautions), candle gazing, chanting Om	**Meditation:** Wake early, candle and meta meditations, nature walks, mantras	**Meditation:** Yoga Nidra, So Hum meditation, Chakra Bija Meditation, forest bathe, wade in natural water
Pranayama: Subtle techniques: Nadi Shodhana, Brahmari, etc.	**Pranayama:** Kapalabhati, Ujjayi	**Pranayama:** Lions Breath, Nadi Shodhana, other long, deep, and cooling breaths

195

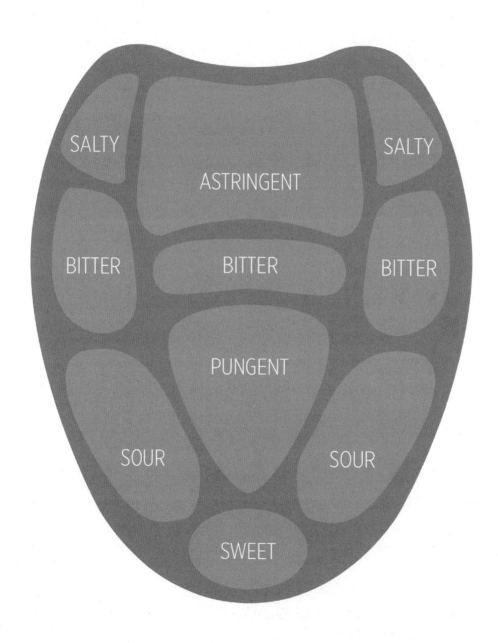

Six Tastes to Include in Each Meal

A balanced meal incorporates the following tastes, introduced to the body in the order below (based on when and where they hit your tongue):

Sweet (Water & Earth)
- ❖ Builds tissues & calms nerves
- ❖ Fruit, grains, natural sugars, milk

Sour (Earth & Fire)
- ❖ Balances acid base, cleanses tissues, increases mineral absorption
- ❖ Sour fruits, yogurt, fermented foods

Salty (Fire & Water)
- ❖ Stimulates digestion, improves taste, lubricates tissues, maintains mineral balance and hydration
- ❖ Natural salts, sea vegetables

Pungent (Fire & Air)
- ❖ Improves digestion, metabolism, and strengthens digestive enzymes
- ❖ Fresh ginger, chili, peppers, garlic, herbs, spices

Bitter (Air & Space)
- ❖ Detoxifies/lightens tissues, antibiotic, antiseptic, and body purifier
- ❖ Dark leafy greens, herbs, spices

Astringent (Earth & Air)
- ❖ Absorbs water, tightens tissues and gives tone to the body, dries fats, stops bleeding
- ❖ Walnuts, green bananas, neem, green tea

Reflection

The World is a Samkhya Stage: Perception, Reality, and Ayurveda

1) What is Purusha?

2) What is Prakriti?

3) Prakriti is characterized by the Gunas. Name the three primary Gunas and their attributes.

4) What is Ayurveda?

5) Ayurveda highlights three main doshas that comprise an individual's body type. Doshas affect the Gunas. Please list each doshas AND its elemental quality.

6) How is Purusha and Prakriti viewed in my own life? Crafting concepts through alternative, artistic means supports the embodiment-process. Here, we'll explore the answer to this question through poetry, be it free style in your unique expression, or use the guide on the following page to support the crafting of various poetic forms. *Here is a beautiful Haiku example from my 16-year-old Yoga student:*

Silent, I though ask

Is life but an illusion?

I watch from above

Poetry Guidelines: A Samkhya Reflection

The Five W's Poem: *Who, What, When, Where, Why*
- ❖ Line 1 - Who or what is the poem about?
- ❖ Line 2 - What action is happening?
- ❖ Line 3 - When does the action take place?
- ❖ Line 4 - Where does the action take place?
- ❖ Line 5 - Why does this action happen?

Haiku: *An ancient Japanese form with no rhyme. Haiku often deal with nature.*
- ❖ Line 1 - 5 syllables / Line 2 - 7 syllables / Line 3 - 5 syllables

Cinquain: *A five-line poem consisting of five, usually unrhymed lines respectively containing two, four, six, eight, and then two syllables.*
- ❖ Line 1 - One word title
- ❖ Line 2 - Two descriptive words
- ❖ Line 3 - Three action words
- ❖ Line 4 - Four feeling words
- ❖ Line 5 - One word, which answers the question, "When I think of the title, I think of...?"

Diamonte: *A diamond-shaped poem of seven lines that is written using parts of speech.*
- ❖ Line 1 - Noun or subject
- ❖ Line 2 - Two Adjectives
- ❖ Line 3 - Three '-ing' words
- ❖ Line 4 - Four words about the subject
- ❖ Line 5 - Three '-ing' words
- ❖ Line 6 - Two adjectives
- ❖ Line 7 - Synonym for the subject

Free Verse: *Poetry without rules or form, rhyme, or rhythm, written in any way you choose to write.*

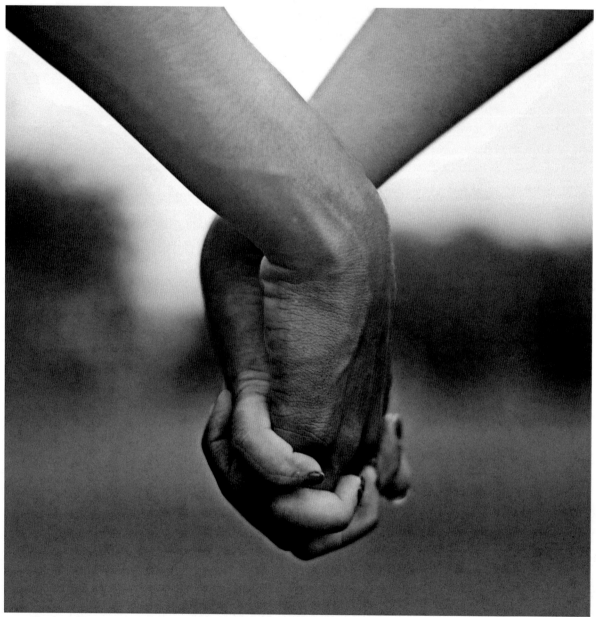

Union

Chapter 5

Upanishads:

Union of the Seeker and the Sought

Historical Timeline

PRECLASSICAL YOGA ERA

INDUS-SARASVATI AGE: 6500-4500 BCE
- SANATANA DHARMA: "ETERNAL LAW"
- INDUS RIVER VALLEY & SEALS

VEDIC AGE: 4500-2500 BCE
- CONSCIOUSNESS EXPLORED
- VIBRATION OF INTENTION & CAUSATION
- CAUSE & EFFECT: MANTRA & KARMA

SAMKHYA YOGA: 8000-100 BCE
- REALITY EXPLORED: PRAKRITI/PURUSHA
- BODY'S CONSTITUTION: DOSHAS
- AYURVEDA

UPANISHADIC AGE: 2000-1500 BCE
- NON-DUALISM OF ATMAN/BRAHMAN
- DISTILLATION OF VEDAS
- MEDITATION

BHAKTI YOGA: 1000-500 BCE
- ADORATION
- HINDU EPICS / UNIVERSAL INSIGHTS
- 3 BRANCHES OF YOGA

BUDDHISM: C. 500 BCE-PRESENT
- INDIVIDUALITY / MONASTIC TRADITION
- MIDDLE WAY
- FOUR NOBLE TRUTHS / EIGHT-FOLD PATH

CLASSICAL YOGA ERA

CLASSICAL YOGA: 75 BCE-100 CE
- THE YOGA SUTRA'S OF PATANJALI
- EIGHT-LIMBED PATH
- HARNESSING THE MIND

ESOTERIC AGE

TANTRA: 600-1300 CE
- 6 + 1 CHAKRA SYSTEM
- WESTERN NOTION OF EMBODIMENT
- SUBTLE BODY (NADIS, CHAKRAS, ETC.)

HATHA YOGA: C. 1300-1400 CE
- MIND V. BODY
- HATHA YOGA PRADIPIKA
- ASANA / BREATH / BANDHAS / MUDRAS

RISE OF MODERN YOGA

SWAMI VIVEKANANDA: 1872-1950
- INFLUENCED RISE OF MODERN YOGA
- INTRODUCED YOGA TO THE WEST

SRI T. KRISHNAMACHARYA: 1891-1989
- YOGA'S EXPANSION
- FATHER OF MODERN YOGA
- MODERN CONTRIBUTORS

Chapter 5

Upanishads: Union of the Seeker and the Sought

1. Overview of Lecture

Chapter 5 explores the distillation of the Vedas embodied in the Classical Upanishads. The key concepts of Atman and Brahman are discussed in comparison with Purusha and Prakriti. Additionally, the essential concepts that are seen in every day modern Yoga classes, such as the power behind the chanting of Om, the energy bodies of koshas and chakras, pranayama, a review of the gunas, and the concept of liberation (Moksha) are examined. We also explore the Five Prana Vayus (movements of Prana) in relation to asana and specific pranayama practices.

2. Learning Objectives: I will...

a) Recognize the Upanishads are distillation of the Vedas
b) Understand and translate the concepts of Atman, Brahman, and Moksha
c) Explore major yogic concepts found within classical Upanishadic texts

3. Pre-lecture Assignments

a) Read the chapter and become familiar with the Reflection questions
b) Read *The Upanishads*, recommended translation by Eknath Eswaran
c) Daily Sadhana - Daily Personal Practice

4. Reflection: *found at the end of the chapter*

The Wonderful Wizard of Oz

(1900) by L. Frank Baum

A point of interest: Baum was a yogi scholar. The book The Wonderful Wizard of Oz was written to show how the Seeker and the Sought are the same, and to help readers discover that all that is needed is already within them; that the gifts they want are already theirs. Each character had to "die" to who they were in order to become courageous, intelligent, and to have heart.

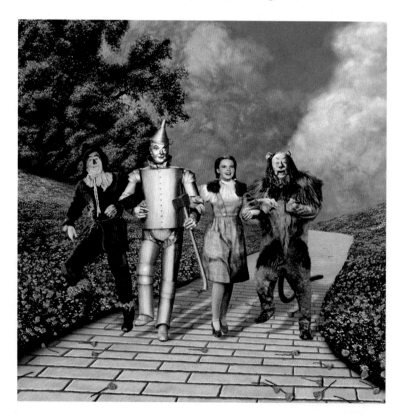

"Your silver shoes will carry you over the desert," replied Glinda. *"If you had known their power you could have gone back to your Aunt Em the very first day you came to this country."* **(And yes, the shoes were silver, only changed to red to show up better in the movie.)**

"But then I should not have had my wonderful brains!" cried the Scarecrow. *"I might have passed my whole life in the farmer's cornfield."*

"And I should not have had my lovely heart," said the Tin Woodman. *"I might have stood rusted in the forest till the end of the world."*

"And I should have lived a coward forever," declared the Lion, *"and no beast in all the forest would have had a good word to say to me."*

"This is all true," said Dorothy, *"and I am glad I was of use to these good friends. But now that each of them has had what he most desired, and each is happy in having a kingdom to rule besides, I think I should like to go back to Kansas."*

"The silver shoes," said the Good Witch, *"have wonderful powers. And one of the most curious things about them is they can carry you to anyplace in the world in three steps, and each step will be made in the wink of an eye. All you have to do is knock the heels together three times and command the shoes to carry you to where you wish to go."*

The Wizard of Oz is showing us that the scarecrow, the lion and the tin man were, in fact, Dorothy in various states, learning how to use her mind, body, heart and soul for her own empowerment; the Wicked Witch being the fear of her ego; the Good Witch being her Self.

What does it mean for you, seen through the eyes of Yoga?

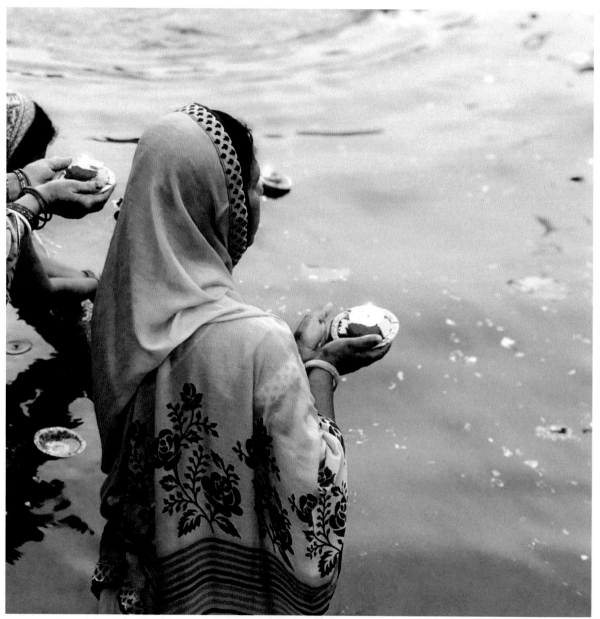

Communion

206

The Upanishads

You are what your deep driving desire is. As your desire is, so is your will.
As your will is, so is your deed. As your deed is, so is your destiny.
~ Upanishads

From every sentence (of The Upanishads), deep original and sublime thought arise, and the whole is pervaded by a high and holy and earnest spirit. In the whole world, there is no study, so beneficial and so elevating as that of The Upanishads. They are destined, sooner or later, to become the faith of the people. It has been the solace of my life – it will be the solace of my death.
~ Arthur Schopenhauer

This path doesn't always hug the ridge tops; it often falls into deep canyons, sometimes moves along the waterways across the valleys, deserts, and the tall peaks of your inner self.
Its direction may not always seem clear as you venture into the wilderness within.
~ Charles Breux

The Vedas, as you know, were instrumental in the development of Hinduism, Buddhism, Christianity, and other religions and philosophies, and are the foundation from which the Yoga Tradition rises. The knowledge within the Upanishads are considered Divine Revelations, called *Smirti* in Sanskrit, and are the oldest source text beyond the Vedas.

The classical *Upanishads* hold the essence of the Vedas, which are distilled into stories, resembling parables. The original books are a collection of 11 manuscripts written by sages. They are unsystematic in nature, giving rise to various traditions and Vedanta schools that are alive today. *Upanishad* literally means to 'sit near, to study at the feet of a guru, a remover of darkness'. Unlike a philosophy that provides explanations or instructions, *The Upanishads* are darshan. *Darshan* is "sight to behold the truth; truth that is seen and experienced and holistically internalized." Its central concept is *non-dualistic*. One's true Self is Divine; the Seeker and the Sought are one.

207

The Upanishads explore the gunas and the dominant doshas (as seen in Samkhya Philosophy), the here and now, how to discover and break free from patterned thinking and behavior, and how to bring everything back into balance. The power of *OM* and *Aum* are also discussed. Upanishadic-era gurus understood there was no separation between Brahman and atman, and the very purpose of a life is to realize the timeless fact that everything is Divine. They strived to see the world through the lens of equanimity.

One who is fully Awake while living is called a *Jivanmukta*. Jivanmuktas taught their students how to be in tune with Purusha/Source by offering tools and techniques from their own experiences. This enlightened being (guru) had personally experienced and internalized a liberating knowledge, Moksha. The guru passed on their transcendent experiences, along with instructions on how to reach this state, to worthy students.

The gurus understood that there was no separation between Brahman and atman; that life was non-dualistic. These sages uncovered how individuals could attain Moksha, a liberation which released them from suffering and the necessity of re-birth, in their lifetime by emulating what worked for them in their own Awakening. Gurus created a system of self-study that was not caste dependent. Their emphasis was on taming the "wilderness within". They helped others to understand how to connect with their own wilderness by tapping into the body, rooting down (through the breath and meditation) to understand the expansion and contraction of subtle energies.

Gurus shared stories demonstrating the oneness of Brahman and atman. Brahman was defined as God being the Conscious, timeless, all-powerful force which controls the universe. Brahman was feminine, masculine, universal. Everything originated from, existed in, and eventually dissolved into Brahman.

All living beings, all flora and fauna, also have an atman. The atman harkens to the soul/Seer. And, if life is indeed non-dualistic, then atman is Brahman. This is the essence of Namaste - that all living things are Divine. People thought, incorrectly, that atman was separate from Brahman, and this caused suffering. **So, why do you misidentify your true Self as separate from the Divine?**

According to *The Upanishads*, every thought or action you take produces karma. Karma sticks to the atman, obscuring the individual's view of his/her true divine nature through maya (illusion) that affects their world-appearance and self-understanding. The atman, with all its karma attached, travels from one lifetime to the next in a cycle of rebirth (samsara).

When you recognize that atman and Brahman are one, the veil of illusion lifts, your true divine nature is understood, and your karmic bonds are dissolved. Without karma, the atman is liberated from samsara at death, never to be reborn again, achieving liberation (moksha).

An analogy is that each soul (atman) is a drop of water in the ocean (Brahman). The point of the Upanishads is to recognize that you are not an individual drop that is separate from the ocean. You are the drop that is a part of the ocean. Another analogy would be that you are a wave in the ocean. The ocean creates the wave, but the wave can't exist without the ocean.

All life is interconnected.

Discomfort can be based on a misconception of who you truly are. You are THE drop and you are THE wave. One way of overcoming your misconception of yourself as Either/Or is to identify where the "vibration" of discomfort is coming from within your body. The stories in *The Upanishads* ask: *Who sees through my eyes? Who hears through my ears? What is it like to taste, feel?* It becomes the process of linking atman back to Brahman, linking the Observed to the Observer.

The Upanishads shine light upon your life's unique potential, encouraging you to LIVE! Your personal experience give rise to your atman's (soul's) magnificence, which lets you become the teacher instead of the victim. The stories show you how to become the light of Love – your true essence. The Upanishad definition of Yoga is both the practice that leads to the liberating insight that atman and Brahman are one, and the experience of being absorbed in that liberating knowledge (*Samadhi*).

The Upanishads offer the first concrete definition of *Yoga*: the restraint of the senses, known as *Pratyahara*. *The Upanishads* state that oneness can be realized in this lifetime, without priests or rituals or organized religion. You are encouraged to look inward while fully experiencing the outward.

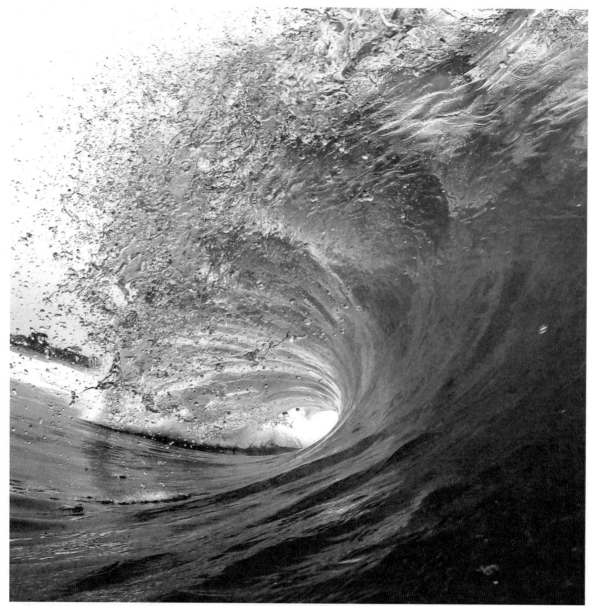

Atman and Purusha

Foundational Concepts

ATMAN and PURUSHA

Atman is Brahman. Brahman is eternal and one
There can be no difference in Brahman.
Atman is Cosmic and universal.

Purusha is Singular. Purusha is eternal and plural.
Purushas are as multiple as there are experiencers.
Purusha is individual but not personal.

Non-dualistic Nature of Atman and Brahman

ATMAN - the essence of YOU. May be represented by a drop of water in the ocean, the microcosm.
Soul, Seer, Deathless Self, Witness, Inner Truth, True Self, Universal Essence & Spirit

Indestructible, yet after the death of the body, it achieves Moksha (release/liberation) by uniting with Brahman or is reborn with the opportunity to overcome samskaras/karma. One who attains the atman experiences bliss. The goal of the atman traditions is the experience of one's own blissful *Sat-Chit-Ananda* – existence, consciousness, bliss – which is the nature of the atman. *Kaivalya* is the highest state of experiencing atman. Kaivalya means aloneness, autonomy, experiencing the state of one's innermost self; the experience of the atman itself.

BRAHMAN - the essence from which YOU came. May be represented by the ocean, the macrocosm.
Absolute Truth, God-force, Independent of space and time, Reality, Prana

Brahman is a term that means the Absolute Truth. Ishvara and Bhagavan can be personal beings, while Brahman is an impersonal being. Yet, direct personal experience is the proof of Brahman's existence.

But the term can go another way, as well. Atman merges with Brahman, like rivers merging to the sea. Once the river merges into the sea, it's not a river or individual thing anymore; it becomes one with the ocean. The atman loses its individuality upon enlightenment and obtains the Absolute, which is Brahman. Brahman is presented in impersonal terms. Other Upanishadic passages suggest the soul retains its individuality, even in liberated states. Here, Brahman is personal; a thinking being that creates. For example, *The Shvetashvatara Upanishad* shows Shiva as the Supreme Ishvara, which is Brahman.

What is Brahman? What is the relationship between Atman and Brahman?
What is the relationship between Brahman and the world?

Adi Shankara, an 8th century Hindu philosopher and theologian, posits that the world is false and is a mirage. How you see the world is a superimposition which only exists in *Avidya*, ignorance. You think there are things like tables and chairs, mountains, and universes.

You think, "I am different than you. I am an individual atman, and you are an individual atman." This type of thinking is from a world of duality.

But in an enlightened reality, there is no world; it's all a false, superimposition. Atman is Brahman without separation, not an individualized monad of consciousness. Everything is the all-pervading Brahman.

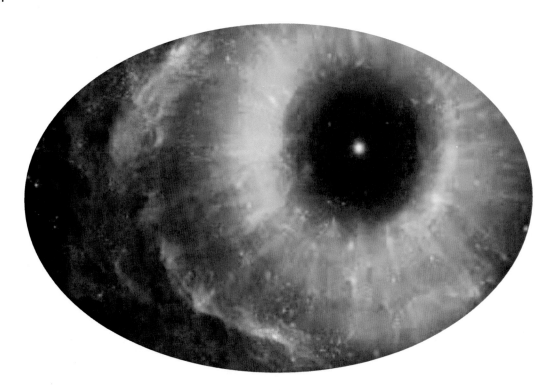

The 11 Classical Upanishads

Isha Upanishad: The Inner Ruler

The Lord is enshrined in the hearts of all

Katha Upanishad: Death as a Teacher

The term "Yoga" first appears here
Concept of "Die 1000 times each day"

Brihadaranyaka Upanishad: The Forest of Wisdom

Description of the Self and the "Unitive State"
Being in the Here and Now

Chandogya Upanishad: Sacred Song

Known as the "sacred song", links Vedas by giving power to sound
Diagram of the subtle body: nadis and chakras arise

Shvetashvatara Upanishad: The Faces of God – shift of an era

Emphasis on a personal God, Yoga, transcendent self as goal of Yoga
Use of deities to overcome boundaries and limitations

Mundaka Upanishad: Modes of Knowing

All major themes of the Upanishads are seen
Knowing when you are out of balance and how to regain balance

Mandukya Upanishad: Consciousness and Its Phases

The Self has four states of consciousness and Koshas

Kena Upanishad: Who Moves the World

"This truth is all the Seeker need discover" / Remembering you are not your Story

Prashna Upanishad: The Breath of Life

Prana and its movements

Taittirya Upanishad: Ascent to Joy

Distinction between pleasure and joy
Exploring the Koshas and energetic bodies

Aitareya Upanishad: The Unity of Life

All reality is consciousness: *prajnam* (wisdom) Brahman

The Lord dwells in the womb of the cosmos,
the creator who is in all creatures.
He is that which is born and to be born;
His face is everywhere.

~ Shvetashvatara Upanishad

You are what your deep, driving desire is.
As your desire is, so is your will.
As you will is, so is your deed.
As you deed is, so is your destiny.

~ Brihadaranyaka Upanishad

The light of Brahman flashes in lightning;
the light of Brahma flashes in our eyes.
It is the power of Brahma that makes
the mind to think, desire, and will. Therefore
use this power to meditate on Brahman.

~ Kena Upanishad

The Self is the source of abiding joy.
Our hearts are filled with joy in seeing him
enshrined in the depths of our consciousness.
If he were not there, who would breathe, who would live?
He it is who fills every heart with joy.

~ Taittiriya Upanishad

Aum stands for the supreme Reality.
It is a symbol for what was, what is,
and what shall be. Aum represents also
what lies beyond past, present, and future.

~ Mandukya Upanishad

Those who depart from this world without
knowing who they are or what they truly
desire have no freedom here or hereafter.
But those who leave here knowing who they
are and what they truly desire have freedom
everywhere, both in this world and in the next.

~ Chandogya Upanishad

Lead me from the Unreal to the Real.
Lead me from Darkness to Light.
Lead me from Death to Immortality.
Let there be peace, peace, peace.

~ Brihadaranyaka Upanishad

What is reality? What is illusion? What happens at death?
What makes my hand move, my eyes see, my mind think?
What can satisfy the human heart?
Does life have a purpose, or is it governed by chance?
Who is the Experiencer of the experience?
Who is the Dreamer? Who is the self and the Self?
What does it mean that nothing is separate, and that God alone is real?

~ Chandogya Upanishad

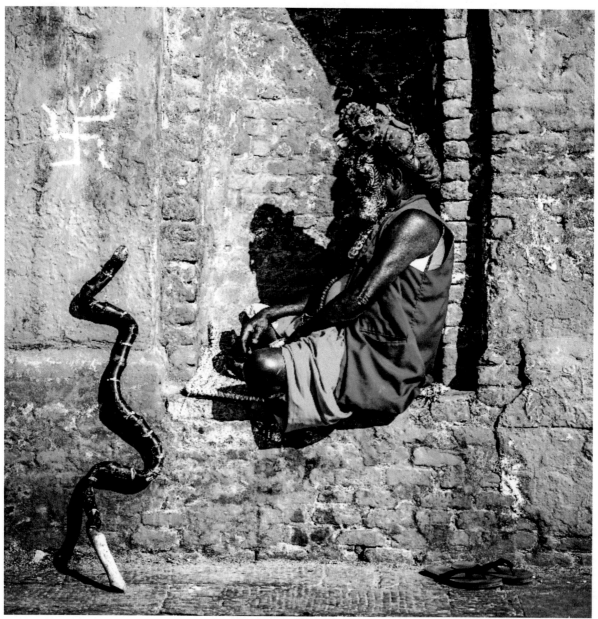

Ascetic Path

218

Guru and Shishya: Teacher and Student Relationship

The Upanishads state that oneness can be realized in this lifetime without priests or rituals or organized religion. You are encouraged to look inward while fully experiencing the outward. Ultimately, Prakriti offers two choices. Prakriti may bind the atman through the attachments of the gunas. This option is a life being lived through reaction; life within the 'storm'. You don't know where your center is; you feel scattered. Or Prakriti may liberate the atman through self-awareness. This option is life being lived through conscious response; life as the 'eye of the storm'. You know when you are pulled from your center, and you know how to then realign.

Gu- means 'darkness' and *-ru* means 'remover'. The term *Guru* literally means 'the remover of darkness'. Through personal experience, the guru has moved from knowingness to the understanding that atman is Brahman. With this knowingness, they are considered a jivanmukta – a person liberated while living. Through their teachings of personal experiences, gurus demonstrate the oneness of Brahman and atman, and they uncover how individuals can become liberated, what tools to use, and how to be in tune with the purusha source self thereby taming the "wilderness within".

A guru will often make his/her energy and spirit available to those who are seeking during special times, called *darshan*. Darshan, or Divine Sight, can lead to significant personal experience by the seeker, which leads to liberation. A *shishya*, or student, is guided every step of the way by their guru.

The student remains mindful that the individual self creates karma, therefore inward work must be done to purify intention. Thoughts lead to words, words lead to actions, actions lead to character, and one's character paves the way for one's destiny. Your inner vibration, which is based on the purity of your loving energy, mirrors your heart to the world. Divinity is both inward and outward. With this knowledge of Self Realization, karma melts away, and moksha is achieved. When you achieve moksha, you live in equanimity, seeing no difference between the mud puddle and the crystal lake, the diamond and the dust. Rather than reject the environment, you choose to see its Divine nature.

219

Philosophical Contributions of the Upanishads

Different Vedanta traditions oriented themselves around the different *Upanishads'* thoughts of both the impersonal and personal Brahman. The Vedanta tradition tries to systematize these *Upanishads*, as they are not a systematic philosophy, but rather say different things in different places. In some places Brahman (the Divine) seems to be a personal being while in others, impersonal. In some Upanishads, the atman merges with Brahman and ceases to be individual, and at that point, atman and Brahman are the same. In other places, there is a distinction of the two, which is the foundation of Bhakti Yoga. Because of these differences, Vedanta has broken up into various illuminating schools.

Seven main Indian Philosophies were established from *The Upanishads*, though there are thought to be many others. However, only six philosophies are considered Vedic, and they are seen as *shad darshans*, meaning six views, six insights, six schools of Vedic Thought. The seventh shad darshan gives rise to Buddhist philosophy, which later breaks from its Vedic foundations.

1. **Nyaya:** Valid knowledge is acquired through logical systems, rules, and criticism.

2. **Vaisheshika:** Analysis of the aspects of reality. Liberation is attained through understanding and analyzing the nature of the world: earth, water, light, air, ether, time, space, atman and mind.

3. **Samkhya:** Categorizes all outward and inward experiences. Knowledge of Purusha is recognized when the gunas, attributes of Prakriti, are balanced.

4. **Yoga:** Practical disciplines of Self Realization found in Patanjali's Yoga Sutras. Raja Yoga of personal transformation through transcendental experience.

5. **Mimamsa:** Freedom through the performance of duty. The correct performance of Vedic rites as the means to liberation, also seen in the honoring of one's dharma.

6. **Vedanta:** The Philosophy of Monism. There is one Absolute Reality - Brahman. Life's purpose is to realize this truth through right knowledge, intuition, and personal experience.

7. **Buddhism (unorthodox Indian philosophy):** Rejects the authority of the Vedas.

Review of Upanishadic Insight

The Classical *Upanishads* are a distillation of the Vedas. They contribute to the modern-day definition of Yoga. Please note there is no reference to physical asanas in *The Upanishads*.

❖ The Seeker and the Sought are the same
❖ Oneness Realization without organized religion
❖ Internalized ritualism: inner sacrifice and worldly renunciation
❖ *Sanyassin* = personal choice in the renunciation of society
❖ *Guru/Shishya* Tradition: teacher/student relationship
❖ *Ashram*: spiritual community under the guidance of a guru
❖ *Aranyakas*: forest teachings of a guru
❖ Ego and the states of consciousness
❖ *Atman*: deathless Self, the microcosm
❖ *Brahman*: Supreme Consciousness, the macrocosm
❖ *Aum*: states of consciousness: Om: reality of the universe
❖ First notion of chakras
❖ *Koshas*: sheaths of energy and consciousness
❖ *Gunas*: *rajas, tamas,* and *sattva*, which comprise Prakriti
❖ *Karma*: individual self creates change
❖ *Dharma*: living one's duty in full Authenticity, also known as ultimate Reality.
❖ *Moksha*: release / liberation
❖ *Samsara*: birth, life, death, rebirth
❖ *Samskara*: pattern, subconscious impression
❖ *Maya*: illusion, veil, blinding one from Truth
❖ *Avidya* (ignorance) / *Vidya* (removing ignorance)
❖ *Namaste*: I bow to the divine in you
❖ *5 Vayus*: Five movements and functions of prana

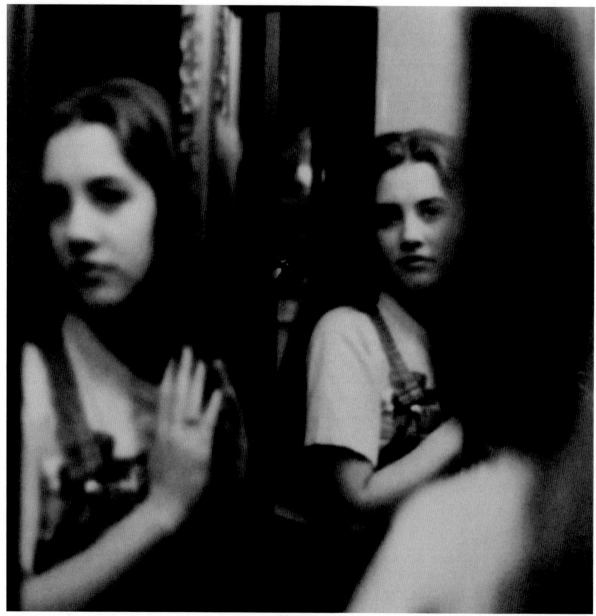

Discovery

222

Finding Authenticity

My oldest friend sent me this once-forgotten picture. I'm 16, most likely skipping school with her - with a clove cigarette nearby, I am certain. Our glorious hangout was Pike Place Market in Seattle, where I eventually moved to and worked a year later. To this day, it is my favorite place in the world. It delights me to intimately know the winding tunnels of shops, the familiar scents of fish and spice and wet concrete. This picture represents how I have spent years sifting through the layers of myself to find my Self.

I'm still in the process. Thank God.

I believe I gain a true heart-connection - *a true authenticity* - through experiences that bring me to my knees and through people that I clash with. *There is something for me to learn in the internal rub.*

I have grappled with spirituality for most of my life. At 16, I was going through my personal trial-by-fire with the concept of God. I was fascinated and enthusiastic and demanded a genuine relationship, but I didn't know what that felt like.

At 17, I was told by church elders that I would 'lead children astray from God', and I was asked to leave my congregation that I grew up with. This stemmed from my 'disrespect' by me questioning my pastor's messages of bigotry – and I lived with my best friends who were gay. My shock of betrayal from my spiritual tribe, and my resulting humiliation, turned to white-hot rage. I quickly learned what authenticity felt like, and to this day, I see how that experience was my greatest gift.

My searing emotions ushered my Embodiment. I was Awakening while I was dying to who I was.

I entered a great transformative process. Behind closed doors or on empty beach shores, I literally screamed every four-letter word known in the English language at my church and at God, again and again and again. To escape being associated with whom I deemed hypocrites, I tried to be atheist, but I couldn't shake the feeling of Divine Grandeur. Where was this unspoken Sweetness coming from in this broken world soothing my broken heart? Then I realized sacred sweetness was coming from inside of me, whole and complete and eternal. Yet this luminous spark needed cultivation to shine, so I polished myself through inquiry.

Who am I? I don't know.

I rolled up my sleeves and ventured to find out who I was. I became a social anthropologist, studying world religions, the history of World Wars, the history of birth control and the feminine mystique, obscure mythologies, and art. I became a Wanderlust, traveling around the world and hitchhiking; sleeping on sidewalks, in palaces, on beaches, and in the arms of one-night lovers; finding sustenance from chunks of bread, cheese, wine, and from prayers in ancient churches and street musicians.

My eyes were opened, and I saw the world wasn't broken.
It's pure Wilderness! For the first time, I tasted color, I felt music,
I embodied poetry, I heard hope, and I smelled stories.

I also learned that life is not linear. Life is like a spiral. To this day, when I think I've healed a massive wound, another 'teacher' comes along - different face, same message - and I'm confronted with similar energy that I thought I healed years ago. I love it when I recognize familiar bullshit. Recognition within itself is the ultimate change-agent for growth and authenticity.

"Ah... yes, old friend. I know *you*. You just have a different face. Thank you, Universe, for loving me so much that you feel that I can be stronger. Thank you, Divine Grandeur, for loving me so much that I have more layers of healing to do and more empathy to embody. I didn't know until now."

When I look upon my 16-year-old self, I see *'Me'*, looking steadily back, and I can say that I am head-over-heels in love with myself. That is the only way I can dance and heal and shine in this world.

Fall madly in love with yourself first, scrapes and all. That is where God resides. All other Love will follow as needed to usher in your divine, authentic relationship with Everything. That is Yoga.

true power is living
the realization
that you are your own
healer, hero, and leader

~ Yung Pueblo

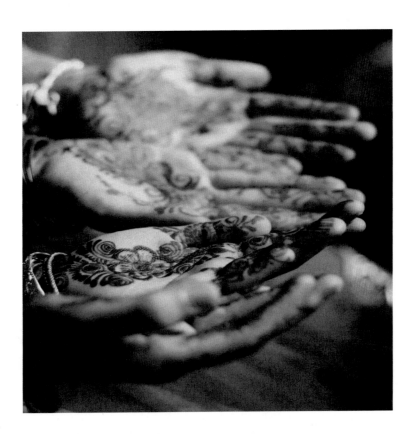

Reflection

The Upanishads: Union of the Seeker and the Sought

1) What are *The Upanishads*? What does the term *Upanishad* literally mean?

2) Describe Brahman and Atman. Compare them to Purusha and Praktri.

3) The Wizard of Oz is based on the concept of *The Upanishads*. The Seeker and the Sought are the same. Fear often stands in the way of you tapping into your magnificence. When you identify your fears - feel where they reside in your body - you are closer to transmuting them.

   a) Identify and write about a few of your greatest fear/s.

   b) State where your pattern/s of fear originated and where the feeling/s of fear landed in your body.

   c) Identify how your fears are limiting your full potential.

   d) How can you transmute them to be a gateway to your greatest strength?

   e) Using insight in this and former chapters, what tools have you developed to allow you to have a different relationship with your fear/s?

4) Create a Vision Board!

Here is my first vision board, created when I was a student in a 200-hour teacher training program. I worked in a public school system and was nervous to teach Yoga in a studio setting. No matter what my fears were, I was striving to ultimately embrace an inner calling.

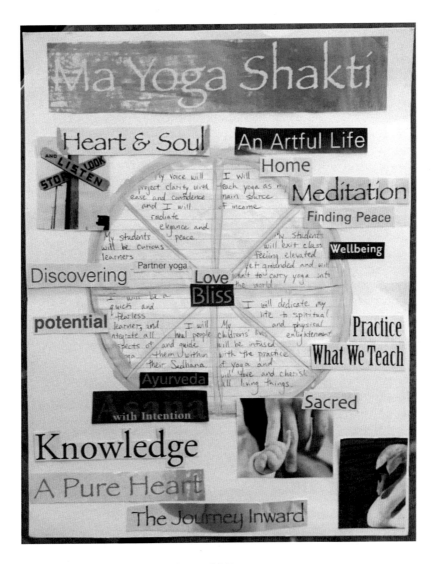

Vision Board Creation

In the study of Yoga, you are focusing on bringing awareness to your *heart's voice* and harnessing your inner power. The power of vibrational energy - the Power of Attraction - is the foundation for it all.

The Creation and Use of Your Board

Vision boards are symbolic representations of the emotional heart. They represent your desire to know God, your ideal life, your purpose, goals, and aspirations. Vision boards ultimately remind you of your potential.

As you create your board, come from a place that is acknowledging your appreciations. Be grateful for the good that you have and believe that more is to come. See yourself as having already embodied your vision.

There are many ways to fashion your board, through a collage format, a pie chart, a grid, etc. Be as colorful and creative as you wish. Most important, be neat and selective and specific so you don't attract chaos.

While creating a board, I like to use a thick piece of paper. Find a size that works for you, keeping in mind that you will have it front and center in your day-to-day life. Please put a date on your board and know that you may create different vision boards as your visions manifest, perhaps a new one each year.

Remember, dive deep into the awakening of your vision! Think of key words and quotes that embody your ideals and serve as personal affirmations. Find pictures from magazines (or Pinterest) that you would like to make a reality in your life. Place a picture of you on your board, one in which you feel most beautiful.

Create a statement for each pie or grid space. State your statement in present tense. "I travel frequently to beautiful places." "I am healthy and full of vitality!" Decorate your statements with correlating pictures. Say your affirmations aloud as well as stating how your life looks and feels. Believe it is already yours.

If you are working to create multiple changes in your life, you may keep a vision board in your workspace as well as your home space. Place your Vision Board somewhere highly visible, perhaps on your bathroom mirror or refrigerator. Share with others to keep the energy fresh, alive, and accountable!

Because you are invoking the Power of Attraction, you must FEEL your visions as reality. Feel your joy, success, abundance, health, and peace throughout your body. Light yourself up from the inside out! You are internalizing the belief that you are worthy and ready! You are moving from a knowingness to an understanding of your worth. Tap into this feeling throughout the day and focus on this feeling during meditation.

Visualize and Manifest Your Potential

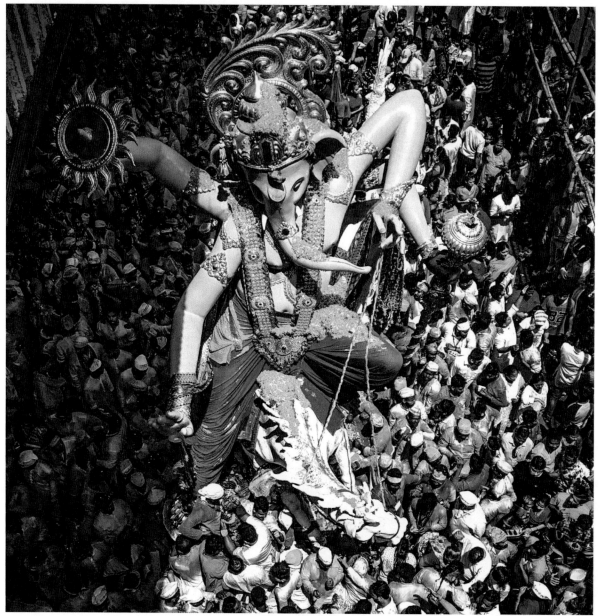

Mirror of the Self

230

Chapter 6

Deities: Symbols of Self

If one offers Me with love and devotion
a leaf, a flower, a fruit, or even water,
I accept it, offered in pure consciousness.

~ The Bhagavad Gita

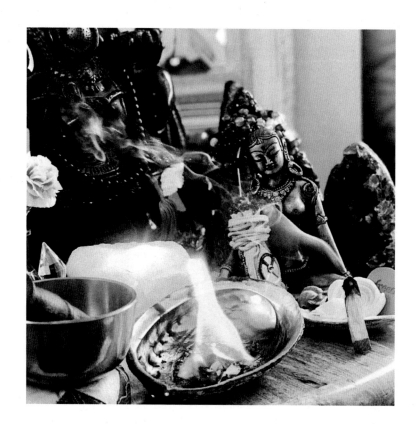

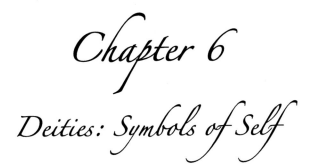

Chapter 6
Deities: Symbols of Self

1. Overview of Lecture

Chapter 6 briefly explores the symbolism of the deities. These aspects of Divinity are foundational spiritual elements of the Yoga Tradition and represent characteristics found in humanity.

2. Learning Objectives: I will...

   a) Understand the symbolism of deities represents the symbolism of our life experiences
   b) Articulate how deity forms are expressed in Hinduism and how deity worship relates to other spiritual practices and religions
   c) Explore Deity Yoga for self-accountability

3. Pre-lecture Assignments

   a) Read the chapter and become familiar with the Reflection questions
   b) Daily Sadhana - Daily Personal Practice

4. Reflection: *found at the end of the chapter*

The Seeker and the Sought

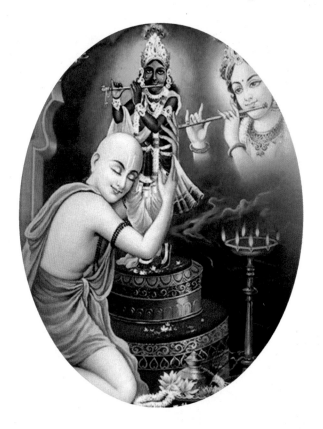

I was in Rishikesh, India, known as *The Gateway to the Himalayas*. The holy Ganges River is alive here, changing her waters from robust greens to crystal clear turquois blues, and her banks offer rich soil or fine white mountain sand. It is a magical place.

That said, my first visit to this land was less than magical. I was in culture shock for the first few days, and I felt defensive and judgmental about the situations and a people I didn't understand. One afternoon, I found refuge in the former home of Swami Sivananda Saraswati, who was a spiritual teacher and Yoga guru. (His former home is open to the public, and people visit to offer prayers and respect.)

I sat in relished silence, leaning against a wall in the bare simplicity of the space, catching my breath from the constant dance of sound and color that enveloped everything in the streets. I observed the incredible diversity of visitors entering the room in silence; the only décor being a massive, floor-to-ceiling, framed image of Swami Sivananda covered in garlands of orange and yellow marigolds, smelling of Nag Champa incense.

My ignorance gave birth to cruel judgment, however, as I saw people quietly fall to their knees and belly, arms stretched out, forehead to the floor in prostrated reverence of the image before them. *They are worshiping a dead guy. Have they no brains and power for themselves!* (Ignorance breeds false righteousness and separation from others, yes?)

So, there I was, in separation and agitation, vibrating with anger and rage over things unnamed and years of unhealed wounds. And like a golden wave of mercy, it all evaporated, in a single moment. I was struck with a force that shook my mind and body and my heart, and I was Divinely gifted Understanding. My icy heart melted, and my rigid body relaxed.

I knew with soul-clarity that I was actually witnessing people bow to their own life-potential, ripe and blooming with non-dominating power and an innate intelligence. That's what gurus do! They remove the darkness of ignorance by setting patient examples of how to live and how to embrace the known and unknown, expressing the understanding that all things are possible within life.

Your deep driving desire is energy radiating from your soul, reminding you that you are capable of achieving anything, especially when that desire serves humanity. The Seeker and the Sought are the same. Behind all images, behind all forms of deities, is the unifying essence of *That*.

I soon found myself in prostration before the garlands, before the beautiful smile on the face of Swami Sivananda, silently weeping with gratitude to the wisdom of my heart, which was finally freed of limitations by the Grace of God, which often shows up in unexpected ways … but always with perfection.

Symbolism of Deities

Mirrors of the Self

Brahman may be compared to an infinite ocean, without beginning or end. Just as, through intense cold, some portions of the ocean freeze into ice and the formless water appears to have form, so, through the intense love of the devotee, Brahman appears to take on form and personality. But the form melts away again as the sun of knowledge rises. Then the universe also disappears, and there is seen to be nothing but Brahman, the infinite. ~ Sri Ramakrishna

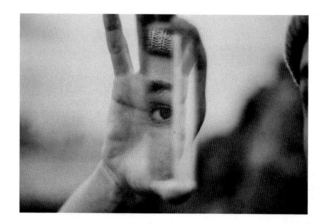

Bhagavan, Yahweh, Elohim, Zeus, Jehovah, Osiris, Buddha, Allah, Huwa, Love, Baha, Satnam, Wakan Tanka, El Shaddai, Gaia, and thousands of other names, known and unknown, are names of God. Within the vast and varied traditions of the Hindu religion, please note that this is a monotheistic tradition where Bhagavan is the name for God, meaning Supreme, Absolute Truth. Brahman is an aspect of Bhagavan, meaning ultimate reality that underlies all phenomena. Brahman is formless but is the birthplace of all forms of visible reality.

In Hinduism, Brahman has many different aspects, or faces. Multiple gods and goddesses represent the various aspects or faces of Brahman, similar to other major religions around the world. Many deities are avatars of Brahma, Vishnu, and Shiva, who are often called The Trinity, or *Trimurti*.

All beings are inherently connected energetically. Deities represent aspects of your human potential. Deity power also offers wisdom, illuminates information about your own innate intelligence, sheds light and bravery to explore your blind spots, and offers ways to expand your consciousness.

What is the message the deity symbol is offering you?

A common question people in the West ask is why do some deities have blue skin? Let's explore this. Why do you see a blue sky and blue water? This is really an optical illusion. Air and water look blue and vast and deep but are actually colorless. Once you see God with your Divine Eye you are self-identified and realized with formlessness, undifferentiated Reality. You rest in God's lap and all wrong ideas of you are removed. You may see yourself and God as you really are. One. When mindful of time, place, and space, your eyes, mouth, and body are reminded that You, too, are of Divinity. Source, God, whatever name you choose is seen in everything. Divinity is not only felt within holy walls but is infused in all things if you have the sight to see.

The deities that are shared in this chapter are some of the most popular yet ancient forms, used in both artistic symbolism while representing inspirations. They are all interconnected from monotheistic traditions of one God, unity, and balance. Deities also tap into the trinities. Like the Christian trinity of Father, Son, and Holy Ghost, Hindu's revere Creator (Brahma), Preserver (Vishnu), Destroyer (Shiva).

In the process of deity worship through meditation, your mind becomes purified, your ego thins away like mist, and superimposition ceases. World-appearance and the illusion-of-separateness vanish in the blaze of Transcendental Consciousness where there is duality - nothing but Brahman, the single, all-embracing, timeless Fact.

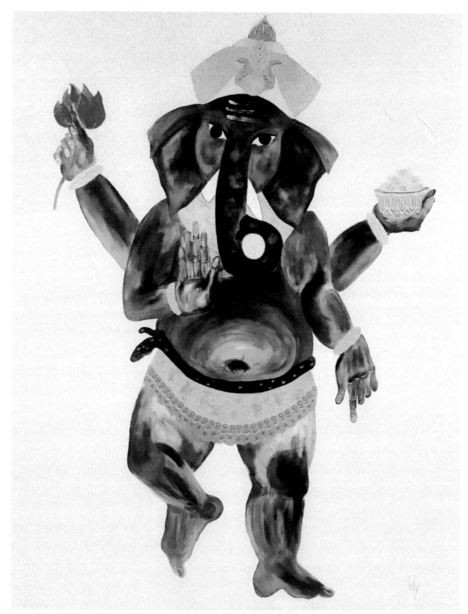

Ganesha, painting by Lily Kessler

Invoking Ganesha

Remover of Obstacles, Beacon of Possibility, Lord of the People

Om Gam Ganapataye Namaha

I offer my salutations to the Remover of Obstacles; the Possibility Illuminator.

Ganesha is honored at the beginning of any yogic pursuit. Most yogic texts begin with an invocation to Ganesha, as he is a gatekeeper of Transcendental, Absolute Knowledge and is referred to as the Lord of Obstacles; the Possibility Illuminator.

Ganesha puts obstacles in your way that are necessary for your transformation, and he also removes them. He is the quality and energy of life that participates in the placing and removing of obstacles. Ganesha's huge body is representative of the vastness of reality that you are looking to encounter through your practice. His crooked trunk is representative of the meandering trajectories through life that takes you to that Moksha, liberation.

Ganesha is related to the root chakra, and he represents harnessing personal energies so you may be powerfully present to the moment, discerning how to dance from moment to moment. He is the eldest son of Shiva and Parvati, and he is the lord of all living things. He has the head of an elephant and the body of a man and gives blessings to important endeavors. Ganesha clears obstacles, as symbolized by the axe that he carries. He often holds a bowl of sweets, a lotus flower, and gives a blessing. He is the scribe of the *Mahabharata* and used his right tusk to transcribe it; hence his right tusk is either missing or partially missing. Ganesha rides a mouse, which represents ego. Ganesha controls the ego, and one who controls the ego has Ganesha consciousness. Rosewood is his mala, and Wednesday is his special day of the week.

Christine Lily Kessler

The Trimurti: Trinity Aspects of Creation

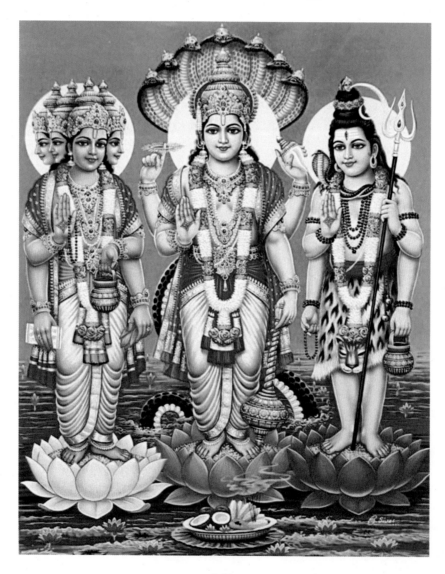

In the Yoga Tradition and Hinduism, God is made up of three forms called the Holy Trinity, or Trimurti. The main aspects of this trinity are Brahma the Creator, Vishnu the Preserver, and Shiva the Destroyer, which are all infused into One.

Gurur Brahma Gurur Vishnu

Gurur Devo Maheshwaraha

Guru Saakshaat Para Brahma

Tasmai Sri Gurave Namaha

Our creation is that guru (Brahma-the force of creation); the duration of our lives is that guru (Vishnu-the force of preservation); our trials, tribulations, illnesses, calamities and the death of the body is that guru (devo Maheshwara-the force of destruction or transformation). There is a guru nearby (Guru Sakshat) and a guru that is beyond the beyond (param Brahma). I make my offering (tasmai) to the beautiful (shri) remover of my darkness, my ignorance; (Guru) it is to you I bow and lay down my life (namah).

❖ **NOTE:** In this chapter, mantras are paired with traditional meanings rather than my own translations, as found in Chapter 2.

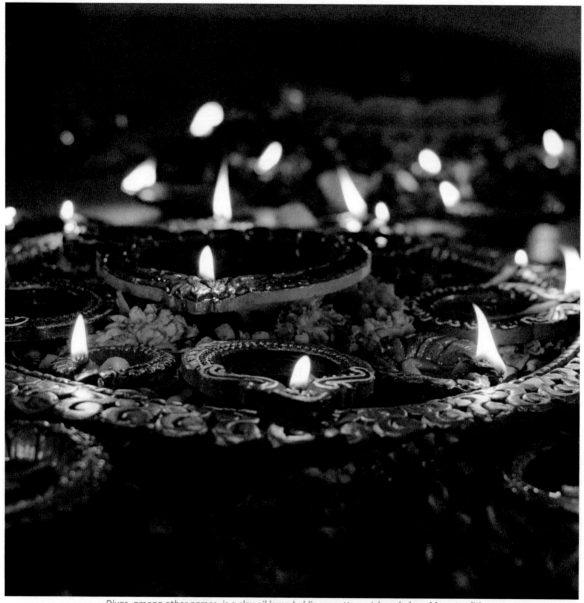

Diyas, among other names, is a clay oil lamp holding a cotton wick and ghee. Many traditions use them in prayer ceremony and other rituals and festival

242

BRAHMA: Creator of the Universe, Knowledge and the Vedas

Om Eim Hrim Shrim Klim Sauh Sat Chid Ekam Brahm
I bow to you, the Supreme One who has brought the conspicuous universe to existence.

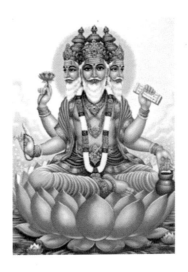

Though Brahma is an aspect of Brahman, Brahman is Absolute Reality as Brahma is a deity known as the creator of the world and all beings. Brahma is called *Svayambhu*, meaning self-born from the lotus that grew out of his navel. Paradoxically, Brahma is also known as the son of Lord Vishnu, who is an avatar of Krishna, which represents the Godhead Personality of Bhagavan, the Supreme Truth. Brahma is among the Trimurti with Vishnu and Shiva. He is regarded as the creative aspect of Lord Vishnu and is regarded as the Lord of Speech and the creator of the four Vedas.

Brahma is often shown sitting on a throne in the shape of a lotus with four faces. These four faces represent the four corners of the universe. Unlike other deities, Brahma carries no weapon. In his four hands, he holds a ladle, the Vedas, a jar of the sacred water of Life from the Ganges River, and a garland of prayer beads (mala). The ladle represents ritual. The Vedas represent knowledge. The water from the Ganges represents pilgrimage. The prayer beads represent meditation. Brahma rides a swan, although he is often shown sitting on a lotus. His wife is Saraswati, the goddess of culture and education.

VISHNU: Preserver of the Universe

Om Namo Bhagavate Vasudevaya
I bow to the Lord who resides in the hearts of all beings.

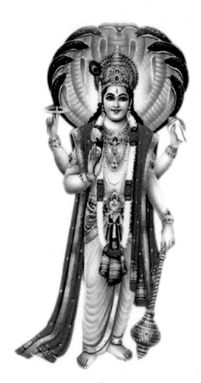

Vishnu maintains the balance between good and evil in the universe and helps people find their *dharma*, their true nature. He has 10 different avatars. His two most popular avatars are Krishna and Rama, and eventually the Buddha. In his four hands, he holds a discus/chakra, a club, a conch shell, and a lotus flower. The club and discus are weapons signifying his power over evil. The conch shell and lotus flower represent purity. Often, devotees of Vishnu paint a V-shape on their foreheads. This symbol signifies Vishnu's footprints. Vishnu rides on an Eagle, Garuda, who is also represented in *asana* (pose). His wife is Lakshmi, the goddess of wealth and prosperity.

SHIVA: Destroyer of Evil, Usherer of Beginnings and Yoga

Om Namah Shivaya
I honor the inner Self, Shiva, the light of consciousness within me.

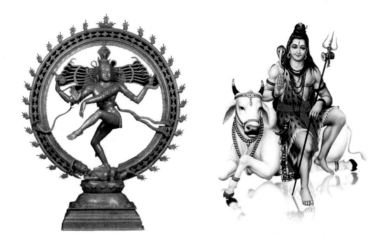

He purifies the universe through destruction. His most common representation is as Shiva Nataraja, Lord of the Dance. As Shiva Nataraja, he is surrounded by a halo of fire representing *samsara*, the cyclic pattern of lives - rebirth, birth, life, and death. Another version of samsara is viewing it as patterns and habits that don't serve you, yet you are stuck in them. The cobras around his neck symbolize *avidya*, internal poison that diminishes your spirit with the misunderstanding that you are not divine, hence, your attachment to samsara, the material world. As he dances, Shiva crushes the mischief causing, dwarf-demon of ignorance underneath his feet. This demon encourages you to create dramas, but Shiva reminds you to be the master of your life. In two of his four hands, he holds a drum and a flame. The drum helps him keep the rhythm of the universe, and the flame represents enlightened knowledge. As long as he keeps dancing, the endless cycle of creation, preservation, and destruction of the universe continues. His hand is raised in a blessing while his other arm gestures toward his raised foot as a promise of his mercy and kindness to his devotees. Shiva is commonly depicted with a trident, a symbol of the Hindu Trinity. Often, devotees of Shiva paint three parallel lines on their foreheads, representing the Hindu Trinity. His wife is Parvati, the mother goddess. Shiva rides a bull named Nandi.

The Feminine Balance of the Trimurti

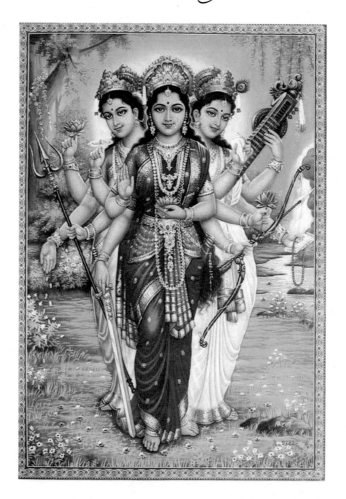

All living beings are comprised of both feminine and masculine energies, comprised of the gunas. Aspects of human nature are represented through qualities expressed within the deities. Deities are artistic representations of the energies of the Divine. Feminine expressions are often called *consorts*.

SARASWATI: Culture, Education, Creativity and Music

Om Aim Hrim Kleem Maha Saraswati Devaya Namaha
The giver of wisdom, intelligence, wealth, destroyer of the enemy,
Saraswati Devi, I bow before you.

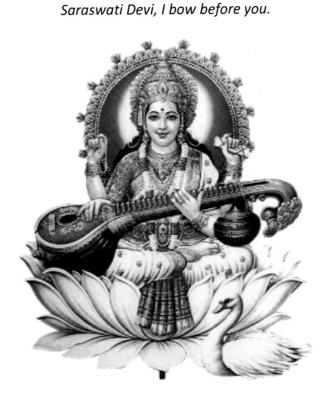

Saraswati is the consort of Brahma and is the first goddess in Hinduism. She plays the *veena* (stringed instrument) with two of her hands and holds pearl mala beads and the Veda's in her other two hands. The mala beads represent meditation. The books represent learning and philosophy. The veena represents culture and the arts. Saraswati is considered very beautiful and rides a swan. People pray to her for a successful education.

247

LAKSHMI: Goddess of Wealth, Good Fortune and Happiness

**Om Sarvabaadhaa Vinirmukto, Dhan Dhaanyah Sutaanvitah
Manushyo Matprasaaden Bhavishyati Na Sanshayah Om**
*I pray to Goddess Laxmi to destroy all evil forces around me
and bless me with a prosperous and bright future.*

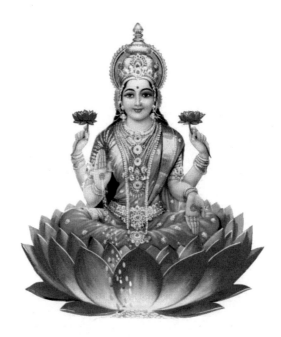

Lakshmi is the supreme goddess of prosperity and good fortune. She emerged from the primordial sea of milk and is the consort of Vishnu. Lakshmi's emblem is the lotus, which she holds in her hands. In another hand, she blesses all creation, and with another, she bestows an endless supply of gold, showering her generosity of holistic wealth on her beloveds. She often is seen with two elephants at her sides, more symbols of wealth. Lakshmi sits or stands on a lotus throne, but does not have a vehicle, such as an animal on which to ride. People pray to her for wealth, fortune, and prosperity.

248

PARVATI: Benevolence, Fertility, Love and Devotion

Sarva Mangala Maangalye, Shive Sarvaartha Saadhike
Sharanye Tryambake Gaurii, Naaraayanii Namostute
*Auspicious Goddess Parvati, consort of Lord Shiva, I adore you, you who love all of
your children. I bow to you Great Mother, who gives refuge to me.*

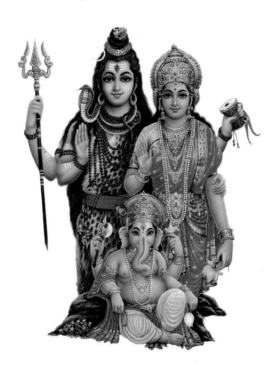

Goddess Parvati is the consort of Shiva and mother of Ganesha. She is a powerful yogini and has many names, some being, Sati, Uma, Kali, Shakti, and Guari. She is the literal definition of the "Power of We" and of sacred partnerships. All female deities are avatars of Parvati, as she is the model of the empowered feminine, the lover, the mother, and she supports the balance of work life and love life.

Other Popular Avatars

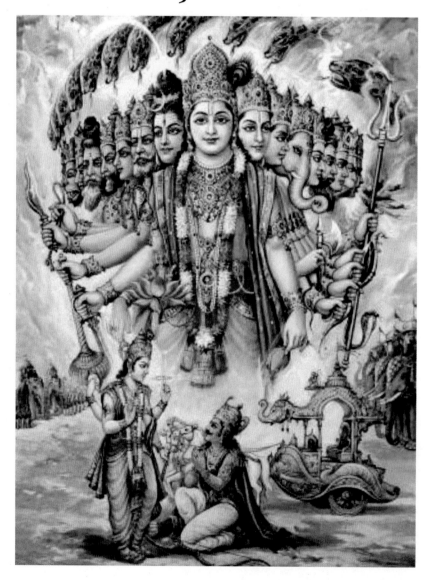

DURGA: Preservation, Energy, Strength and Protection

Om Dum Durgayei Namaha
Protect us from harmful energies.

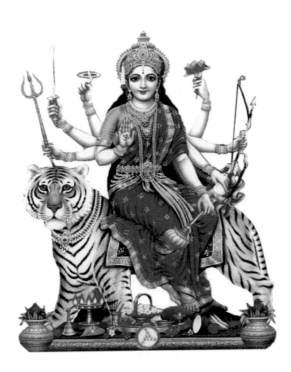

Durga is an avatar of Parvati, and her name means "invincible" in Sanskrit. Durga is the goddess of war and battles against suffering and injustice for mankind and animals. She has eight arms. In five of them, she holds weapons (a sword, a discus, a club, a bow, an arrow, and a trident). In the remaining two, she holds a conch shell and a lotus flower, representing purity. One hand is in a mudra of teaching (being receptive yet discerning). Durga teaches the art of war and the responsibility of duty. People pray to Durga for strength, and she rides a tiger or a lion.

251

KALI: Death, Time and Change

Om Kring Kalikaye Namah
Bring us into pure consciousness.

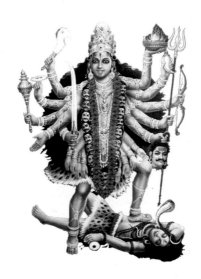

Kali is an avatar of Parvati and is the fierce form of the mother goddess. In her four arms, she holds a sword with blood on it, a trident, a severed head, and a bowl of blood. She wears a necklace of severed heads or skulls and a skirt made of arms. She dances on top of her husband Shiva, who is protecting the world from her intense power. Kali is the Divine Mother, fully devoted to her children, despite her appearance. And she's full of beautiful symbolism. Her three eyes represent past, present, and future because she is the devourer of time - a Goddess of Birth and Destruction. The red eye is also that of astute concentration and raw power willing to be used. Her tongue shows how she devoured the demon, Raktabija, whose blood created demons. Her skull necklace, comprised of the demons of ignorance, represents infinite knowledge. Her nudity shows freedom from illusions as well as her holistic transparency. Kali holds a sword of higher knowledge which severs that which binds, the bowl of purity and protection, and the head of false consciousness. She provides blessings to all.

HANUMAN: Courage, Devotion and Self-Discipline

Om Shri Hanumate Namah
Bestow upon me power, strength, and stamina.

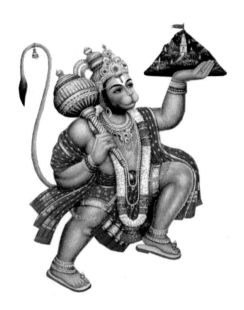

Hanuman makes his appearance in the epic text, *The Ramayana*, where he is commander of the monkey army and first meets Rama. There are three common depictions of Hanuman. In the first, he holds a club and a mountain, representing his strength. In the second, he is also opening up his heart, and inside his heart are Rama and Sita, representing his strong devotion. In the third, he is hugging Rama, representing his devotion. Hanuman rides the wind and people pray to him for strength, comfort, and to help them become better devotees. Hanuman is a popular deity in Bhakti Yoga. His genesis story explains why he has forgotten that he embodies Divine Gifts, but these gifts are revealed in 'time of need', which reflects human potential. Everything we need is within us; we embody Divine Gifts. Hanuman is also known as the Demon Destroyer, and can be called upon for protection.

KRISHNA: Protection, Compassion, Tenderness, Love and Yoga

Om Sri Krishnah Sharanam Namah
Relieve all grief and miseries in my life and mind to restore peace.

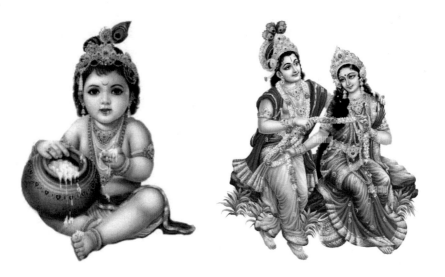

Krishna has various forms and is the most revered Godhead Personality of Supreme Truth, which is Bhagavan. Krishna is an avatar of Vishnu, and his name in Sanskrit means "the dark one" and "all-attractive one". Krishna is viewed as one of the most important gods in India. He has two common depictions. In the first, he is seen as Maakhanchor, a mischievous baby knocking over a butter bowl and breaking rules, representing his playfulness. In the second, he represents all encompassing love as a young man playing his flute and winning the hearts of *gopikas*. Gopikas are represented by women who look after cows. However, they truly represent the highest of devotees with their willingness to hear God's voice and see God's presence in all things. Innately, they will stop everything to be with Krishna/God. They live in the bliss of Infinite Love, wisdom, and devotion. These pure-hearted women are teachers of Divinity by their life-example, as they are unconditional devotees to Krishna. However, Radha won Krishna's heart, and their shared love is said to have begun the Bhakti movement, which is the Hare Krishna Movement. People pray to Krishna for good fortune.

A Deity Yoga Practice

A Practice for Self-Accountability and Compassion

"Do everything you have to do, but not with greed, not with the ego, not with lust, not with envy but with love, compassion, humility and devotion." ~ The Bhagavad Gita

Deities are reflections of human nature, invoking the Divine within. Deity Yoga is a practice to cultivate deep peace as you rise to meet your Authentic Self by releasing habitual patterns. A Tantric practice, taken from Buddhism, is to embody the energy of a deity. Your projections and internalizations as the deity are not outside of who you are. Rather, deities project qualities which are a part of your innate human nature. Humans are ever-transforming spiritual beings, having a spiritual experience on a spiritual plane. Your human experience is *all* spiritual.

The mind is drawn towards having a physical symbol for the heart to love, hence Deity Yoga. This deity may be a Tantric deity, such as Tara or Manjushri, or you may embody the essence of Jesus, Parvati, Buddha, or Quan Yin.

Deity gender is irrelevant. See beyond the deity-symbol and embrace its full essence, void of form. Embody this deity's energy until your thoughts and behaviors naturally align. You may send energy to yourself or others by generating compassion, loving kindness, and other virtues. If you understand that anyone can serve in this way, it can be a lovely, humbling blessing to invoke the deity, your larger Self.

TRY IT - When you are waiting in a long line or find yourself in a busy space, invoke an internal calm and healing presence. Be the change. I travel often, for example, and I practice rooting and radiating my energy on planes, or even when I am at a busy grocery store. It takes only one person to upset a group by a snide comment, a roll of the eyes, or a bold burst of frustration. To counteract, sit or stand tall. Quietly deep breathe. Smile from your lips and eyes at another person. Chant a mantra silently to yourself. Your vibration will uplift your environment and alter the trajectory of any negativity.

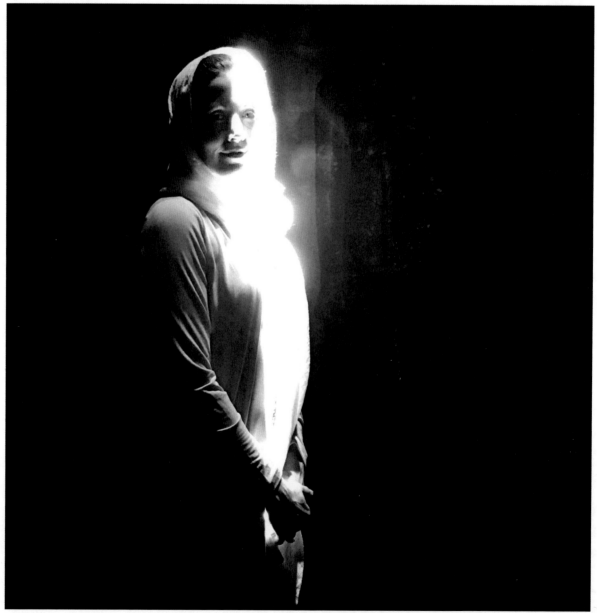

Crone

Claiming the Crone

By Lily Kessler

They tried to kill you
    Goddess
They took your face away
    with stones and hammers
    fire and bullets

They changed your name from Powerful
    to old, ugly and
    bad tempered

They burned you alive
    again and again and again and again
    because of your intelligence and sensuality
    your ability to voice your opinion
    your beauty
And you're refusing to be possessed
    by the dogma of an unsophisticated mind
    of those who separate
    and use the name of God as a weapon

You, who listens to the wind
You, who smells the rain
You, who tastes the green
Having always recognized yourself within Its
    rhythms

Claiming your Self
Standing in the center of your Wholeness
Unity with other realms beyond Vision
Ah, your sharp mind doesn't tolerate fools
        you Independent Female Goddess
You know your Intuition is
        your greatest Wealth
        your inherent Strength
Not to be compromised
        as a puppet of others who feel lack
You Virago Female Warrior
        Full Moon Wisdom Center
Crone

They try to call you weak and unworthy
When your hair becomes white
When your hands become skilled
When overwhelming compassion grows in your heart

They try to make you a cannibal
        Woman against Woman
        nails scratching faces
Clipping the wings of
        others who dance to their own heartbeat
To be the last gladiator standing
        alone and hungry
        just like them

They try to silence and shame your
  communion with your Holy Moon Blood
Where you were once fed honey
  in the Red Tent of Rest
  now condemned to Ritual Impurity Laws
Yet even with this knife in your back
  fertile blood still runs down your legs
  nourishing your footsteps
Ah, in the still of the night
  I smile as I see you enter the temple to offer yourself
  to the lingam
  prayed over unaware by the priests
  in their morning rituals which they thought
  you were banned from
Women unite take back the night

REMEMBER

You are the Radiant Full Moon
  Wise Crone
You lay the seeds
  for your daughters to dance
  among wildflowers
  reminding them of their holy wildness
  that is to be held forever sacred
  and joyous
And free

REMEMBER

> *You are the Lover that shifts with the winds*
> > *dancing with Life/Days-Yet-To-Be-Explored*
> > *not stagnating under swallowed oppression*
> > *cursing your dried breasts*
> > *or filling them with plastic*

> *Nor are you drinking the Poison of Doubt*
> > *that questions your very worth*
> *Instead*
> > *your smile lines glow*
> > *your perspectives soar*
> > *you bury loved ones*
> > *and your hair becomes the color of starlight*

REMEMBER

> *You are the Virago the Powerful*
> > *the Goddess*
> > *the Baba Yaga*
> > *the Eve*
> > *the Charity*
> > *the Formidable*
> > *whose very nature is Knowledge*

> *You are the most valuable gift of*
> > *our human race, being humanKIND*
> > *Crone, You*

The older you become
The brighter you shine
Coaxing sap from roots
You
Energizing Nymph
Nourishing Tide on the Moon
You

REMEMBER

A woman who knows herself is dangerous
in the minds of the Scared
who can't stand their own reflection
their own Magnificence
the Light of their Glow

You who can change and love yourself
can change the world into a new creation
Not to be recognized
but direly needed

You give birth
through the fertile soil of your experiences
through your triumphs and sorrows
through your discernment
Nourishing life with your tears of joy
and anguish
and awe of it All

REMEMBER

You are the Full Moon not the wane
Remember who you are, Diana
  leader of the Great Hunt
   with wild hounds at your heels passionately
Enraptured by your intrinsic freedom
Your uninhibited heart

May you be blessed to grow old
May you carve space for age
  to settle in your bones
May you look another woman in the eye and
  remind her she is beautiful

May you know the fleetingness
  and importance of a life well lived
  comfortable in your own skin
  which is the Truth of Beauty

REMEMBER, CRONE

The night is your playground
  to ignite your fire

Reflection

Deities: Symbols of Self

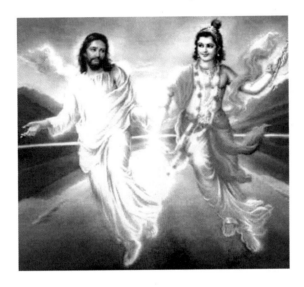

The Gita says, "Do everything you have to do, but not with greed, not with the ego, not with lust, not with envy but with love, compassion, humility and devotion."

In Deity Yoga, you are rising to meet your Authentic Self. Your projections and internalizations as the deity are not outside of who you are. Rather, deities are reflections of human nature, and invoke the Divine within. Humans are ever-transforming spiritual beings having a spiritual experience on a spiritual plane. Your human experience is *all* spiritual.

This reflection is simply to observe how your daily sadhana is going. Consider if you need to incorporate the practices of mantra, japa, or puja into your daily living.

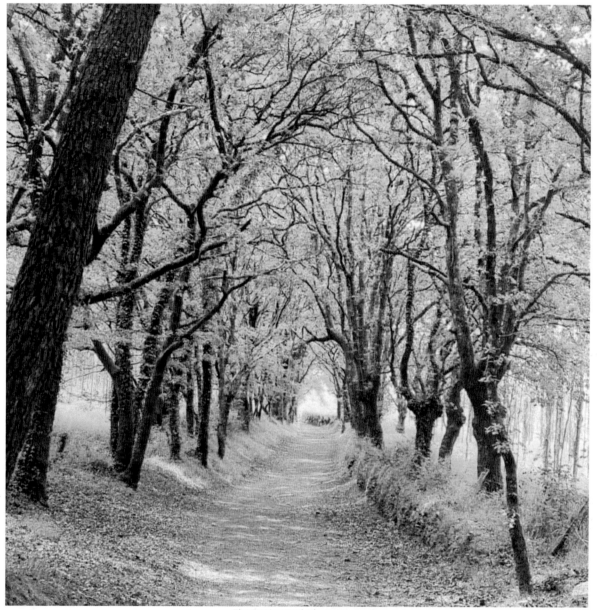

The Camino Trail Pilgrimage, Spain

Chapter 7

Bhakti Yoga: The Hero's Journey and The Path of Devotion

Historical Timeline

PRECLASSICAL YOGA ERA

INDUS-SARASVATI AGE: 6500-4500 BCE
- SANATANA DHARMA: "ETERNAL LAW"
- INDUS RIVER VALLEY & SEALS

VEDIC AGE: 4500-2500 BCE
- CONSCIOUSNESS EXPLORED
- VIBRATION OF INTENTION & CAUSATION
- CAUSE & EFFECT: MANTRA & KARMA

SAMKHYA YOGA: 8000-100 BCE
- REALITY EXPLORED: PRAKRITI/PURUSHA
- BODY'S CONSTITUTION: DOSHAS
- AYURVEDA

UPANISHADIC AGE: 2000-1500 BCE
- NON-DUALISM OF ATMAN/BRAHMAN
- DISTILLATION OF VEDAS
- MEDITATION

BHAKTI YOGA: 1000-500 BCE
- ADORATION
- HINDU EPICS / UNIVERSAL INSIGHTS
- 3 BRANCHES OF YOGA

BUDDHISM: C. 500 BCE-PRESENT
- INDIVIDUALITY / MONASTIC TRADITION
- MIDDLE WAY
- FOUR NOBLE TRUTHS / EIGHT-FOLD PATH

CLASSICAL YOGA ERA

CLASSICAL YOGA: 75 BCE-100 CE
- THE YOGA SUTRA'S OF PATANJALI
- EIGHT-LIMBED PATH
- HARNESSING THE MIND

ESOTERIC AGE

TANTRA: 600-1300 CE
- 6 + 1 CHAKRA SYSTEM
- WESTERN NOTION OF EMBODIMENT
- SUBTLE BODY (NADIS, CHAKRAS, ETC.)

HATHA YOGA: C. 1300-1400 CE
- MIND V. BODY
- HATHA YOGA PRADIPIKA
- ASANA / BREATH / BANDHAS / MUDRAS

RISE OF MODERN YOGA

SWAMI VIVEKANANDA: 1872-1950
- INFLUENCED RISE OF MODERN YOGA
- INTRODUCED YOGA TO THE WEST

SRI T. KRISHNAMACHARYA: 1891-1989
- YOGA'S EXPANSION
- FATHER OF MODERN YOGA
- MODERN CONTRIBUTORS

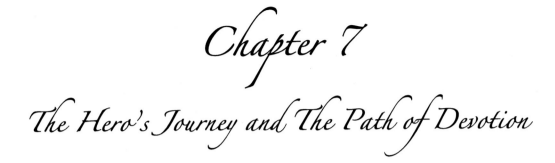

Chapter 7
The Hero's Journey and The Path of Devotion

1. Overview of Lecture

Chapter 7 examines Bhakti Yoga, the Yoga of Devotion, which is the most popular form of Yoga practiced throughout the world. We explore the vulnerability of courage, bravery, compassion, and interconnection through examining the stages of the Hero's Journey. The seminal text of Bhakti Yoga, *The Bhagavad Gita* in relation to Atman and Brahman, is also addressed, along with the power of mantra and kirtan. A comparison of Bhakti Yoga to the two other forms of Yoga highlighted in *The Gita*, being Karma Yoga and Jnana Yoga, are presented.

2. Learning Objectives: I will…

a) Understand the basic components of a Bhakti Practice
b) Recognize my Hero's Journey/s and interpret how *The Gita* is an allegory
c) Recognize the three types of Yoga - *Karma Yoga, Bhakti Yoga, Jnana Yoga*

3. Pre-lecture Assignments

a) Read the chapter and become familiar with the Reflection question
b) Watch Film: *Finding Joe*
c) Read *The Bhagavad Gita*, recommended translation by Eknath Eswaran
d) Daily Sadhana - Daily Personal Practice

4. Reflection: *found at the end of the chapter*

Joseph Campbell

1904 - 1987, Comparative Mythologist, Writer and Lecturer

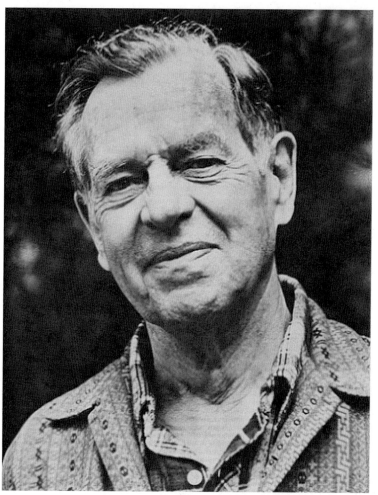

Joe

The Hero's Journey

Joseph Campbell independently studied mythologies and religions. He claimed that great epics and myths found in cultures around the world, including *The Bhagavad Gita*, share a common structure called a monomyth, which is now known as *The Hero's Journey*.

The Hero's Journey is based on the notion that the Universe unfolds opportunities within each person's life by interrupting a linear existence. This interruption is needed to break open one's innate potential. In this process, one can choose to be a victim of circumstance or choose to learn through courageous vulnerability, empowered by compassion and empathy. All stumbling blocks faced can become steppingstones in which compassion for others is learned. Campbell believed that there are Guardians within everyone's life whose purpose is to keep individuals, tribes (and the world), safe and unchanged, so the Hero is misdirected and limited in self-expansion.

Heroes embrace adventure and remain open to recalibration, a realignment and clarity of the calling of the heart. This requires a death because accepting adventure leads to dying a thousand times; the Hero dies to who they think they are to embrace who they truly are. Each time an attachment is released, there is a death, only to be born into a greater life. Therefore, dharma is honored.

The Hindus believe that dharma is duty, and that duty changes with time and commitment. The Buddhists believe that dharma is the ultimate reality. For both, it is non-attachment; to be in the world as much as possible; to be in duty with a full heart, but not attached to results (Both/And).

The Bhagavad Gita is the sixth book of *The Mahabharata*, the Holy Text within the Hindu philosophy. *The Gita* was passed down verbally through the millennia and was compiled and printed in 1970. The 18 chapters of the Mahabharata explain dharma and explore the relationships to Prakriti, the gunas, and the concept of non-attachment. The elements within each chapter are how to follow dharma in a non-dharmic world; the ability to follow the heart, even though that decision could break the heart. Individual growth occurs when you alter yourself from the inside out, and the outside in. This alters your words, your character, and your destiny.

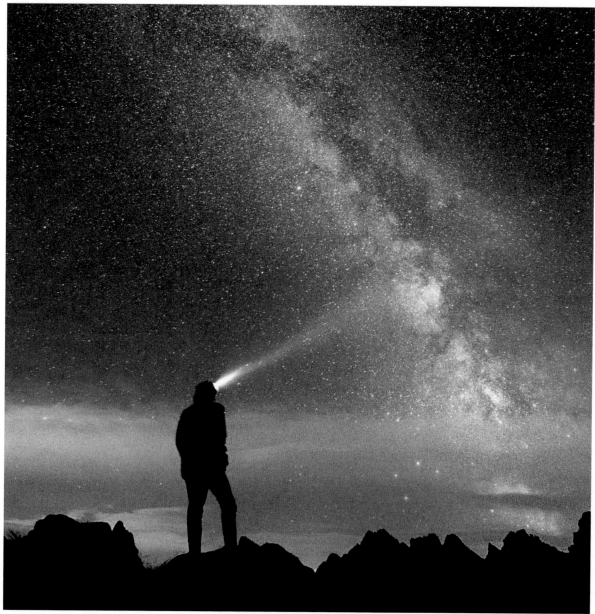

Embracing the Unknown

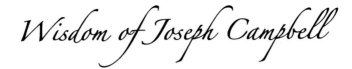

Wisdom of Joseph Campbell

- ❖ You must let go of the life you have planned, so as to accept the one that is waiting for you.

- ❖ You enter the forest at the darkest point, where there is no path. Where there is a way or path, it is someone else's path. You are not on your own path. If you follow someone else's way, you are not going to realize your potential.

- ❖ Follow your bliss, don't be afraid, and doors will open where you didn't know they were going to be. If you do follow your bliss, you put yourself on a kind of track that has been there all the while, waiting for you, and the life that you ought to be living is the one you are living.

- ❖ It is by going down into the abyss that you recover the treasures of life. Where you stumble, there lies your treasure.

- ❖ Opportunities to find deeper powers within yourself come when life seems most challenging.

- ❖ The goal of life is to make your heartbeat match the beat of the universe, to match your nature with Nature.

- ❖ What each must seek in his life never was on land or sea. It is something out of his own unique potentiality for experience, something that never has been and never could have been experienced by anyone else.

- ❖ When you quit thinking primarily about yourself and your own self-preservation, you undergo a truly heroic transformation of consciousness.

- ❖ I don't believe people are looking for the meaning of life as much as they are looking for the experience of being alive.

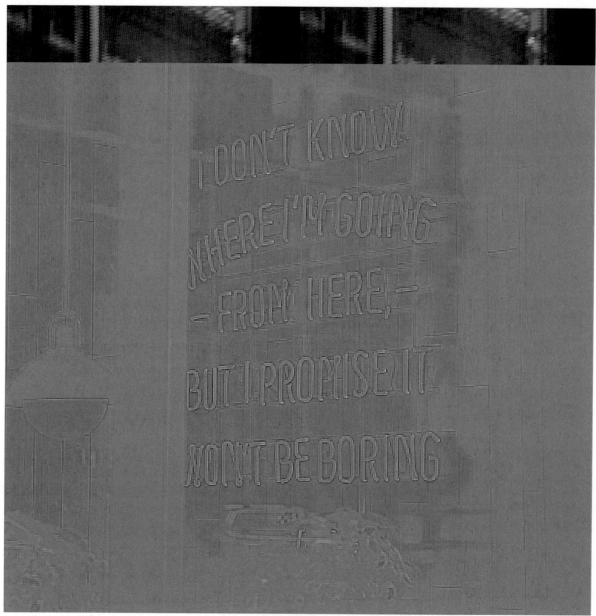

Finding Dharma

The Hero

Myths are clues to your spiritual nature,
and they can help guide you to a sacred place within
where you might unlock the creative power
of your deeper unconscious self.

The Labyrinth

You will never be alone in an adventure because heroes of all kinds have come before. ~ J. Campbell

The *labyrinth of consciousness* is inherently known by each of us. Oftentimes, you may find yourself trapped inside the maze of your mind because of limiting perspectives and beliefs. As a result, you may only see the impediments in front of you and become frustrated by your inability to discern the path leading to an enhanced life.

Ancient yogis understood that each person creates their own obstacles through a limiting narrative of one's own life story. But yogic insights also offer tools that transcend perspective and consciousness; the maze of life becomes clearer. Rather than seeing only the walls in front of you, a beautiful labyrinth design emerges.

A labyrinth is within you where you may become temporarily stuck on a dead-end path or become thrust into the abyss of the unknown. In an alternative perspective, everything is a teacher, an opportunity to see the bigger picture of life and to rise above the obstacles, emerging from the labyrinth as a hero for humanity.

273

The Hero's Deed

There are two types of deeds than can be undertaken while on The Hero's Journey.

The Hero's Journey is a deed that has been undertaken by many, many people, as the hero can be anyone who has given their life to achieving/becoming something bigger than themselves. Doing so often requires a type of death and resurrection – a cycle of departure, fulfilment, and return.

The first type of deed is physical, such as physical acts of heroism – for example, giving yourself/sacrificing yourself for another, or for a higher cause. The physical deed can also be seen in a simple initiation ritual in which a child has to give up their childhood to become an adult. They must *die* to their juvenile personality and psyche and come back as a self-responsible adult. This is a fundamental experience that everyone must undergo, emerging from physical and psychological dependency, into one of self-responsibility and maturity.

The second type of deed is spiritual. The spiritual deed of heroism is learning/experiencing a supernormal range of human spiritual life, and then coming back to communicate your knowledge to others. Like every Hero's Journey, it is a cycle; a going and a return.

The story of Buddha and Christ are perfect representations of the spiritual Hero's Journey. Though their births are roughly 500 years apart, both traditions are like mirrors to the other. Buddha and Christ undergo three temptations. Christ faces temptations in the desert, and Buddha faces temptations in the forest. Both of their journeys lasted a long time until clarity emerged. And like Buddha, Christ overcomes these temptations and returns to choose disciples who help him establish and teach a new way of consciousness based on what was discovered during the journey.

Similar spiritual journeys were undertaken by Moses, Muhammed, and others. In each case, the hero sacrifices their individual needs and shares the higher levels of consciousness and wisdoms obtained through their journeys for the greater good of all humanity. All major religions teach that the trials of the Hero's Journey are a significant part of achieving spiritual consciousness - that there is no reward without renunciation.

To be a hero, you must stop thinking of your own self-protection. You must lose yourself, give yourself, to another. This is a trial, an initiation within itself, offering a huge transformation of consciousness, as all myths offer a transformation of consciousness. You think one way then transform to think another way.

The Adventure and the Dragon

Reality as it is known must be altered for life to continue.

The Hero's Journey can be a serendipitous adventure, as the achievement of the hero ultimately becomes one for which they are ready. This is an initiation which is used as a ladder for further skill development. The hero stands on the edge of the unknown and embarks into the outlying spaces. In so doing, the adventure evokes a quality of the hero's character that they didn't know they possessed.

The first stage in the Hero's Journey is leaving the *norm*, which is controlled and what is known. Once the journey begins, the hero may be confronted with the "dragon" that lives in the abyss, where the norm no longer is.

In life, this confrontation can take the form of an unexpected loss of a job, the loss of a loved one, or personal injury of any sort. This stage of the journey can be seen as either a spiral of suffering or the beginning of something new to create. At this point, the hero may be cut to pieces and descend into the abyss in fragments, eventually to be resurrected. Or … the hero may find his hidden power, slay the dragon, assimilate his new-found power, and claim a more authentic relationship with his true self, seeing the world in a more encompassing reality.

As you move through the journey of your life, all limitations, whether self-imposed or imposed by forces perceived as outside your control, become your "dragons."

Achieving this shift in what you perceive as "reality" requires an understanding that consciousness does not reside in the brain, but instead is inherent in the "gut" – in the humanity of your entire body.

275

The brain is a necessary, but secondary, organ of a total human being, and it must not be allowed to always be in control.

The logical, ego-driven desires of the brain can become the controlling power of the dragon within its own lair. When the brain puts itself in control, it has gone over to the intellectual side. Society operates under this control. This illusionary *Lila*, this labyrinth of life, can eat you up and relieve you of humanity, or it can offer a contrast to highlight the nobility of human potential within the dragon's lair of society.

You must not be attached to changing this external system, yet you may live within this system while resisting its impersonal claims. (Like Jesus teaches, "to be in this world but not of it") To realize your full potential, the brain must submit and serve the gut; your intuitive sacral center, which is the ultimate body-brain connected to the liberated states of consciousness and less suffering. This is the way to navigate the labyrinth.

Revealing the Hero

Tool: Invoke Gratitude

The Upanishads says that the Seeker and the Sought are the same, so whatever you can dream for yourself, begin it. The boldness of the Hero's Journey has genius, power, and magic in it.

If you don't listen to the voice of your own spirit and heart, and insist on maintaining a certain 'program', you will find yourself off center, falling into a samskaric-patterned life which is *not* the life the body and spirit are interested in.

The world is filled with people who have stopped listening to themselves. In my own life, I've had many opportunities to commit myself to a system and obey its requirements. Those who question rules, roles, or norms established by society, or other tribal ways of thinking, are sometimes considered dangerous and may be secluded. Yet, the hero exists and operates beyond the boundaries of confining norms, in turn providing inspiration for others to break free of their own boundaries.

Anaïs Nin said, "And the day came when the risk to remain tight in a bud was more painful than the risk it took to blossom." This is the beginning of your journey. The hero's potential is within every person, but it takes risk. Your life evokes your character, and you learn more about yourself the older you become. Strive to put yourself in situations that evoke your higher nature. It is important to explore, embrace, and be brave enough to discern knowledge from all experiences.

Such exploration can result in a new balance and harmony. If you are willing to examine the true sources of what brings you *true joy* - not just the impermanent happiness of *pleasure* - you may find yourself on a new path towards that joy.

For example, do you find joy in your job, or is it simply the means to a financial end? The same question can be asked about relationships, where you live, and almost any meaningful aspect of your life. Not that immediate change is always required. But engaging in the exploration, asking the questions, can help ease anxiety and help put you in accord with the opportunities in your life. Doing so also may allow you to identify the positive values of what may otherwise be perceived as negative in society. You can say yes to the adventure of living, and no to the "dragons" that seek to keep you captive in the lair.

Psychologically, the dragon is your own binding to your ego. In other words, you are caught in your own dragon cage. Your fears are the dragon yet, seeing beyond them, can help slay it. The real dragon is in you; the ego holding you in. What I want, what I believe, what I think I can do, what I think I love, what I regard as the aim of my life, etc., can be too small. The environment in which you live is too limiting, and it is reflected by your inner dragon.

Following Your Bliss

How do you slay the dragon? *Follow your bliss.*

Find where your bliss is and don't be afraid to follow it. For example, there is either enjoyable work that you are doing because you choose to do it, or you don't enjoy your work. The mentality of *"I can't do/change that"* is your dragon.

What do you find on the journey (when you are brave enough to begin)? A quiet place of rest within yourself. This is a center out of which you may respond to situations, not merely react to them based on your previous memories of how you acted in similar situations in the past. This is the sacred, innate place where creation and fulfilment of your vision arises. You embody the feeling of actualization and wholeness, which is the trajectory of the energy of your inner calling. Athletes, dancers, etc. know this state of consciousness (often referred to as being in the zone"), which is a yogic state of consciousness. Yet, if action arises only in the field of the mind, you are not performing in alignment of your center. Therefore, tension arises. Until and unless you find your center, you cannot act with the fullness of your being.

Buddha talks of Nirvana and Jesus talks of peace. *Nirvana* is a consciousness that comes when you are not compelled by desires, fear, or social commitments. You hold your center and act from this place. Buddha shows you there is a way beyond fear, but you must first clarify your state of mind, even during the turmoil of samsara (your life experiences).

The hero knows that all of life is a meditation, and most of it isn't intentional. The Hero's Journey brings you to a level of consciousness that is spiritual and helps provide an understanding of how to hold your consciousness on a particular level. The journey eventually allows you to up-level the foundation from which you consciously and spiritually reside. This is the revelation, the gift, of the slayed ego-dragon.

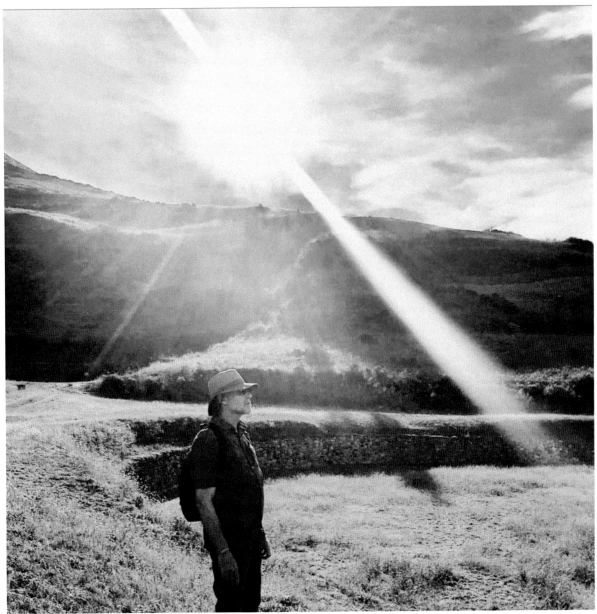

Aligned, Peru

Stages of the Hero's Journey

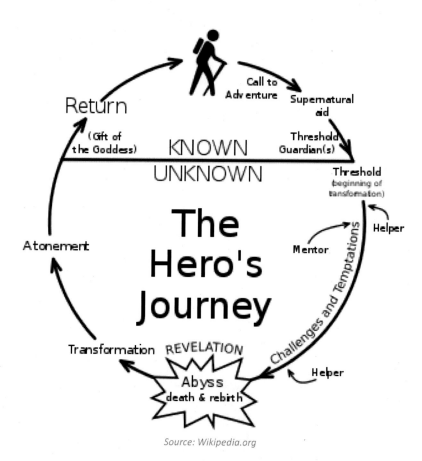

Source: Wikipedia.org

The Hero's Journey ultimately allows you to save yourself, and in doing so, allows you to help save the world. A vital person, by nature, revitalizes, and brings fruition to life. When you are brave enough to heed your calling and embark on your path, others may then find the courage to begin their own Hero's Journey.

Ordinary World:

Most people are content with the status quo because it is a predictable system. They believe in the five-sense world and feel threatened if others, especially loved ones, want to change their comfort boundaries. The Beyond is dangerous, uncivilized, full of undesirables, and is to be avoided at all costs. Guardians, members of the tribe, are those who believe they are doing the Hero a great service by diminishing the Hero's ideas.

The Birth:

A manifestation of Divinity as You. You are the Hero.

The Call to Adventure:

This call is as deep as the atman and allows the process of expansion to begin. Ultimately, this calling, this longing, is the need to return Home. The spiritual path will progress only if it is heeded. It is a summons to live in the Now and to claim your life. To answer the call, the Hero must go on the journey. It's living Authentically by honoring dharma, one's truth.

The Refusal of the Call:

The Hero's focus turns to worldly interests. The Hero loses the power of affirmative action if the call is not heeded. If you don't live your dharma, you become a victim, you ache with dissatisfaction, and you experience a life out of alignment.

Crossing the First Threshold:

The journey begins as the Hero approaches the threshold, a region unknown and which may hold the power to change forever what is predictable and known.

Belly of the Whale:

The whale represents the personification of all that is in the unconscious. Water is the unconscious. The creature in the water is the dynamism of the unconscious, which is dangerous and powerful and must be controlled by the consciousness. The Hero steps over the threshold only to suffer/experience the death of his ego. The warnings offered by the Guardians appear to have been correct. However, the ego's death must happen for the Hero to be reborn. This is the most life-centering, life-renewing act possible. Like the snake shedding its skin, all attachment must be shed.

The Road of Trials:
Here the Hero endures a series of trials, culminating in what's often referred to as The Dark Night of the Soul. *The Gita* shows the horror of Reality where the Hero encounters monsters, inner demons, limiting beliefs and prejudices, all of which are based on the energy of fear. However, the Road of Trials must be endured as a crucible necessary to purify the Essential Self. The Hero may be assisted in this part of the journey by the supernatural (amulets, wands, swords, fairy godmothers, protective wizards). The importance of symbolic reassurance is that protective power is always present in the sanctuary of the Hero's heart.

The Epitome:
The Hero leans into the void and experiences the Divine state of the Witness Self. It is the climax of the journey as the Hero is freed from suffering and prejudice, allowing the Hero to be free from attachment but rooted with clarity and focus. Both/And.

The Boon:
A benefit, advantage, and/or blessing. Symbolized by the Holy Grail, the boon is taken for immortality and may become an obstacle if the Hero does not use it with integrity and upmost care.

The Return Threshold:
Having received the boon, the Hero returns to share the experience and knowledge gained during the journey. The status quo has changed, and the Hero may be perceived as dangerous. The Hero must demonstrate the value and benefits of change.

The Return:
The Hero becomes master of two worlds, Purusha and Prakriti, and moves freely between both like a cosmic dancer with one eye out and one eye in. The boon transforms the world, but the Hero must be willing to release it because its benefits cannot be experienced through attachment to the boon itself. Expansion can only occur through non-attachment, even to a great gift.

"You've changed."
Two of the best words
You will ever hear.

~ Cara Alwill Leyba

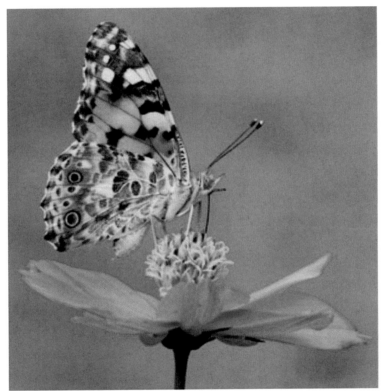

Always Change

The Hero's Journey: Condensed

∞

Stage One: The Threshold and Call to Adventure

You find yourself on the threshold of a great choice. The journey begins when the challenge arises, and you are called to Adventure. You may either accept this challenge or find you have no other choice than to engage. This may not necessarily be a physical journey, but a journey within yourself, as you no longer can live the way you are living. You must challenge your routines, family, friends, and innermost desires to re-establish or remove your place within those relationships.

Stage Two: The Innermost Cave

The journey is not an easy task. It is a journey of changing your perspectives, shedding your skin, dying to who you think you are. You must die a thousand times so you may live. You must shed who you thought you were (ego), in order to become who you truly are (in order to become your authentic self). You enter a deep, uncharted psychological cave that threatens the very foundation of everything you thought was true. The Innermost Cave is the place of greatest danger and is the most terrifying part of the Hero's Journey. It truly is the Great Unknown, and therefore, you are faced with the threat of failure. Yet, there is no choice but to go within. Once you are in, you must be steadfast and rely on your intuition. Here, you must be willing to let your ego and all its layers of protection die. But most importantly, you must be willing to be born again as a stronger version of who you are.

Stage Three: The Seizing of the Sword

The Sword is a boon and comes in the form of a once-hidden quality of strength that you never knew existed until it is needed in a time of great need. Your greatest strength is found in the place of your greatest weakness. You rise to the occasion and do things you never knew you could do. The beauty of your supposed weakness and fear is that it paves the way for your strengths to emerge. Only through trial can you tap into your greatness. The Journey is choosing strength, rather than remaining a martyr or a victim. When you choose strength, when you seize the Sword, the ascent (the rebirth) begins. You have slain the monster of fear in the Innermost Cave.

Stage Four: The Rebirth

The final stage of the journey is the re-emergence, which is inwardly triumphant. You had to die to who you thought you were, seize the newfound Sword of Strength, and become reborn into a stronger version of yourself. Yet, you cannot return to your beginning point because you are changed, spiritually and psychologically. Instead, you return to a vantage point with knowledge gained in a lesson that was experienced and internalized, prepared to meet more of life's challenges. This strength is also called the elixir. The elixir arms your courage, and lets you know you can navigate future challenges because many more Innermost Caves await exploration.

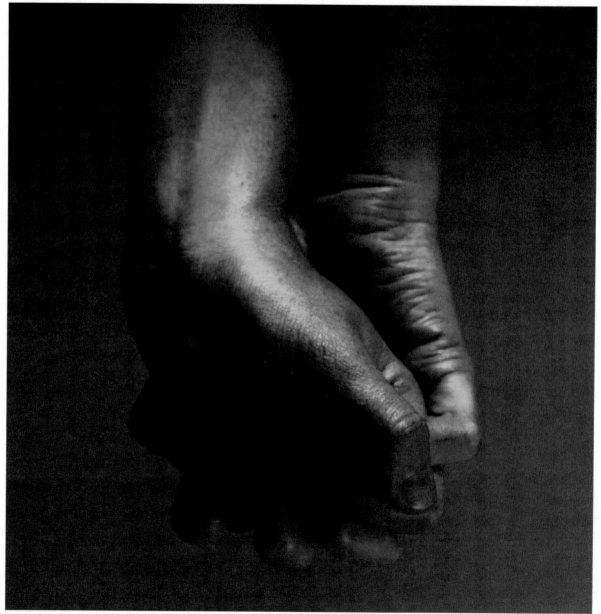

Hold My Hand

286

Hold My Hand

By Lily Kessler

Hold my hand and I'll hold yours.
Side by side we'll stand to face this great Gaping Wound that now
gushes generations of sickness, of blame, of blindness
into the light of day to be seen. Into the light of day to be healed.

Hold my hand and I'll hold yours.
Let's agree to not pick up the rock at our feet.
Hold my hand tight when I want to throw rage back and hurt those who hurt me.
Remind me that hatred doesn't discriminate and it's always hungry.

Hold my hand and I'll hold yours.
Our shared strength will allow this Great Tsunami to break against us
again and again until it cries itself to sleep
empty and exhausted ready to be soothed with lullabies of
the truth of Wholeness, the beauty of Diversity
our connection to Everything.

Hold my hand and I'll hold yours.
Together we celebrate Humanity's courage
expressed through vulnerability and humbleness.
We teach our children curiosity, the art of dialogue, and accountability;
And that Love requires Bravery to see ourselves in all beings.

We are strong enough to put the rock down.
The simplest peace offering is a great blessing upon the world.

A Yoga Perspective on the Hero's Journey

The privilege of a lifetime is being who you are. ~ Joseph Campbell

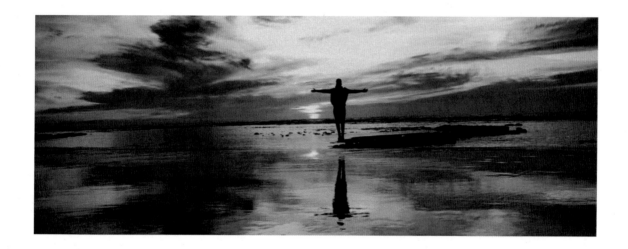

Personal: To find clarity, you must be vulnerable and allow yourself to recognize doubts and fears. You must be open to coincidences and cultivate the ability to view your journey with greater scope. Here, be willing to shed layers of the ego and embrace the brave understanding in the notion that *this is for me, it's not about them*. When you follow your bliss, you follow your own Truth, your dharma.

In Pose & Practice: If the pose is feeling unavailable or you are feeling reluctant, allow yourself to feel the strain and breathe. This is a normal feeling. Open yourself up to a new normal, a new belief system. Allow your body and spirit to respond with the inquiry of *'Why do I feel this way?'* Be Witness to the answer. This is the alchemy of *tapas*, the curious burning of labels and boundary walls. Turn anger, or whatever stagnant energy you are experiencing, into something positive and expansive that will feed the energy of Love.

Yearning for a new way will not produce it. Only ending the old way can do that.
You cannot hold onto the old all the while declaring that you want something new.
The old will defy the new; the old will deny the new; the old will decry the new.
There is only one way to bring in the new. You must make room for it.

~ Neal Donald Walsch

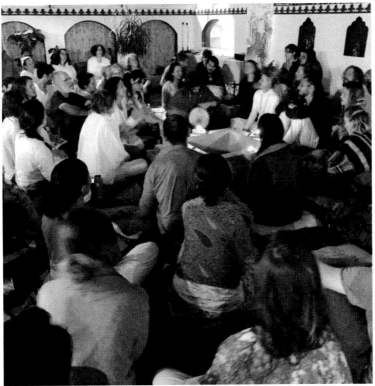

Bhakti Kirtan (Rishikesh, India)

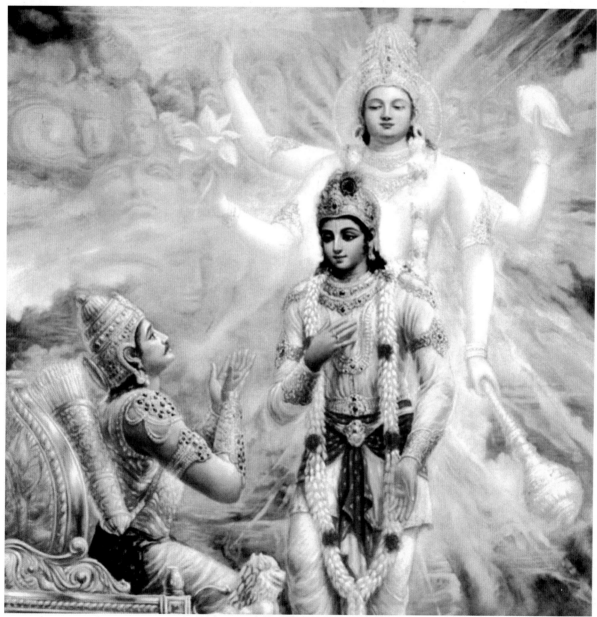

Krishna reveals Himself to Arjun, Google Images

Spiritual Yoga

When you do things from your soul, you feel a river moving in you. ~ Rumi

Real Love is possible only when you see everything as yourself. ~ Sri Swami Satchidananda

When you drink the water, remember the spring from where it came. ~ Chinese Proverb

As vast as God is, there is also a great vastness of heavenly states, which appeal to different people in different ways; in other words, *to each their own*. Therefore, there are different schools in the Yoga tradition to meet varied human tendencies. This begs the questions: How do you practice? What is your focus? Is it about the atman and the self-realization of *Ishvara* (another name for the Ultimate Purusha)? Or is it about the journey to Bhagavan? Simply put, liberated states vary – not one size fits all.

In all the traditions of Yoga, the highest state of the atman is defined by a *merging* or *focus*. There is a name for this state of liberation: Moksha. Yoga practices connect you with a higher truth. And there are many different Yoga traditions that have different understandings as to what that higher truth is. But the starting point is the atman – the deep-level, inner-most Self.

It is important to note that the goal within some Yogic traditions is not adoration of God, but rather to experience your own, ultimate atman. This is considered a non-dual tradition. Non-duality is the recognition that, underlying the multiplicity and diversity of experience, there is a single, infinite, and indivisible reality, whose nature is pure consciousness, from which all objects and selves derive their independent existence. This reality is the foundation of peace.

Upanishadic gurus recognize that atman and Brahman are the same. Likewise, the goal in Classical Yoga is to experience your own nature as object-less, or Pure Consciousness. Additionally, the concept of *svarupe vasthanam*, explored in Patanjali's *Yoga Sutras*, is the ego's absorption into the true Self, where consciousness is conscious of its consciousness. This non-dual goal begins as a dualistic practice where the Seer and the Seen are separate. As atman merges with the absolute truth of Brahman, all differentiation merges and contributes to Unity Consciousness, rather than being a mere perception or concept of Oneness.

In Samkhya and Vedanta philosophies, the deep level self is *not* the physical body or the mental self. Yoga, within itself, is a function of mental activities. But Self is beyond the mind. Just as fire is different from its sparks and smoke, the body is connected to the Purusha, but is not the Purusha. The Seer is the atman, which is different from the mind and intelligence, internal organs and senses, and sense objects, all of which is Prakriti.

Other traditions say there is a supreme atman that is distinct from your individual atman (eternally, metaphysically, and ontologically distinct). The goal is to understand that this deeper or higher atman exists – a supreme atman that pervades all the universes and sustains all beings. As a result, the goal is not to be absorbed in your own blissful *svarupa* (your own nature) for eternity, but rather to ultimately have a loving relationship with Bhagavan, which opens a whole journey in the spiritual landscape of possibilities. This loving relationship with God is called Bhakti Yoga. *Bhakti Yoga* is the *Yoga of Devotion* (*Spiritual Yoga*) and is the most practiced form of Yoga, based on service, truth, and love.

This timeless tradition accepts the non-dual teachings within *The Upanishads* and *Yoga Sutras*. Yet unlike Patanjali, who tries to still the mind with the mind to stand within the Self, Bhakti practitioners are not trying to still the mind. They are focusing the mind on one thing; contemplating and thinking about Bhagavan. Bhakti incorporates multitudes of devotional practices that merge a devotee with Bhagavan in the temple of their heart, which is Yoga.

The practitioner is called a *Bhakta*, who focuses on having a personal relationship based on the adoration of God, making this a dualistic practice in which a connection is being sought between "subject" and "object". Consciousness of atman (subject) is connected to a distinct, separate Supreme Consciousness, which is Bhagavan (object). Bhakti Yoga is the practice that supports a personal relationship with Bhagavan; absorbing the mind in Bhagavan. Here, the mind is filled with bliss, which is ultimately expressing true love of the Divine.

A relationship between the two is needed for the bestowing of love and devotion to occur. (Note, the feminine form of Bhagavan is *Bhagavati*, and is represented by Goddesses such as Kali, Sarasvati, Durga, and others.) This journey to Bhagavan is the practice of Bhakti Yoga. This spiritual process of Bhakti Yoga takes the atman beyond the gunas, beyond karma, and beyond samsara, which is the concept of rebirth and cyclicality of all life, matter, and existence, and is a fundamental belief within many Indian religions. In other words, Bhakti is a process that will liberate the atman through the form of a loving relationship between the practitioner, Bhakta, and a form of Bhagavan or Bhagavati.

Humility is key and is considered the key to the heart of Bhagavan. When you become humble you are ready to "hear" or receive. Then what? The world of name and form vanishes, and the sense of an individualized self evaporates. All that remains is pure, infinite, all pervading Consciousness.

Bhakti has associated mental practices, which including various forms of meditation, japa, and contemplations on Bhagavan. Many devotional traditions in India are rooted in 18,000 Puranas. The Puranas are Hindu religious texts woven with intricate layers of symbolism in stories, legends, and lore that discuss cosmology, astronomy, music, dance, genealogy, geography, yoga, and culture. The Bhagavata Purana is a revered text which examine the forms of Bhagavan, self-knowledge, salvation, and bliss.

What form does Bhagavan take? Whatever form(s) captures the heart of the practitioner and allows you to experience Ishvara. In India, sometimes these forms are inherited in family and cultural traditions. For generation upon generation, a family may worship a particular form of Krishna, Shiva, Narayana, or in east India, the form of Kali or another Goddess. Even though there are various forms of Bhakti based on family and regional traditions, Krishna and Shiva Bhakti pervade the whole of India.

Ultimately, at its deepest level, Bhakti is love. You may fall in love with a form of God/Ishvara that has nothing to do with family or region. And there is always the possibility that your soul finds Bhakti and in unique forms lifetime after lifetime. There are no rules and regulations. It is a matter of the heart ... the heart of each practitioner/devotee.

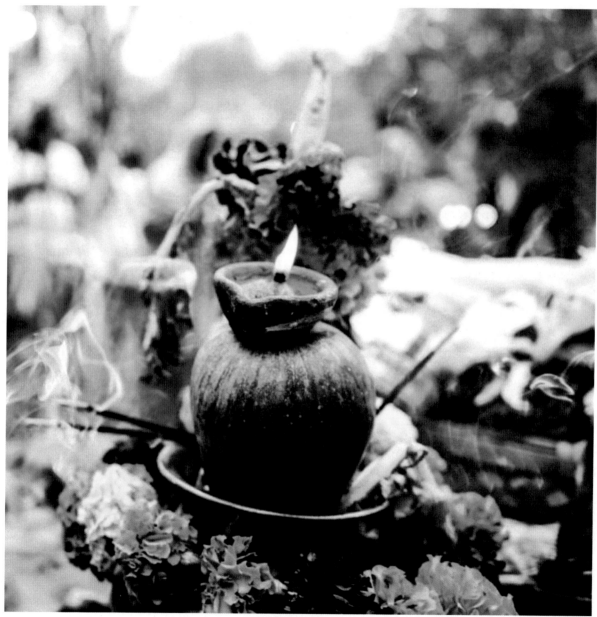

Wide World of Bhakti

Aspects of Bhakti

Bhakti practitioners believe that the Universe is based on the concept of *Lila*, the Divine Play of Life and Illusion. The Yogi who has achieved realization of Bhagavan, the Supreme Personality, has moved beyond the ego and illusion and has attained the topmost level of transcendental knowledge. The path to this knowledge is Bhakti.

The Bhakti Movement's point of origin is unknown, though it is claimed to have begun in the southern region of the Indian subcontinent around 1000 BCE. The tradition spread north and east and peaked between the 15th and 17th Century. Even today, Bhakti Yoga is the most popular form of Yoga in the world.

Personal Relationship with Bhagavan

Brahman is present throughout the entire cosmic existence, and it is the great unifying and sustaining life force of all beings. *Bhagavan* is the eternal, personal form of Supreme Truth. *Krishna* is the supreme Personality of Bhagavan. Krishna/Bhagavan is the Absolute Truth, and is an eternal, sentient being which *The Bhagavad Gita* names the Cause of all Causes. This Truth is fully cognizant of every subatomic point of subspace throughout all creation. In other words, impersonal Brahman is like a ray of the sun, shining the Supreme Truth of Bhagavan, which is Krishna, the Supreme Personality of Godhead.

Some Yogic practices merge with the formless, impersonal Brahman. This is the goal explored in *The Yoga Sutras*. *When the spinning mind is calm, the Seer abides in His own nature.* But Bhaktas think this goal is an incomplete realization of the Supreme Truth.

"The impersonalist and the meditator are also indirectly Krishna conscious. A directly Krishna conscious person is the topmost transcendentalist because such a devotee knows what is meant by Brahman. His knowledge of the Absolute Truth is perfect, whereas the impersonalist and the meditative yogi are imperfectly Krishna conscious." ~ Bhagavad Gita 6:10 Purport

A personal relationship to Bhagavan is the focus in Bhakti Yoga. A transcendentalist devotee always keeps his or her mind on Krishna and sees Krishna everywhere, in all forms. Bhakti Yoga incorporates many gods and goddesses within its tradition, primarily focusing on Vishnu and Hanuman. Bhaktas can also be called Vaishnavas, as they believe Krishna is the avatar of Vishnu. Rama is also an avatar of Vishnu, so is Christ and Buddha. Vaishnavism is one of the major Hindu denominations. Devotees of Bhakti engage in a personal relationship with Lord Krishna.

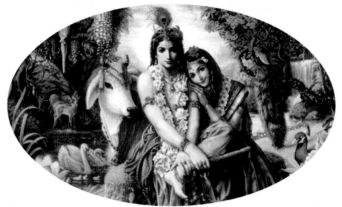

Krishna & Radha

Saint Meerabai was a 16th-Century mystic and Bhakti poet who compared her relationship with Krishna to the relationship between the union of Krishna and Radha, Krishna's consort. In the Bhakti Tradition, Lord Krishna and Radha represent the world's most passionate lovers, and they represent the balance of masculine and feminine energies. Importantly, Krishna is Bhagavan, and Radha represents the individual atman/soul and the embodiment of Love toward Krishna.

Radha is also a Supreme Goddess representing the three main potencies of God: *Hladini* (immense spiritual bliss), *Sandhini* (eternality), and *Samvit* (existential consciousness). Various devotees worship Radha because of her merciful nature and her relationship with Krishna. Radha is also sometimes depicted as Krishna himself, split into two, for the purpose of his enjoyment. Ultimately, it is believed that Krishna enchants the world, but Radha enchants even him. Therefore, she is the Supreme Goddess of all, and together, they are called Radha-Krishna.

Bhaj: To Share

Bhakti comes from the Sanskrit word *bhaj*. *Bhaj* has various meanings including: share, receive, give, enjoy, serve, attend, adore, in flow with. This suggests an intimate, two-way relationship between the deity and the devotee. Throughout human history, Bhagavan has been expressed in a myriad of forms and worshiped in innumerable ways. Inspirations of Bhagavan exist throughout the world making God accessible and perceptible in vastness, creativity, and possibility.

Human nature craves a relationship with a tangible figure for the mind to comprehend and the heart to revere. When one practices Bhakti Yoga while focusing on a particular deity or image, such as Krishna, one is ultimately connecting to Bhagavan through that deity or image through the consciousness of Brahman.

Ultimately, Bhakti is something you do, and can be expressed in a set of actions performed with a certain emotion of a loving, surrendering, humble disposition. For example, Bhakti embraces the practice of *japa*, a meditative repetition of a mantra on a divine name.

In the japa practice, Bhagavan doesn't care about pronunciation (or mispronunciation), but cares about pure, loving devotion while chanting mantra. This loving devotion is the invocation that reveals the essence of Bhagavan within the practitioner. Bhaktas chant to reveal intimacy and sweetness and playfulness. There is even space to honor mischievousness, which is expressed in Baby Krishna, who delights in his devotees and allows them to be sweet, curious, and childlike, rather than rigid.

Hare Kṛishṇa Hare Kṛishṇa Kṛishṇa Kṛishṇa Hare Hare

Hare Rāma Hare Rāma Rāma Rāma Hare Hare

This japa mantra is often used in Bhakti.

Puja: Ceremonial Ritual

Common forms of Bhakti Yoga involve a *puja*. A *puja* is a ritual done at home, in temples, or in other intimate settings. Rituals within a puja symbolize communion with Divinity. Your body is a holy vessel. Your body can experience marvels and can remind you that you are one with this Divinity. The external experience is internally shared with Bhagavan; you become the reflection of your worship.

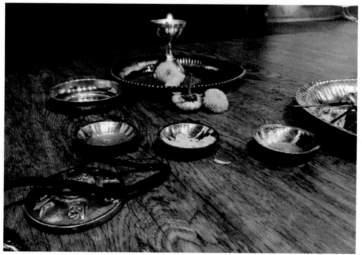

Shala Puja

A common form of puja involves the senses – a *darshan*. Darshan has various meanings that include sight and viewing. This implies that a shared, reciprocal experience occurs between Bhagavan and the devotee. What you experience, Bhagavan experiences, and vice versa.

Inviting a bell to ring invokes sound to remind one to be in the present moment. Food is offered as a tangible means of taste and sharing. Fire is present and represents a give and take relationship as well as an honoring of the ever-transforming nature of life. Incense is often used representing smell and touch.

Worship

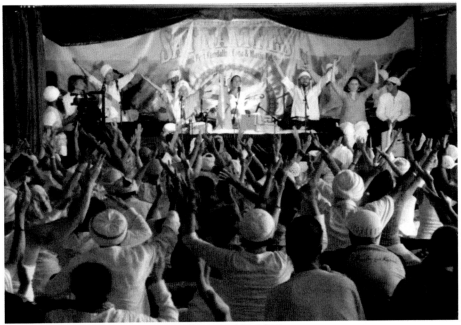

Kirtan at Sat Nam Fest

Another expression of Bhakti Yoga is enjoyed through *kirtan* (group call and response) or *bhajan* (devotional song). These are performed in a group setting at a home or temple and are becoming more popular in various venues in the West. In this musical and high-vibrational setting, devotees sing the name or names of Bhagavan, allowing their hearts to overflow with nourishing, connecting vibrations.

Bhakti Yoga and the Bhagavad Gita

The seminal text of Bhakti Yoga is the celebrated *Bhagavad Gita*.

"You have the right to work, but never to the fruit of work. You should never engage in action for the sake of reward, nor should you long for inaction. Perform work in this world, Arjuna, as a man established within himself – without selfish attachments, and alike in success and defeat. For yoga is perfect evenness of mind (Chapter 2, 47-48)."

The Bhagavad Gita has served as the template for a wide variety of mythologies and stories defining The Hero's Journey, as described by Joseph Campbell.

The Gita is considered an *Upanishad*. An Upanishad is based on a guru giving a student Divine guidance to support Self Realization. An Upanishad embodies the psychology of the Hero's Journey. This process is how the student, the seeker, is transformed and emerges the Hero of their authentic Divine nature.

To begin this path to understand yourself deeper, a shift in perception is needed. Your greatest strengths may once have been labeled as your greatest weakness. As expressed in *The Bhagavad Gita*, the Hero's Journey shows that vulnerability can provide clarity, allowing you to see how doubts and fears can be steppingstones, not stumbling blocks.

Dharma is a key concept in *The Bhagavad Gita* and in any Hero's Journey. Dharma means both 'duty' and 'uncolored reality.' *How do I act authentically in an unauthentic world? How do I best serve the world at this stage in my life?* Uncolored reality is not having a story or expectation that is attached to any situation. Tapping simultaneously into the body and heart becomes key. *Does what I'm doing make me feel expanded or contracted?*

Divinity is expansion and is the big YES in moving forward. Quickening is the contraction after the expansion. This allows you to integrate what might otherwise be experienced as disparate thoughts and feelings. When you feel the longing to expand and you say yes to yourself, you are ready to begin the Hero's Journey.

This is a very different notion of moksha. In the Bhakti traditions, you are given a beautiful, spiritual body to have these relationships expanded, with God. The Krishna stories are meant to offer a glimpse of what those relationships might look like.

Five general principles of Bhakti Yoga

❖ Divinity is all
❖ Serve Divinity by serving humanity
❖ All people are equal
❖ Caste distinctions are superstitious practices that are detrimental to society
❖ Filling the mind and heart with the Divine is more authentic than religious ceremonies or going on pilgrimages

A Practice: Seven questions in Bhakti Yoga that focus the mind

❖ What should be "heard"?
❖ What actions should be performed?
❖ What should be remembered?
❖ What should be worshipped?
❖ What should be avoided?
❖ What mantra/japa should one have?
❖ What dharma should be honored?

301

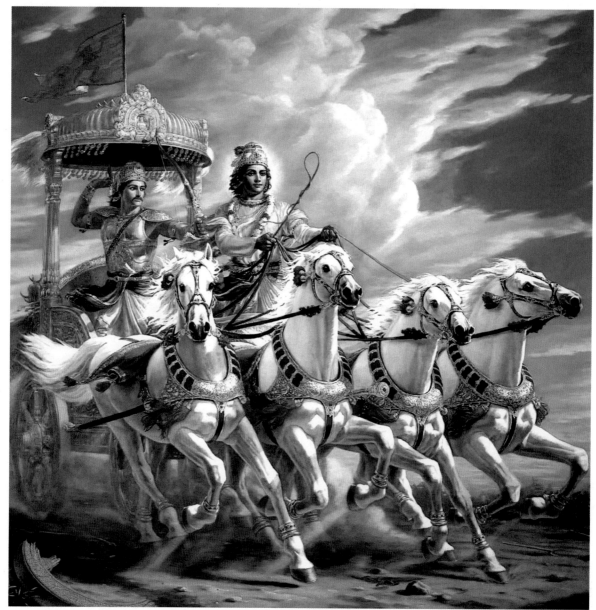

The Bhagavad Gita

The Bhagavad Gita: Jewel of the Mahabharata

The Gita gives us not only profound insights that are valid for all times and for all religious life. Here spirit is at work that belongs to our spirit. ~ J.W. Hauer

Renunciation of the fruits of action is the center around which the Gita is woven. It is the central sun around which devotion, knowledge, and the rest revolve like planets. ~ Mahatma Gandhi

Love God with all your heart and love your neighbor as yourself. ~ Jesus Christ

Bhaga is Sanskrit for Lord of Love. *The Bhagavad Gita* means The Beloved Lord's Love Song. It is profoundly philosophical and is considered a universal gospel answering all the spiritual questions of humankind. It has remained a beloved text for many generations, is regarded as the first full-fledged Yoga scripture, and is Bhakti Yoga's seminal text. Though scholars disagree on the dates when the story itself takes place, many believe it occurred roughly around 3140 BCE as a part of The Mahabharata, while others posit the story appears in 400 CE.

The Mahabharata is an epic Sanskrit poem of ancient India and is important in the development of Hinduism. It is made of nearly 100,000 couplets and is seven times the length of the Iliad and Odyssey, combined. *The Mahabharata* is divided into 18 sections, or chapters. Authorship is attributed to the sage Vyasa.

The Bhagavad Gita is the 18th chapter of *The Mahabharata*, with 18 chapters within it, hosting over 700 stanzas. This is considered one of the first books on *Bhakti Yoga* (Path of Service), *Jnana Yoga* (Path of Knowledge), and *Karma Yoga* (Path of Action). *The Bhagavad Gita* is a song written in rhymes in Sanskrit, which is often lyrically sung. Out of these 700 stanzas, over 100 of them teach that suffering is caused by desire, which is rooted in ignorance and *raga* (passion).

303

The Gita is a profound study and journey through different facets of Yoga. It's about finding Stita Pragna. *Stita Pragna* is an equanimous person who is unmoved by anything in life; happiness and sorrow, death and birth, love and hatred, war and peace, difficulty and ease simply have no effect. Equanimity overcomes fears, primarily the fear of death. Lord Krishna describes these qualities as being the highest pinnacle of human nature.

The Bhagavad Gita teaches that peace can be attained even in the middle of intense activity through Yoga. One is to do their dharma, their duty, with balanced mind through wisdom, devotion, and selfless service. This is service to others, which is therefore service to Bhagavan, without having to fulfill any particular goal. In other words, act for action's sake without expectation.

The Gita teaches how to attain perfection in this lifetime, giving greater ease and gracefulness in every situation in life. There is advice on how to handle situations internally; truly being brave enough to examine the source of what is upsetting you and to go to a place beyond it. Deep Bhakti is the essence of *The Gita*, and it is filled with metaphors. It holds a dialog between Lord Krishna/Bhagavan and Arjuna (great warrior king/atman) on the battlefield of Kuru. Many consider this the Battlefield of Life, however it is showing us a way of living in the Field of Life, also known as Lila. Lila, the grand play and illusion of life, is a very powerful theme throughout the texts.

The Gita is a story of two families that are forced into battle with one another. The warring families of the *Pandavas* and *Kauravas* represent positive and negative human dispositions, the negative being "blind" and ignorant to Truth. This battle continues today within each human life. People are often blind to truth and are attached to the results of their actions.

The battle takes place at *Kurukshetra*, the Sanskrit name of a holy place that literally means darkness, light, destroy, and transcend. This is the Hero's Journey, as something must be destroyed to be transcended. This is a transformation in consciousness. What you are really destroying is the ego that doesn't see or feel the oneness with others.

The Bhagavad Gita is a poem and allegory. Its central question reflects the daily journey of a human being. Its primary theme is dharma, and it gives advice for how one should respond to conflicts of dharma. *"How do I live my life?"* or *"How do I act ethically in an unethical situation? How do I follow my dharma in an un-dharmic world?"* These questions are answered in a circular manner, again and again. *"Let go. Be in the world but not of it."*

The Upanishads and *Yoga Sutras* are steeped within the essence of *The Bhagavad Gita*. Seeing and experiencing the presence of Brahman in everything is Yoga. By letting go of attachments and desires, the mind is purified to its natural state, *svarupa*. One can be active in the world with the mind immersed and inspired by the Divine; with the heart expanding toward bettering all living creatures by doing what should intrinsically be natural – to live authentically, peacefully, without fear.

Ultimately, *The Bhagavad Gita's* message is that peace is at hand. Yogic work is in the realignment of thoughts and actions, allowing grounding peace within the heart. In this state, you are at home with Brahman, shining the rays of Bhagavan's Supreme Truth that your heart and God are always one. This is where your strength lies; the Field of Life opens doorways toward freedom.

Sri Krishna said, "No one is as dear to me as the one who imparts this Knowledge. It is my hope that you one day, if not already, impart the Gita's teachings to others." This is the blessing of being a teacher of Yoga.

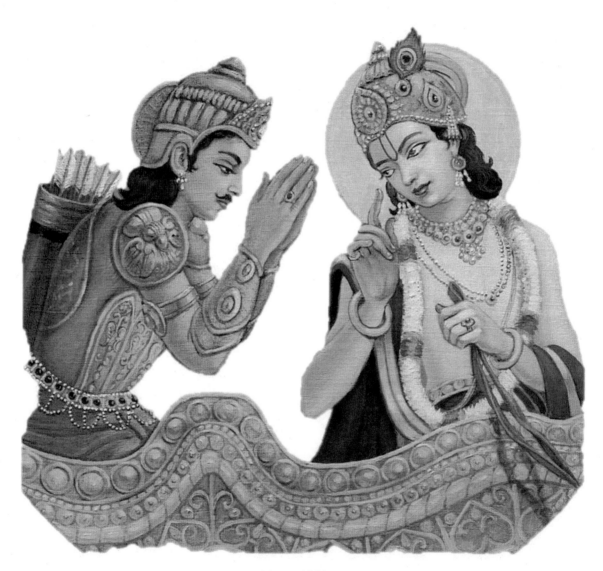

Arjuna and Krishna

The Gita: A Nutshell Summary

There are times in life when you feel you are lost within yourself. That is when *The Gita* helps bring the mind into one-pointedness where it can remember what its original role is.

King Bharata of the Kuru Dynasty was faced with a conflict of dharma when he had to decide whether to pass his kingdom on to his blind elder son, Dhritarastra, or his younger son, Pandu. He knew Pandu would be a better king, but the laws of dharma dictated that a kingdom should be passed to the eldest son. The laws of dharma also dictated that you cannot have a blind king. (Dhritarastra's blindness is both physical and metaphorical for not seeing truth.) Bharata decided to pass the kingdom to Pandu, and Pandu ruled very well, but he died suddenly at a young age. Pandu's sons were too young to take the throne. Therefore, the blind Dhritarastra became king, and he banished Pandu's sons from the kingdom for fear they would threaten his power. In time, the kingdom fell into disarray under King Dhritarastra's rule. The sons of Pandu grew up and realized that they must follow their dharma and return to the kingdom, fight their uncle and cousins, and reclaim the throne.

The Bhagavad Gita is set on the battlefield of Kuru on the eve of the battle between the Pandavas (sons of Pandu) and the Kauravas (sons of Dhritarastra). The battlefield itself is a metaphor for the field of dharma. The head of the Pandavas is Arjuna, eldest son of Pandu. The head of the Kauravas is Duryodhana, eldest son of Dhritarastra. The text is primarily a dialogue between Arjuna and his charioteer (Krishna), as they survey the battlefield in preparation for the following day's battle between the Pandavas and Kauravas armies. The conversation between Arjuna and Krishna is dictated to King Dhritarastra by his omniscient minister, Sanjaya.

Dharma is questioned. As Arjuna looks out over the battlefield, he realizes that fighting means that he will have to battle his own cousins and even his guru, who will be fighting on the side of the Kauravas. Arjuna has a sudden conflict of dharma. He's a Kshatriya (warrior caste), and his dharma is to fight for the good of the kingdom, but the laws of dharma dictate that he must not kill family members or his guru.

Humans don't like change. Human nature is to keep things the way they have always been. Due to the impending change, Arjuna is in despair. He is overwhelmed by confusion and despair, and he tells his charioteer that he will not fight. Throughout the course of their dialogue, Arjuna relates to the charioteer as a friend, then a teacher, and finally the charioteer reveals his divine nature as Krishna.

The warrior is one who may not be free of fear, but who has the courage to face that fear. Krishna advises Arjuna that there will always be conflict in the external world and the way to respond is through Yoga, a process of turning inwards to connect to divinity and then returning to the external world of conflict to act. Krishna then presents three types of Yoga: Karma Yoga, Jnana Yoga, and Bhakti Yoga. Krishna's Bhakti Yoga synthesizes earlier waves of Yoga spiritual practices into one coherent system.

To experience Yoga, one must live their dharma and protect the qualities of the mind by awareness of the ever-changing gunas; the ropes of existence that drive Prakriti. The gunas are saatva (balance/harmony), tamas (heaviness/dullness), and rajas (activity/passion) and they govern the forces of Prakriti that control the cosmos. Finding peace in action will burn off karma.

Karma during Vedic times referred to ritual action, offerings to the Vedic deities through fire sacrifice. Krishna takes the idea of karma as ritual sacrifice and extends it to all actions. He teaches Arjuna Karma Yoga, the Yoga of Action. This implies that action can bring one closer to the divine. Krishna advises Arjuna to act, but in a certain way. In other words, as a human, his role is to do his duty in service to God, work off any negative karma and end the samsaric cycle. Arjuna should act according to his dharma, and without attachment, surrendering the results of his actions to the Divine.

Jnana during the Upanishadic period referred to the knowledge that the individual atman was really the same as Brahman. Krishna tells Arjuna that the practice of Karma Yoga leads to the liberating knowledge that you are a precious and unique expression of Bhagavan. Being absorbed in this knowledge of the true Self is called Jnana Yoga, the Yoga of Knowledge. One does not need to renounce the world and become an ascetic to experience Jnana, as one was required to do during the Upanishadic period. This knowledge is available to everyone regardless of caste or gender, which harkens to Buddhist teachings.

Dhyana, during the Classical Yoga Period, was referred to as Meditation. Krishna advises Arjuna to meditate on the knowledge of the true Self. This is Dhyana Yoga, the Yoga of Meditation. Through Dhyana Yoga, one becomes absorbed in the true knowledge of the Self.

Different Yoga styles suit different temperaments. After reinterpreting Karma, Jnana and Dhyana, Krishna reveals how these types of Yoga are encompassed in the supreme Yoga, which is Bhakti Yoga. In Bhakti Yoga, every action in one's life becomes an opportunity for devotion.

For the Bhakti Yogi, all actions in life are done as offerings to Krishna/Bhagavan. The Bhakti practitioner surrenders everything, with great focus, to the Divine. When one practices Bhakti Yoga consistently, one can trust their impulses in any given ethical/dharmic conflict. Thus, the question of 'what is the correct thing to do (the correct dharma)?' becomes a non-issue. In other words, through journeying into the inner world of the true Self and communing with the divine there, one can then enter back into the world of the external with divine intuition of how to act.

According to Krishna, a person should choose the deity that one feels most connected to for the practice of Bhakti Yoga. All deities are simply manifestations of Bhagavan. Whichever deity a person chooses, that deity chooses the person back and loves the person with as much love as the person offers. The deity and the devotee share in the experience of divine love. Ultimately, the individual Self is divinity itself.

Your Dharma

Go where the way opens as it may lead to your dharma. The Sufi's say, "Remain unmoving until the right action occurs." The ancients say discrimination of your dharma comes through meditation.

What is *Dharma*? Is dharma associated with rules? A duty in life? A *Calling*? A profession? At the cosmic level, dharma refers to the underlying order in nature. At the basic human level, it refers to behaviors being in accordance with that order. It's the life you have come into with your natural, unique skills and talents, your own personality, and that which you are responsible for (your karma). Any action that does not make you feel afraid or restless is a path to understanding your dharma, which is your life purpose.

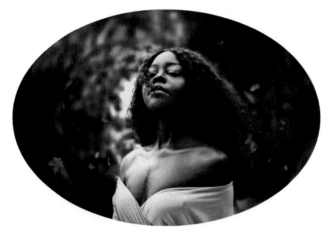

Yogis say there are no accidents for anything in life. You have a vibrational attunement that mirrors other vibrations; like attracts like. Another perspective is that you come into the world through an atman/karmic-contract to see what life on Earth is like, with opportunities to help others; opposites attract. This life on Earth is chosen by your previous actions in your previous lives. This dictates the body type you take on, the endocrine system you take on, your thinking mind, your family members, etc.; you've agreed to everything to "up-level" your atman.

Dharma brings you back into the world according to your past karmas. Dharma and karma go together. You can define it as seeing your part in the play of the nature of the world. You see it as what is right for you in this world, at this time, in the fulfillment of your own destiny. To honor dharma, you must follow the dictates of your atman's Calling. There is motivation, an ease, a flow, a flourishing, and a creative expression when you are aligned with your dharma. If these aspects are not present, appreciate that clarity is coming to you in the contrasts.

At one time, children followed in the footsteps of their parents. But maybe that child had an incredible passion to be something different, an artist, or poet, or musician, rather than running the family business or corporation. Some teachers are even teaching Yoga, and it is not their dharma. It could also be a business or activity that is *adharma* (out of accord with their dharma). Adharma opens you to disharmony, unfulfillment, and often a rootedness in ego.

Remember, it is a privilege to teach, and it must be an undeniable calling of your heart. If you choose to teach any aspect of the Yoga Tradition, you must be very clear and humble in your intentions.

In *The Bhagavad Gita*, there are two forces of light and shadow that are in battle. What I find interesting is that even those fighting in the 'light' could be embracing adharma, while those fighting in the 'shadow' could also be embracing dharma. Some are meant to be warriors while others should not be on the battlefield.

Understanding dharma is an opportunity to rise beyond labels and know life is Lila – a divine play. What is considered good or evil has larger influences in the tapestry of karma and the universe. You must see beyond the labels and understand that all events happen to refine the atman. Your role as a conscious human being is to awaken to your dharma; opening yourself to your own Hero's Journey.

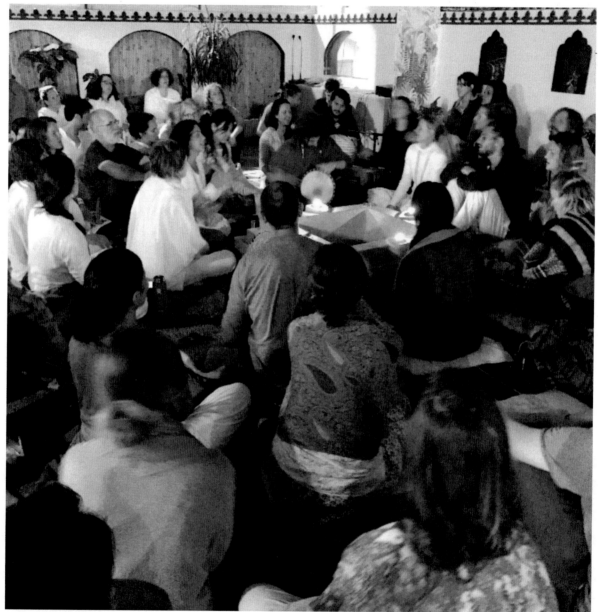

Bhakti (Devotion to the practice of Yoga), Rishikesh, India

Types of Yoga in the Bhagavad Gita

It is appropriate to blend these yogic qualities to gain a holistic understanding of the Practice.

KARMA YOGA - union of action

Yoga of Perfected Action and Service springs from the belief that people carry karma, and karma can be eliminated by doing selfless service for good. Ultimately, every action has an equal and opposite reaction. You strive to think and act in ways that liberate your karmic bonds, and if you empathetically do work that serves to help others rise, then your karma also is allowed to rise. Karma Yoga was made popular by *The Bhagavad Gita* and was the primary inspirational text for Gandhi. "The best way to find yourself (Highest Self) is to lose yourself in the service of others." Mother Teresa exhibited this with her work with orphans in Calcutta. "You may not all be able to do great things, but you can all do small things with great love."

BHAKTI YOGA - equanimity

Yoga of Devotion, Emotion, and Love is a form of Yoga that allows the Yogi to see everything through the eyes and the heart of the Divine. Bhakti is often invoked through japa, and this Yoga is the most practiced form of Yoga in the world. The practice is to see everything, everyone, and the Self as a manifestation of God, but Bhagavan/God is distinct. The practice is the adoration of the Divine. Additionally, one is constantly thinking of Bhagavan in the way as a lover thinks of his beloved. Bhakti practitioners, Bhaktas, repeatedly chant the name of the Divine to feel a merging with Divinity.

JNANA YOGA - will & intellect

Yoga of Perfected Wisdom that fully utilizes the right use of the mind. The main practice is meditation, experiencing deep self-inquiry and mindfulness. The Zen tradition is a derivation of Jnana Yoga. The intellect reasons that Yoga is your natural state, and it strives to set aside false identities by understanding that atman and Brahman are one and the same. Intellect supports the meditative introspection of "Who am I?" In turn, "I Am." *So Hum. Sat Nam.*

313

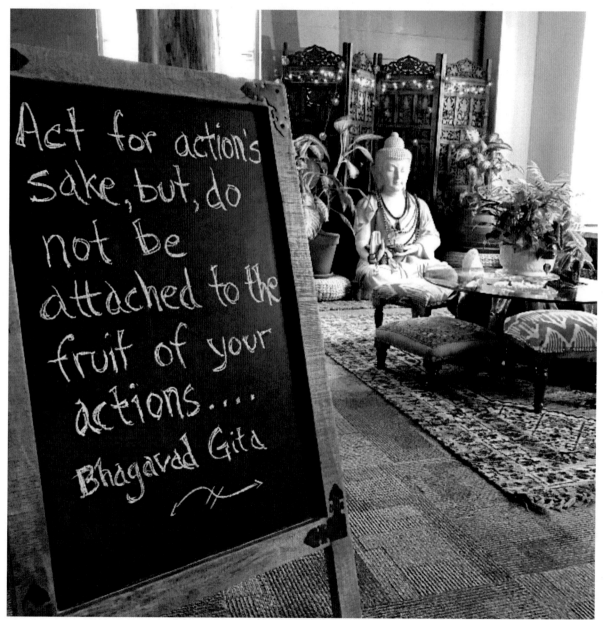

Unattachment

Unattachment

The mind needs an anchor point, and fear is often that anchor point. Think of your biggest concern, here and now. Now, what was your *last* biggest concern? What was the biggest concern before that one? There will always be an anchor point of fear if the *samskara/vasana* (mental impressions/desires) is present to welcome it.

Ultimately, when you fear, you fear you are going to lose something. You fear you are going to lose your body. You fear you are going to be injured. You fear what people think of you, which is insecurity. But fear is ignorance, *Avidya*, based on your ego, which is called *Asmita*. If you are absorbed in the *kleshas* (which are hinderances to enlightenment, including ignorance, attachment, and aversion), you feel fear. The fear of death is the largest fear, and it can take on different forms such as jealousy, claiming objects/ideas/people/places as 'mine', lack of abundance/scarcity, fear of change, always being in a state of want, unsatisfaction, blame, etc.

You can choose what to do with your mind. You can think with your body and absorb your mind in Lila and *chitta vritti* (fluctuations of the mind) over fears. But you tend to solve one fear and allow another one to immediately arise. This is a tormented life.

A healthy alternative is to absorb your mind in Yogic teachings which constantly reinforce that you will be okay as things change, because you are a pure atman. This is precisely what *The Gita* teaches. *The Gita* says you are not the body but trust the body's messages. Absorbing your mind in *The Gita* will ease your fear and ignorance, unattaching from the body/mind and going to a place beyond your ego. That place beyond is eternal where you can never be harmed; you are immune to criticism; you are immune to all the things you might be fearful of.

But reestablishing new mind patterns takes hard work. Bhakti Yoga practice focuses on the combined practice of mantras with the japa practice of *Ishvara Pranidhana*. This is the devotion to your higher self with the surrender of the individual ego.

315

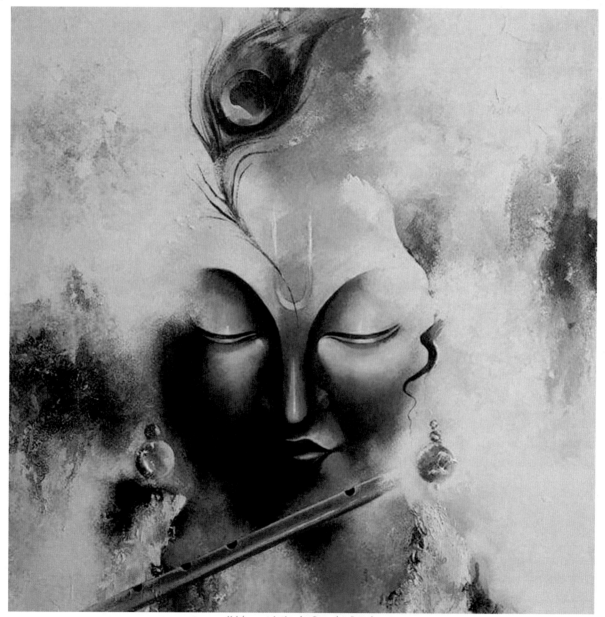

Krishna, painting by Basudev Basak

Reflection

Bhakti Yoga and the Hero's Journey

The Hero's Journey is a journey of human potential, which is an invitation for holistic, spiritual growth. Every person will be invited at some point to consciously begin this journey. Some people choose to embark on the Hero's Journey, while others do not. You can engage in many small and large Hero's Journeys throughout your life.

1) Reflect on life-changing events. Choose a past challenge/opportunity and write about it using the Four Stages of the Hero's Journey as a guide.

2) What is Bhakti Yoga?

3) What are the three types of Yoga as seen in *The Bhagavad Gita*? From a universal lens, briefly describe how they are related in daily living and thinking.

4) In *The Bhagavad Gita's* Book 2, stanza 47 states, "You have a right to your actions, but never to your actions' fruits. Act for the action's sake. And do not be attached to inaction." Ghandi lived his life with *The Gita* as his guide. He said the *Essence of The Gita* is found in Book 2, stanzas 55-72. The concept of non-attachment is a major *Gita* theme.

Consider the following:

❖ What does it mean to be unattached to the fruits of your actions?
❖ Consider what you are attached to and list them.
❖ If you feel anxious, what are you afraid of?
❖ Why has this fear-pattern been created? What are the effects of it in your life?

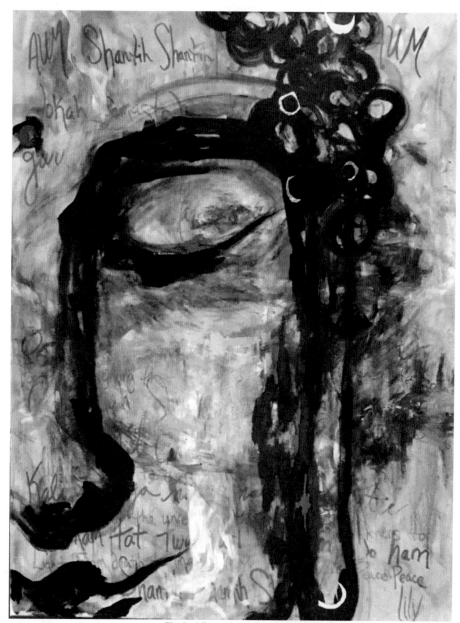

The Buddha, painting by Lily Kessler

318

Chapter 8

Buddhism:

Dancing Along the Middle Path

Historical Timeline

PRECLASSICAL YOGA ERA

INDUS-SARASVATI AGE: 6500-4500 BCE
- SANATANA DHARMA: "ETERNAL LAW"
- INDUS RIVER VALLEY & SEALS

VEDIC AGE: 4500-2500 BCE
- CONSCIOUSNESS EXPLORED
- VIBRATION OF INTENTION & CAUSATION
- CAUSE & EFFECT: MANTRA & KARMA

SAMKHYA YOGA: 8000-100 BCE
- REALITY EXPLORED: PRAKRITI/PURUSHA
- BODY'S CONSTITUTION: DOSHAS
- AYURVEDA

UPANISHADIC AGE: 2000-1500 BCE
- NON-DUALISM OF ATMAN/BRAHMAN
- DISTILLATION OF VEDAS
- MEDITATION

BHAKTI YOGA: 1000-500 BCE
- ADORATION
- HINDU EPICS / UNIVERSAL INSIGHTS
- 3 BRANCHES OF YOGA

BUDDHISM: C. 500 BCE-PRESENT
- INDIVIDUALITY / MONASTIC TRADITION
- MIDDLE WAY
- FOUR NOBLE TRUTHS / EIGHT-FOLD PATH

CLASSICAL YOGA ERA

CLASSICAL YOGA: 75 BCE-100 CE
- THE YOGA SUTRA'S OF PATANJALI
- EIGHT-LIMBED PATH
- HARNESSING THE MIND

ESOTERIC AGE

TANTRA: 600-1300 CE
- 6 + 1 CHAKRA SYSTEM
- WESTERN NOTION OF EMBODIMENT
- SUBTLE BODY (NADIS, CHAKRAS, ETC.)

HATHA YOGA: C. 1300-1400 CE
- MIND V. BODY
- HATHA YOGA PRADIPIKA
- ASANA / BREATH / BANDHAS / MUDRAS

RISE OF MODERN YOGA

SWAMI VIVEKANANDA: 1872-1950
- INFLUENCED RISE OF MODERN YOGA
- INTRODUCED YOGA TO THE WEST

SRI T. KRISHNAMACHARYA: 1891-1989
- YOGA'S EXPANSION
- FATHER OF MODERN YOGA
- MODERN CONTRIBUTORS

Chapter 8

Buddhism: Dancing Along the Middle Path

1. Overview of Lecture

Chapter 8 explores Buddhism and the concept of Self. The history of Buddhism, the Four Noble Truths, and the Eightfold Path are highlighted. Buddhism is tied to and contrasted with Vedantic Philosophies, and it sets the stage for Classical Yoga and the Tantric Era. Ultimately, this chapter looks at how Buddhism manifests itself though a life of compassion-in-action and devotion-in-motion.

2. Learning Objectives: I will…

a) Develop an overview of historical Buddhism development
b) Understand the Four Noble Truths and the Eightfold Path
c) Compare the Eightfold Path with the Ten Commandments and the Eight-limbed Path
d) Recognize the similarities and differences of Yoga and Buddhism

3. Pre-lecture Assignments

a) Read the chapter and become familiar with the Reflection questions
b) Read *No Mud, No Lotus*, by Thich Nhat Hanh
c) Recommended Film: *The Story of Siddhartha*
d) Daily Sadhana - Daily Personal Practice

4. Reflection: *found at the end of the chapter*

Overview of Buddhist Beginnings

Our exploration of Buddhism begins with the life and teachings of Siddhartha Gautama (563 BCE - 483 BCE) who, through his life experiences and learnings, became the Buddha. The term *Buddha* means awakened or enlightened. Siddhartha lived in what is modern-day Nepal and was of royal birth.

The teachings of the Buddha explored in this chapter spread across the Indian subcontinent, across China, Tibet, and Korea to Japan, and ultimately the West. At one historical point, Buddhism was nearly extinct on the Indian subcontinent. Today, Buddhism has developed into a worldwide religion/philosophy with many interpretations. All have their roots in Buddha's teachings.

Siddhartha

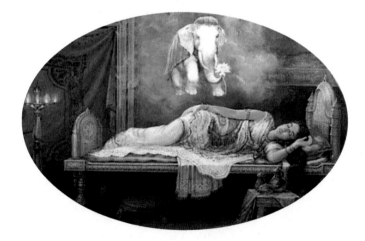

Siddhartha Gautama was born into a royal family as Warrior Caste in Kapilavastu, in the area now known as Nepal. His father was the ruler of a city state. His mother was also of the ruling class and was involved with the Vedic ceremonies and priests.

Prior to his conception, Siddhartha's mother, Maya, dreamed that a white elephant with six tusks "touched" the side of her body and she became pregnant with a son. Upon awakening, she summoned the Brahmans (the priests) to interpret her dream. They confirmed that she was pregnant, after many years of childlessness, and predicted her son would be a world changer using one of two paths: he would either be a great warrior and king or a great teacher.

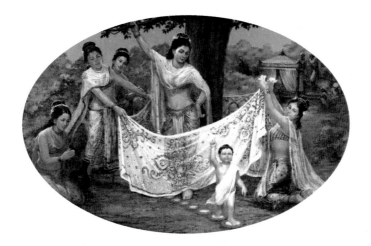

During the journey to her family's home to deliver the child, Maya gave birth. Her son was born from the side of her torso where the elephant's tusk touched her in her dream. (This symbolism indicates a "clean" birth, like that of Christ.) According to legend, the baby immediately showed enlightened characteristics, such as his ability to walk. It is said that he took seven steps, and seven lotus flowers bloomed where his feet touched the earth. Maya died seven days later.

Siddhartha's Awakening

Siddhartha's ambitious father wanted his philosophical and tranquil son to be a king. So, the king isolated Siddhartha in the luxurious family palace. Siddhartha spent his early life surrounded by creature comforts and protected from any of life's realities. All this was done by the king to help ensure the prophesy of his son becoming a king was fulfilled, instead of the prophesy that he would become a great teacher. The artificial nature of Siddhartha's surroundings, however, could not transform his inner nature, which sought to explore the reality of both the external and internal worlds.

When Siddhartha was 29 years old, he took his first tour outside of the city walls to meet his subjects. Despite the efforts of his father to "sanitize" the city, for the first time in his life, Siddhartha saw the three forms of suffering his father had tried to conceal from him: old age, sickness, and death. Siddhartha was overwhelmed by the knowledge that he too would eventually grow sick, old and die. For the first time, he was aware of the transitory nature of life and the impermanence of all material things.

He also saw an *ascetic* covered in ash. (An *ascetic* is a person who dedicates his or her life to pursuing contemplative ideals, and they practice extreme self-denial or self-mortification for religious reasons.) Siddhartha saw this skinny, naked, and dreadlocked man, and stopped to talk with him. The ascetic genuinely seemed to be living without attachment to material things, and he seemed undisturbed by thoughts of illness, old age, and even death. Siddhartha was told that the ascetic's path was the way to end life's suffering and rebirths, through the practice of non-attachment.

Following these experiences, Siddhartha decided to become an ascetic based on his desire to end the cycle of *samsara* (the cycle of birth and death). In the cover of night, he left his wife and newborn son to experience the path of what it takes to achieve *moksha* (liberation). He denied his royal position and broke caste to search for a state of peace.

Siddhartha entered the *guru/shishya* (teacher/student) relationship with various teachers, yet he superseded all his teachers in knowledge, and he was still unsatisfied. In turn, many of his teachers renounced their guru roles to become his students. The guru thus became the shishya once again.

Siddhartha enhanced his extreme *tapas*/austerity further and further by self-mortification, deprivation of all comforts, as well as life-necessities. He became the most ascetic of the ascetics. This was a complete opposite of his life in the palace, which was considered *bhoga* (worldly indulgence). Despite his great swing of the pendulum from one end of the spectrum to the other, Siddhartha did not find what his heart was calling for.

The deprivations caused Siddhartha to lay dying on the banks of a river, too weak to move. According to one legend, a child came upon Siddhartha in this weakened state and offered him a bowl of rice. The bowl of rice nourished him. He then placed the empty bowl in the river water, and it floated upstream. Siddhartha took this as a sign that the Middle Path was the way. He then understood that neither extreme austerities nor extreme luxuries are beneficial for spiritual growth. "When you conquer yourself, you may then conquer reality."

The Forming of the Buddha

All of the disciplines and austerities he went through didn't help until he sat under the pipal tree (later known as the Bodhi tree) to meditate on the truth of life. He vowed not to arise until he found an answer. "I will not move until Truth reveals itself." In this state, he was exposed to the elements, yet a cobra sheltered him, and the earth rose up to protect him because he was needed by the world.

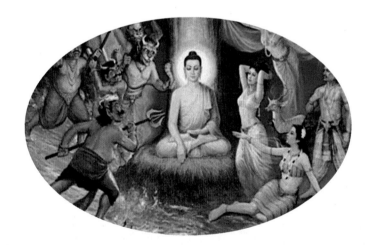

While in a meditative state, Siddhartha contemplated his life and experiences. He thought about the nature of suffering and fully recognized its power came from attachment. In an epiphany, Siddhartha came to realize that suffering was caused by the perceived need for permanence in a world that is impermanent.

One suffered because one was ignorant of the fact that life itself was *change*. One could cease suffering by recognizing that, since this was so, attachment to anything in the belief it would last was a serious error which only trapped one in an endless cycle of craving, striving, rebirth, and death. Buddha knew that if he conquered himself (his ego), he conquered reality.

After 49 days of meditation (or much, much longer in other historical perspectives), and at the age of 35, Siddhartha was "awakened". From that time on, he was known as *Buddha*.

Enlightenment

At this time in Indian history, conventional society was a country of city-states with armies and armor, rigid class systems, and wars. Nature was exploited due to the dawn of the Agricultural Revolution. Wealth and cities were vied for by warrior rulers. Buddha, himself, was born to a warrior class, but he chose to conquer himself, and therefore conquer reality. Buddha knew happiness was possible for everyone, here and now. However:

Buddha saw: *people chasing power and dominion that he knew they would only lose when they soon died. Life after life, people would suffer due to their negative acts that only sought power and dominion life and life again.* ~ Jewel Tree of Tibet, 2005, Robert Thurman

Buddha asked: *"How can I break them out from routine patterns and the social collective of predestined, domesticated norms that they are caught in? How can I show them their heart is an engine of bliss and their brain an instrument of deep wisdom?"* ~ Robert Thurman

In response to the practices of warring and enslaving, Buddha counseled kings. He asked them to simply *harm less* when they engaged in activities that caused suffering. Buddha saw that there must be a process toward peace, rather than full condemnation of warring and enslaving, which would close doors to any eventual reasoning and compromise. To expand peace, Buddha emphasized one should practice daily meditation and honor the Middle Path.

The Middle Path

Buddha taught the Middle Path in an age where severe asceticism was common. (The Middle Path is exampled here through allegory: *When you pull a string too tight it will snap. If you let it be too slack, it won't play.*) Ultimately, the Middle Path honors the capacity of the individual and emphasizes individualism. Buddha's teachings are referred to as *Dharma* which, in this case, means cosmic law and reality. Like the teachings of *The Upanishads*, Buddhist teachings also are based on the premise that an individual is entirely responsible for the consequences of their thoughts, which result in their actions, and ultimately create their reality.

As stated in *The Dhammapada*:

*Your life is shaped by your mind; you become what you think. Suffering follows
 an evil thought as the wheels of a cart follow the oxen that draw it. Your life
is shaped by your mind; you become what you think. Joy follows a pure
thought like a shadow that never leaves. (I.1-2)*

The individual is therefore fully responsible for their level of suffering because, at any point, they can choose not to engage in the kinds of actions, desires and/or attachments that give rise to suffering. Buddha emphasized the need to analyze the mind. Buddha also knew that trying to create artificial limitations on people creates a barrier to self-transformation, therefore suffering remains. He encouraged individual questioning and supported the bravery it takes to break away from conventional, traditional, and even religious ideas.

The Monastic System

Buddha taught that every human has access to divine qualities, and through the practice of meditation, every person has the potential to experience Nirvana.

Buddhism is generally credited with the widespread establishment of the monastic system. This system originated on the Indian subcontinent because it was one of the wealthiest areas in the world at that time. A nun or monk would be supported by the collective to escape from the collective, and a monastery welcomed people regardless of their gender or caste. This monastic institution (and its renunciates) became the *Sangha*, a doorway to happiness.

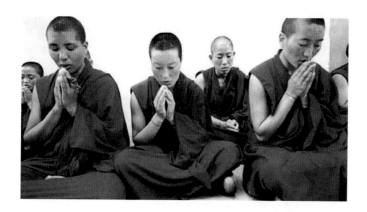

Buddhism is generally credited with the widespread establishment of the monastic system. This system originated on the Indian subcontinent because it was one of the wealthiest areas in the world at that time. A nun or monk would be supported by the collective to escape from the collective, and a monastery welcomed people regardless of their gender or caste. This monastic institution (and its renunciates) became the *Sangha*, a doorway to happiness.

This first monastic system was called *Sangha Jewel*, and its concept caught on like wildfire in India and beyond, eventually expanding to other religious traditions. As the monastic system grew, harmony grew within communities, as people had a chance to both give and receive. New ideas merged with old ideas to establish the foundation for a peaceful change within society.

The path of the Buddhist became three-fold:

1) Buddha (inspiration): Follow the teachings of the Buddha.
2) Dharma (scripture): Dharma, reality, revealed within the Four Noble Truths.
3) Sangha (community): Associate with inspiring others to support you on your path.

The principles and tenets of Buddhism were written in local languages instead of Sanskrit. Doing so further established a common ground for Buddha's teaching, allowing the common person, regardless of sex or gender, to engage in self-study.

Spiritual communities come in many forms throughout cultures and religions worldwide.

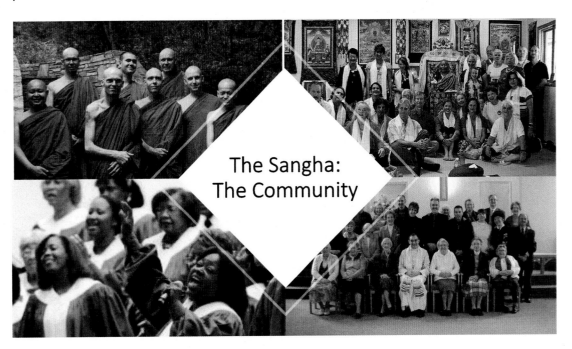

The Sangha:
The Community

Four Noble Truths

*What, monks, is the truth of suffering? Birth is suffering, decay, sickness
and death are suffering. To be separated from what you like is suffering.
To want something and not get it is suffering. In short, the human personality,
liable as it is to clinging and attachment brings suffering.*

~ Tom Lowenstein

The Four Noble Truths illuminate the causes of suffering as they truly are in Prakriti, not as you are conditioned to see them. They simply acknowledge the concept of *dukkha*, which literally means suffering, or can be interpreted by some as the feeling of unfulfillment.

Major forms of suffering stem from:

1) The physical body

2) The living beings from (mosquito, family, invading armies, predators, etc.) and

3) All other forms of misunderstanding and ignorance, attachment, and dissatisfaction

**After recognizing suffering exists, the Eightfold Path then serves
as a guide to live life without attachments.**

1. Suffering Exists

Happiness is temporary. Everyone suffers. You misidentify Reality with reality.

2. There is a cause of suffering: 12-Link Chain of Causation

1. Suffering begins at birth
2. There is a will to be born
3. One wills oneself to be born due to mental clinging to worldly objects
4. One clings to objects due to a thirst to enjoy fleeting pleasures
5. Previous sense experience drives one toward momentary pleasure
6. Contact of senses with objects causes these sensuous experiences
7. Experiences are perceived from 6 organs of cognition and the mind, which depend on the body
8. Body and mind constitute the perceptible being
9. The perceptible being is initial consciousness
10. Consciousness identifies with karmas and past impressions, or samskaras
11. Karmas influence consciousness due to ignorance
12. Ignorance causes attachment, pain, and misery late in life until death

3. There is an end to suffering

Attachment will end, suffering will end.
Understand the nature of life and enjoy life in the here and now.

4. Follow the Middle Path and the Noble Eightfold Path

Embrace the joys of life and don't be indulgent nor austere.

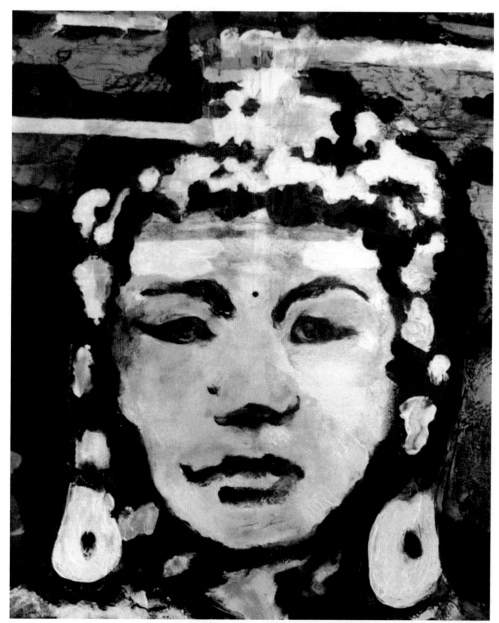

Inner Buddha, painting by Lily Kessler

The Noble Eightfold Path

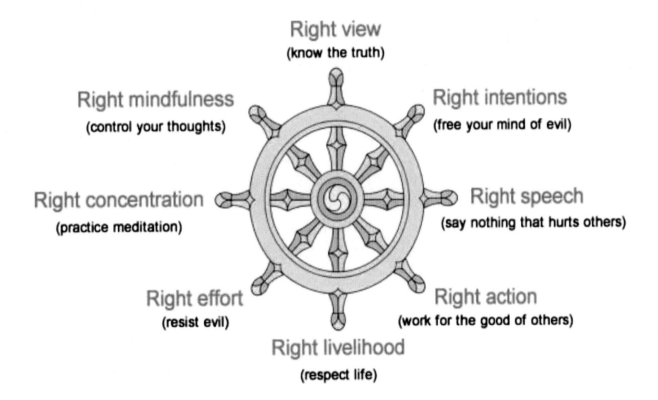

Right view
(know the truth)

Right mindfulness
(control your thoughts)

Right intentions
(free your mind of evil)

Right concentration
(practice meditation)

Right speech
(say nothing that hurts others)

Right effort
(resist evil)

Right action
(work for the good of others)

Right livelihood
(respect life)

Buddha gave a list of simple ethics, much like other moral codes. Unlike authoritarian religions, however, the Buddhist Eightfold Path is a recommendation or a guideline for all aspects of life, which are intended to be integrated into everyday living. The Eightfold Path is considered the foundation of the Middle Path, yet it is not a sequential process. Each step on the Path offers self-discovery and promotes contemplation.

Three Jewels of the Eightfold Path

Wisdom, Ethical Conduct, Mental Discipline

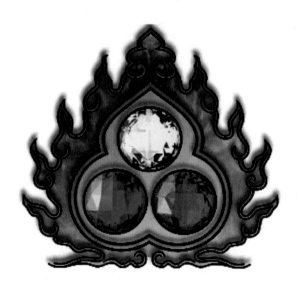

Wisdom

Right View / Right Understanding of the World
Moral Law of Karma / Cause & Effect: Every action (by way of body, speech, and mind) will have karmic results, be it wholesome or unwholesome

Right Intentions
Aspire to rid yourself of immoral thoughts and qualities

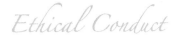

Ethical Conduct

Right Speech
Abstaining from lying, from divisive speech, from abusive speech, chatter, and gossip

Right Action
Abstaining from taking life, from stealing, and work to better yourself and society

Right Livelihood
Your work affects your mind and heart, and these livelihoods must be avoided:

- Business in weapons – avoid instruments for killing
- Business in human beings – slave trading, prostitution
- Business in meat – includes breeding animals for slaughter
- Business in intoxicants – manufacturing or selling intoxicating drinks/drugs
- Business in poison – producing or trading in a product designed to kill

Concentration / Mental Discipline

Right Effort
Make a continual effort to abandon all harmful thoughts, words, and deeds

Right Concentration
Be deliberate and alert to your state of mind

Right Mindfulness
Develop through mindful breathing, through visual objects, and mantras

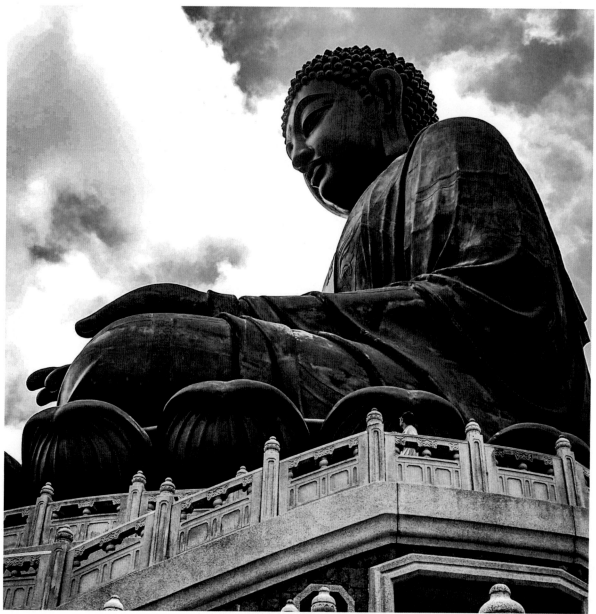

Reveal

336

Buddhism: A New Way of Thinking

**The act of making an agreement with yourself
to pursue an inward calling.**

*Buddhism is a series of methods and arts of
opening doors to reality that fit with any
particular person's location and place.*

It can emerge as Christianity.

*It can emerge as Judaism or humanism, nihilism,
even if temporarily in some special cases.*

*It isn't that it consists of some rigid view,
some orthodox ideology, and some dogmatic
religion.*

*There is no fixed institution or "religion" that
can be pinned down exactly as the referent of
Buddhism.*

~ Robert Thurman

Involution Toward Evolution

Inhale: *Who am I?* * Exhale: *I don't know.*

My greatest freedom is found by dismantling who I think I am; dissolving my attachments. I am evolving through an involution.

India is a country that is my teacher and a great unraveller of my identity. She is a difficult place to reach and for many, she is a difficult place to explore because she is ultimately a mirror that identifies personal attachments. If you cling to daily patterns and norms, you will suffer greatly in India. If you choose to surrender, you will find grace and be embraced within her dance of color, shaken up in her bewildering wildness, given rest in her holy stillness, and life as you know it will be utterly changed.

Experiencing change is a universal promise. Residing in the spirit of hope and grace is practicing Yoga. In its midst, your focus must be on gratitude. Gratitude is liberation. You must not resist, but instead, *lean into change*. Yoga is changing the trajectory of energy into empowerment.

Things in your life are changing. If you are not seeing and experiencing blessings here and now, the only one in the way is you. It's that simple. The world is your inner mirror, and how you choose to view it is your choice, alone. In other words, you must discern what has power over you. Suffering will always lay the foundation for compassion to bloom - if you chose it. This transformation-by-fire opens eyes and hearts to unity.

How are you handling your suffering? How are you viewing your suffering? Yoga is not about avoiding or being immune to miseries or sorrows. Yoga is about having one eye out and one eye in. You must allow yourself to authentically feel what you feel. But here is the key ... you must know the emotion is fleeting and find blessings within it to liberate yourself from further suffering. You must find the Gift and claim it.

I was sick in my ashram bed in a cold and damp room. Instead of spiraling into woe, I practiced Yoga, which was a focus on Gratitude. I felt grateful that I was able to brush my hair and clean my face. In contrast, a woman outside the ashram didn't have arms to clean her face or dress herself. Gratitude. Gratitude. Gratitude.

The rain and damp was inescapable. My scarf was soft and warm. The noise was unavoidable. The collage of sounds became a living Om.

Gratitude is the ultimate practice of Yoga, living in the here and now. Yoga-off-the-mat is the Living Yoga, claiming compassion, empathy, and ease, even in the space of dis-ease. It is returning to your sacred center, again and again, when you recognize you have stepped out of alignment. Live with discernment to redefine and appreciate all the glories and aspects of your life, which are ever-changing, as the Universe does things for you, not to you.

Buddha? Buddha?

This is my mantra when I people-watch. Everyone carries potential to be Living Compassion. In the philosophy of 'rebirth', you are wending your way to the same goal of interconnectedness. It brings my soul peace to know that eventually all people, no matter where they are in their soul's evolution today, will one day be a living sanctuary; an example of Love. We must all grapple in the dark to walk with steadiness in the Light. The Practice is to see a bigger picture.

"Ah yes. I see you now. Buddha. Me. Namaste. Same/Same."

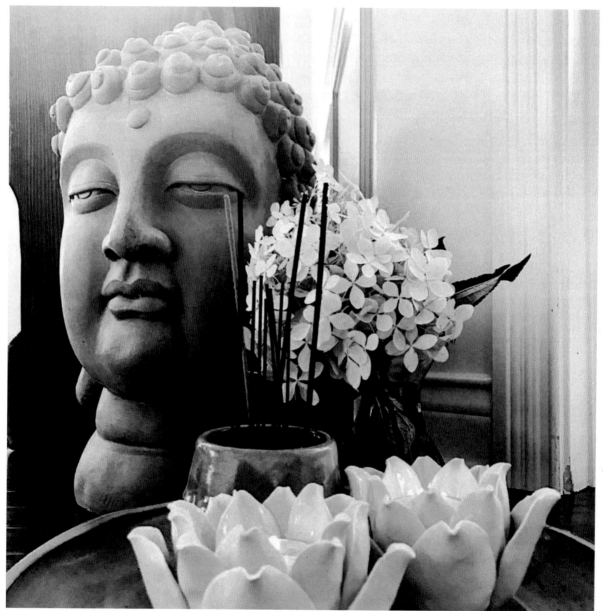

Home Altar

Reflection

Buddhism: Dancing Along the Middle Path

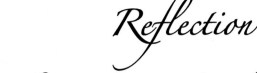

1) What are the Four Noble Truths? List the elements of the Eightfold Path.

2) The essential characteristic of Buddhism is a path that leads to enlightenment, where you may become a Buddha, an awakened being liberated from the world of samsara (the cycle of death, and rebirth) to which life in the material world of Prakriti is bound. In Buddhism, a foundational key element is following the Eightfold Path.

   Describe what it means to follow the Middle Path. Give examples of how you are personifying this concept in your life.

3) Can a non-Buddhist practice Buddhism?

4) The following exercise is an internal exploration of the heart:

   Consider that each person is a perfect being in the here-and-now moment, as everything in life is a learning opportunity. Cultivating appreciation and compassion for all forms of life is an intrinsic piece of Yoga; by seeing Buddha in the face of everything and everyone. Whether in this lifetime or in a future one, you will enter the Buddha-State, where you are a great teacher; a great source of comfort and wisdom, with great reservoirs of compassion and non- dominating power.

   Go on a people-watching expedition. Walking down a street, shopping in a mall, sitting at a cafe, etc., look at the many faces you encounter. Perhaps your mantra will be, "Buddha?" to each person you see. Consider if this mantra is a great equalizer and harmonizer of the world around you.

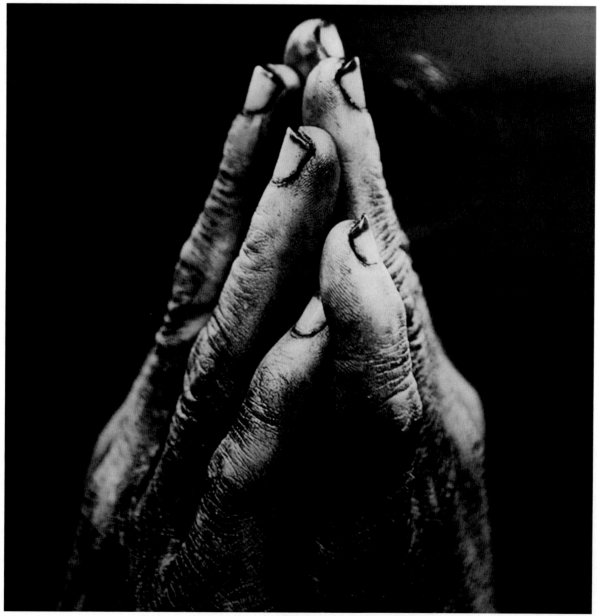

Prayer

342

Chapter 9

Classical Yoga:

Sacred Sutras, Sacred Promises

Historical Timeline

PRECLASSICAL YOGA ERA

INDUS-SARASVATI AGE: 6500-4500 BCE
- SANATANA DHARMA: "ETERNAL LAW"
- INDUS RIVER VALLEY & SEALS

VEDIC AGE: 4500-2500 BCE
- CONSCIOUSNESS EXPLORED
- VIBRATION OF INTENTION & CAUSATION
- CAUSE & EFFECT: MANTRA & KARMA

SAMKHYA YOGA: 8000-100 BCE
- REALITY EXPLORED: PRAKRITI/PURUSHA
- BODY'S CONSTITUTION: DOSHAS
- AYURVEDA

UPANISHADIC AGE: 2000-1500 BCE
- NON-DUALISM OF ATMAN/BRAHMAN
- DISTILLATION OF VEDAS
- MEDITATION

BHAKTI YOGA: 1000-500 BCE
- ADORATION
- HINDU EPICS / UNIVERSAL INSIGHTS
- 3 BRANCHES OF YOGA

BUDDHISM: C. 500 BCE-PRESENT
- INDIVIDUALITY / MONASTIC TRADITION
- MIDDLE WAY
- FOUR NOBLE TRUTHS / EIGHT-FOLD PATH

CLASSICAL YOGA ERA

CLASSICAL YOGA: 75 BCE-100 CE
- THE YOGA SUTRA'S OF PATANJALI
- EIGHT-LIMBED PATH
- HARNESSING THE MIND

ESOTERIC AGE

TANTRA: 600-1300 CE
- 6 + 1 CHAKRA SYSTEM
- WESTERN NOTION OF EMBODIMENT
- SUBTLE BODY (NADIS, CHAKRAS, ETC.)

HATHA YOGA: C. 1300-1400 CE
- MIND V. BODY
- HATHA YOGA PRADIPIKA
- ASANA / BREATH / BANDHAS / MUDRAS

RISE OF MODERN YOGA

SWAMI VIVEKANANDA: 1872-1950
- INFLUENCED RISE OF MODERN YOGA
- INTRODUCED YOGA TO THE WEST

SRI T. KRISHNAMACHARYA: 1891-1989
- YOGA'S EXPANSION
- FATHER OF MODERN YOGA
- MODERN CONTRIBUTORS

Chapter 9

Classical Yoga: Sacred Sutras, Sacred Promises

1. Overview of Lecture

Chapter 9 explores the origins of Classical Yoga, primarily focusing on *The Yoga Sutras of Patanjali*. The Five Kleshas, the Yamas, and the Niyamas are identified and examined in relationship to the Eight-Limbed Path.

2. Learning Objectives: I will…

a) Understand the mythology surrounding Patanjali, the Father of Modern Yoga
b) Identify the 5 Kleshas
c) Decipher how the 5 Yamas and the 5 Niyamas are played out in daily life
d) Compare the Yamas and Niyamas to the Noble Eightfold Path

3. Pre-lecture Assignments

a) Read the chapter and become familiar with the Reflection questions
b) Read *The Yoga Sutras of Patanjali*, recommended translation by Sri Swami Satchidananda
c) Daily Sadhana - Daily Personal Practice

4. Reflection: *found at the end of the chapter*

Yoga Sutras of Patanjali

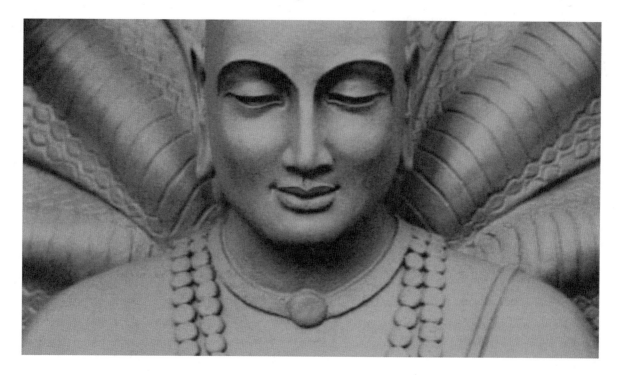

The Yoga Sutras of Patanjali were written in a highly scholastic style, which may be likened to a modern-day technical manual. The condensed information included in the Sutras are essentially a potent, transformative form of minimalism.

Classical Yoga is The Yoga Sutras, and The Yoga Sutras are Classical Yoga. It is the restraint of the mind; the mind is restrained from being in a "horizontal" reality (Prakriti/Ego/Karma), allowing it to become more focused, grounded, rooted, and in its authentic "vertical" nature (Purusha/Atman). Yoga helps you see your own true nature. The lifelong study of one's true nature is called *Svadhyaya*.

Classical Yoga is dualistic and Vedantic and has its origins in Samkhya philosophy. Unlike the Samkhya tradition, though, Classical Yoga is a dualistic philosophy and incorporates a theistic element, acknowledging the existence of a divine force. This divine force is referred to in The Sutras as *Ishvara*, which can also be thought of as *Brahman*, or Absolute Truth. The Sutras explore this relationship with divinity by providing methods and practices to raise consciousness.

The Yoga Sutras are a backward-looking text, meaning that it is systematizing the practices of Yoga that have been established for several hundred years, upward to a millennium. Scholars do not believe that anything was added into The Sutras. The Sutras were based on authoritative oral summaries from the Samkhya Era that consisted of many generations of thought and debate. This gave rise to evolutions of divergent commentaries that were ultimately encapsulated in various written texts. One text that represents the epitome of these commentaries is The Yoga Sutras, which were written in the opening centuries of the Common Era (approximately 75 BCE-100 CE). The Yoga sage Patanjali Maharishi is generally credited with having written The Sutras, and his text became an authoritative darshan of the Yoga tradition.

The Sutras are considered one of the most comprehensive scholastic texts describing the practice of Yoga. There is no "situation" in The Sutras. It is a practical system and approach to the practice in that there is no plot, no characters, and no dialogue. There is no mirror of history within it. It has no time or location, nor does it place judgments. One can bring one's own mythology and story to it. Instead, The Sutras are a collection of steps to self-mastery and unity. They provide a way to understand that the root of suffering is not the obstacles that obstruct us; suffering is caused by not accepting the present reality. The Sutras thus provide a systematic approach to the philosophy and practice of Yoga, making the practice both a goal and a means to achieve that goal, simultaneously. The Eight-Limbed Path of the Yoga Sutras is the awareness of your relationship to the macrocosm of the world, distilled into the microcosm of the Self.

The 196 Sutras, in four *padas*, or books, distill the wisdoms of the Vedas and the Upanishads. The Sutras define Yoga as "the stilling of the fluctuations of the mind." These fluctuations make one believe that one's true identity is Prakriti, not Purusha. This misidentification of the Self causes mental impressions to form, further binding one to Prakriti, and in turn, rebirth. The Sutras further depict the nature of consciousness and how the mind leads a person to either bondage (from every limiting context) or liberation. Liberation is not moksha or nirvana, but non-distinguishing *Kaivalya*, meaning Unlimitedness and Oneness (a concept first encountered in the Upanishads).

Since The Sutras traditionally had to be memorized by an elite, small group of male Brahmanas, Sanskrit scholars who began study early in life, the average length of a sutra is six words. As noted, the Sutras are a scholastic text in the sense that they are considered "incomprehensible" if read on their own by a lay person. Rather, the teachings of the Sutras must be "unpacked" through commentary and with the guidance of a teacher, or *guru*.

The highly practical methods within The Yoga Sutras describe an Eight Limbed Path (*ashtanga*) which attains the conscious state of liberation. Each limb on the path removes the veils that obscure the layers of one's being. This path combines practices in systematic ways through controlling the body, desires, and emotions. The components of the Eight Limbed Path are the ethical principles of the world (*yamas*), your inward journey to connect to wholeness (*niyamas*), seated posture (*asana*), enhancing prana through controlled breath rhythms (*pranayama*), withdrawal of the senses (*pratyahara*), concentration (*dharana*), meditation (*dhyana*), and absorption with Consciousness (*samadhi*) that lead to Kavalia. *Kavalia* is a state of one's innermost self, experiencing atman. It important to note these limbs are not sequential stages of development. They are entry points into an expanded sense of self. The authentic self is then strengthened through experiences, choices, and interpretations, resulting in a life of wonder.

Patanjali accepts that an individual is the essence of one God, therefore Divinity cannot be found by searching outside. Achieving unity with God requires exploration within oneself, in the depths of one's own being. Duality dissolves by overcoming ignorance, absorbing into the pure consciousness of an unadulterated Purusha.

Please note, there is no record of modern *asana* (postures) at this time. The term asana was first used in The Sutras denoting how to sit comfortably to prepare to engage in meditation.

Maharishi Patanjali, who?

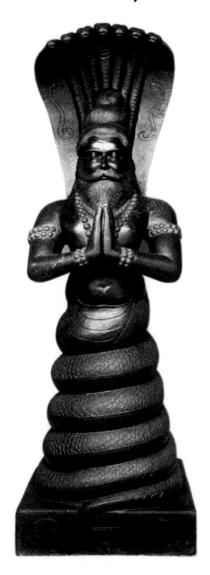

Maharishi Patanjali is known as the Father of Modern Yoga, who elaborated upon and synthesized the principles of Yoga for the benefit of the world. He is considered the author of *The Yoga Sutras*.

Patanjali is derived from the Sanskrit word *pa*, meaning "descended from heaven" and *anjali*, which is the mudra of a prayer, with palms and fingers gently pressing together. According to Patanjali, Yoga leads to freedom from suffering, and the Eight-Limbed Path is the way. Each limb helps expands consciousness within internal reference points, moving from an outer awareness to an inner awareness, transforming ego into spirit. Expanded perspective is the result; and in this space, you can see larger pictures within any situation.

Patanjali, according to speculation, lived 200 years before Christ. However, his existence is not documented, and though some believe that Patanjali did indeed exist, he is widely accepted as a mythological being who represents aspects of human potential, similar to deities. When *The Yoga Sutras* immerged, multiple texts with similar systematic approaches toward enlightenment were circulating. It is simply speculated that *The Yoga Sutras* were the most popular and therefore withstood the test of time.

Tradition says Patanjali is actually Shesha, the thousand-headed cosmic serpent upon which Vishnu reclines when creating the Universes. This is all Lila of course, as Vishnu doesn't need to recline on anything. Yet each head of Shesha is reciting the glories of God/Vishnu/ Bhagavan, each speaking its own glories, never saying the same thing, never repeating itself. Shesha is completely serpent, yet in mythologies surrounding Patanjali, he is half man, half serpent.

Patanjali brings Yoga for the mind, grammar for speech, and medicine for ills of the body. These are gifts of humanity, and therefore he is considered a sage. At the same time, he is considered a cosmic and transcendent presence. He is a form of Vishnu, which includes the gorgeous form of Shesha.

It is noteworthy that many inspirational figures have births that are otherworldly and full of symbolism. It is also interesting that traditional, vaginal births do not harken to the glory of the inspirational figure at hand. The Buddha was born from a side of his mother's torso. Christ's mother was a virgin. Patanjali fell from the heavens. In one version of Patanjali's birth, Gonnika, a yogini and devotee of Lord Vishnu, prayed for years for a child, as she was barren. Lord Vishnu recognized her devotion and asked Ananta, his beloved cosmic serpent, to incarnate into a human. One day, as Gonnika's cheeks were wet with tears, her upturned palms in Padma Mudra, lotus mudra, Vishnu answered her prayers. A tiny celestial aspect of Ananta fell into her hands. Who was she to question God's blessing? This *bija* of Ananta, this divine potential, was nurtured with nourishing love. In time, a baby boy emerged who became one of the world's greatest teachers.

In the Vedic tradition, snakes are revered. The symbolism of the snake represents kundalini energy, knowledge, and keen awareness. When the hood of the cobra is raised, she is present, alert, and has piercing consciousness. In various world religions, the snake also represents knowledge, yet is considered evil. Why? Because knowledge naturally invokes personal empowerment. Through empowerment, change occurs. Many people and ruling powers are fearful of change. The mythological image of Patanjali can be seen to represent the concept that the knowledge you seek is inherent within you; that knowledge is embedded within you. Seeker and Sought are the same.

Patanjali as an incarnation of the thousand-headed serpent Ananta, also known as Shesha, controls time and has the power to preserve and annihilate creation. Ananta supports planets of the universe on his hoods while singing praises to Vishnu, who reclines on his back, floating in the primordial sea of existence and potential. Like Patanjali, Ananta represents non-duality. Non-duality is the essence of the Vedas. Like Patanjali, you have the potential to attain ultimate Oneness, as each person has potential to be a facet of pure Divinity.

Patanjali is a symbolic representation, a reminder, that you are able to rise beyond the shackles of the fluctuations of your mind. These fluctuations create false "stories" based on your conditioned ways of thinking, which are often steeped in the energy of fear. This fear causes great emotional turmoil within you. Fear is simply a heavy energy with the potential to be a great teacher. *Yogas Citta Vritti Nirodha* is the second sutra in *The Yoga Sutras*, meaning, "When the fluctuations of the mind are stilled, you experience Yoga". Yoga is self-clarity, void of story, which controls and perceives experiences. A stilled mind has one eye out and one eye in, being both at home in the Divine human heart and at home in the Divine human world. This non-dualistic experience is the energy that Patanjali promised.

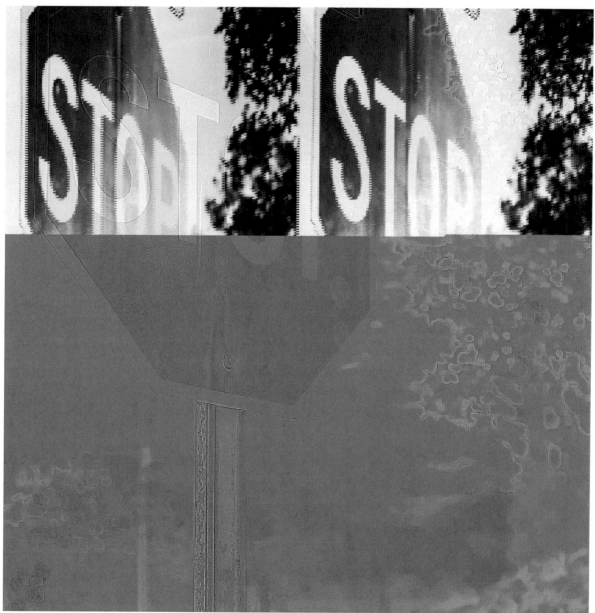

Nirodhah

352

Nirodhah

Patanjali examines the mind and consciousness through the methodological *Yoga Sutras*. Here, the term *nirodhah* is a foundational concept that must be highlighted. **Nirodhah is a Sanskrit term meaning to stop, block, restrain.** In practice, you *nirodhah* (stop or still) the mind when you make the commitment to a regular meditation. When you practice stepping back from the mind in the morning, you can more easily step back from agitation experienced during the day. This is not a goal of Yoga, but it is a very welcomed side-effect.

What is the goal of Yoga?

Different traditions have different goals for different tendencies. In regard to the Sutras, the goal is *Yogas Chitta Vritti Nirodhah*. In other words, the goal is to restrain the thoughts. Why restrain? To recognize your True Nature. As wholeness is divinely recognized, there is freedom from desire.

Yogas: Yoga / Chitta: Mind / Vritti: Thoughts / Nirodhah: Restrain

Remember, a *vritti* is an activation of a samskara. A *vritti* is a thought coming from memory, coming together to create thinking. Vrittis are caused by *kleshas* (afflictions/obstacles that cause human suffering). Meditation stills vrittis, and it takes practice. So be gentle with yourself in your practice.

Sometimes when I am meditating, I suddenly think of checking an email or other random thoughts that pull the symphony of my system in an unexpected direction. I used to act on these impulses, justifying the stopping of my meditation to honor a supposed intuition-hit. What a tricky mind I have! In the growth of my practice, I have experimented with harnessing my thoughts, which takes every effort I have. However, *the initial thought wave of recognition to stop the mind's trajectory is nirodhah.*

The nature of nirodhah witnesses the thought, stops you from going further into the whirlpool of the thought, and pulls you back into meditation. Nirodhah prevents other samskaras from arising. Nirodhah takes focus and willpower, yet it also strengthens focus and willpower.

The Five Kleshas: The Obstacles that Bind

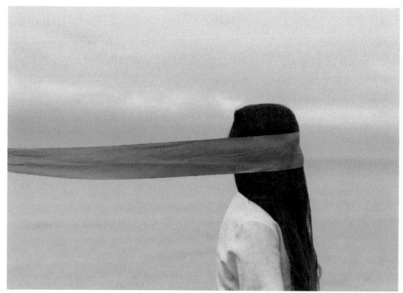

Kleshas That Bind

What is the ego? The ego is comprised of labels. Labels are learned belief systems that are embedded in the ego of *Though Shalt/Though Shalt Not, Them/Us, Victim/Judge*. Only you can choose to change your belief systems.

According to any Yogic path, the purpose of life is inquiring into truth. Karma are reactions accruing from body/mind desires, and you can't find joy through body/mind desire. Remember, joy is everlasting while pleasure is fleeting and arises from body/mind attachment.

Both Vedic and Buddhist philosophies outline five afflictions that cause human suffering. In the second chapter of *The Yoga Sutras*, called *The Sadhana Pada*, Patanjali outlines the same five afflictions (five "obstacles") that are described as being the roots of suffering. These obstacles are called *kleshas*.

354

Recognizing their influence in your life and then taking steps to overcome them will lead to liberation, or moksha.

The kleshas are **ignorance, egoism, attachment, aversion,** and **clinging to life.** These kleshas bind you to the endless cycle of birth and rebirth of samsara, trapping you in the maya, the illusion of prakriti. However, prakriti gives you what is needed to support you on your journey to liberation. But you must overcome ignorance.

All other kleshas arise from ignorance, which is called *avidya,* as does the ego, from which comes desire. Ignorance breeds a certain kind of ego which generates desires and kleshas. Based on the karmic body that you have, that body has certain things that feel good, and certain things that feel bad, and so you try to seek the things that feel good. There are the *ragas*/desires and memories of the things that were once experienced in the past that felt good, and then there are the *dveshas*/aversions, of things that didn't. This generates the ego.

The opposite of avidya is *vidya*, which means knowledge. Vidya says, "I am atman, not mind/body."

The *vrittis*, thought waves, are driven by the undercurrent of the kleshas. In other words, vrittis are caused by the kleshas. Focus and effort are needed to still these mental fluctuations, which various Kriya Yogas explore.

Nirodha is the ultimate state of non-doing. This is to stop the mind from "vritti-ing" thoughts. Thoughts lead to desires, which lead to actions, which lead to experiences, which continue the samskaric cycle. Yoga is to free the mind of desires.

Sutra 2.2 states, "The goal of Yoga is not to obtain something that is lacking: it is the realization of an already present reality. Yoga practice removes the obstacles that obstruct the experience of samadhi, or the state of complete absorption." In Sutras 2.3 through 2.11, each of the kleshas are described in a manner that allows you to discern their characteristics and thus overcome their adverse effects. As a solution to overcome suffering, *The Yoga Sutra's* offer assimilated steps in its Eight-Limbed Path.

1. (2.4) Avidya ~ Ignorance, taproot of all kleshas

Ignorance is the field for the other mentioned after it, whether they be dormant, feeble, intercepted or sustained. Ignorance is regarding the impermanent as permanent, the impure as pure, the painful as pleasant, and the non-Self as the Self.

Ignorance is the core element of human suffering because it blinds you from knowing your true Self. You must be open to the possibility that your world is not always what it appears to be on the surface, and that you are not necessarily limited by your perceived physical "reality".

Ask yourself, "Am I seeing things clearly?"

❖ *Am I mistaking the impermanent for the permanent?*
❖ *Am I mistaking the impure for the pure?*
❖ *Am I mistaking the pain for pleasure?*
❖ *Am I mistaking the self as the Self?*

2. (2.6) Asmita ~ Ego, false identity

Egoism is the identification of the power of the Seer with that of the instrument of seeing.

I-am-ness is the identification of the ego. The ego is your internal and external image of yourself and how you see the world, based on the false projections of your protective personality. Your Authentic Self is blurred with ego-created projections and stories.

Do your behavior patterns reflect yourself or your Self?

❖ *Consider keeping track of your patterns of behavior and their power over you. Did you learn them from your childhood experiences? Were they developed through rebellion or in response to a particular experience?*

❖ *Consider how you compare yourself to other people. What are your relationships with objects and food? What are your responses and reactions?*

❖ *Are you able to recognize your conditioned behaviors? Are you able to disassociate from any such behaviors?*

3. (2.7) Raga ~ Attachment

Attachment is that which follows identification with pleasurable experiences.

Desires and attractions hold you in patterns. You are attached to aspects of companions (friends, partners, pets), objects, food, technology, etc. Needing and wanting these aspects is a part of being human, but not when you cling to them, associating your value and worth in relation to them. When these aspects are inspiring and not obsessed over, you experience lightness and happiness. You must learn to accept the realness in the moment and consider if you are loving or loathing yourself through each moment.

How can you determine your attachments?

❖ *What is your mind drawn to? Where do you feel it in your body?*

❖ *How do you feel being drawn to it? Expanded or constricted? It is a habit/addiction?*

4. (2.8) Dvesha ~ Aversion

Aversion is that which follows identification with painful experiences.

Dvesha may be seen as repulsion or avoidance or a feeling of dislike towards something. This is ego-driven. If you cannot physically avoid dislikes, you suffer. If you cannot mentally avoid dislikes, you suffer. To step outside of the ego's comfort zone creates expansion and rootedness into your Authentic Self. The feeling of friction is an invitation to lean into the rub, rather than resist it. Leaning in to see the 'why' behind the friction supports the removal of your protective personality stories. This helps you connect your internal patterns, so you are more at home in both your inner and outer world.

What would it feel like…

❖ *… if you were to step back when you are drawn to challenges?*

❖ *… if you were to step forward instead of avoiding challenges?*

❖ *… to identify one habit and change it to better claim your power?*

5. (2.9) Abhinivesha ~ Clinging to Life

Clinging to life, flowing by its own potency, exists even in the wise.

This is your will to live and is connected to your instincts. You know you will die, but you fear death and see it as a loss of connection involving deep loneliness. You suffer because your past experiences dictate how your future is lived. This is living in the energy of Fear. You also may cling to the tribal patterns of society and culture that may misidentify and abuse your Authentic Self.

Consider:

- ❖ *Prioritizing your care of people, obligations, and self-care needs that are important to you. Complete them, so you don't owe people or yourself anything and so you may feel a sense of freedom.*

- ❖ *Become a clean slate. Express appreciations, love, ask for forgiveness.*

- ❖ *Asking yourself, "Who am I?"*

SUMMARY

Kleshas are derived from ignorance, bound by the ego. The ego is your protective personality, and it is a living energy that thrives on ignorance and fears change. A major step toward dissolving the kleshas is simply to acknowledge where they influence your life. Remember, life flows more like a spiral than a linear line. You may overcome an aspect of a klesha then be revisited by it again and again. This is an opportunity to polish your Authentic Self again and again, layer after layer.

Explore where your patterned emotions live within your body. As you explore, it is essential to reside in compassion with yourself. Begin by acknowledging the facets of how each klesha plays out in your life. Know that everything has served you for your greatest Good and appreciate how you once protected yourself but no longer need to. Pay attention to your thoughts and your words, in turn, your actions and your habits. Fly and fall, again and again, as you work on removing your kleshas. Witness how it becomes easier and easier to navigate as you release your patterns. This is a part of your life journey! The kleshas are truly doorways to your freedom.

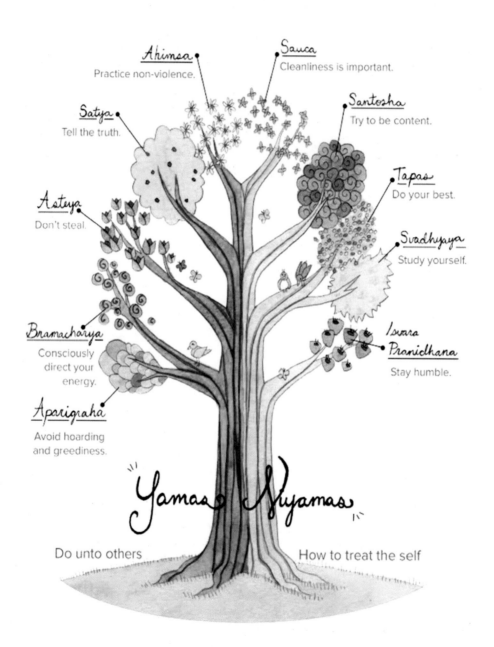

Ahimsa
Practice non-violence.

Sauca
Cleanliness is important.

Satya
Tell the truth.

Santosha
Try to be content.

Asteya
Don't steal.

Tapas
Do your best.

Svadhyaya
Study yourself.

Bramacharya
Consciously direct your energy.

Isvara Pranidhana
Stay humble.

Aparigraha
Avoid hoarding and greediness.

Yamas Niyamas

Do unto others

How to treat the self

360

Ashtanga Yoga: The Eight-Limbed Path

1) **Yamas:** *Rules of Social Behavior, "Do unto others…"*
   - ❖ **Ahimsa:** nonharming, generosity toward your heart and therefore to others
   - ❖ **Satya:** truthfulness and integrity of intention, thoughts, words, actions
   - ❖ **Asteya:** non-stealing, abiding in generosity and honesty
   - ❖ **Brahmacharya:** moderation and balance of energy
   - ❖ **Aparigraha:** non-possessiveness and non-attachment

2) **Niyamas:** *Rules of Personal Behavior, "How to treat the self…"*
   - ❖ **Saucha:** purity, refinement of inner and outer environments
   - ❖ **Santosha:** contentment, living in the blessing of the here and now moment
   - ❖ **Tapas:** austerity, dedication, purifying heat
   - ❖ **Svadhyaya:** self-study, analyzing inner and outer worlds
   - ❖ **Ishvara-Pranidhana:** surrender to Divinity in all things through the Japa Practice

3) **Asana:** *Posture.* Originally meaning 'comfortable seated pose', not series of movements.

4) **Pranayama:** *Breath Control.* Harness mind through breath.

5) **Pratyahara:** *Withdrawal of the Senses.* Opening connection to Divinity.

6) **Dharana:** *Concentration.* A focused meditation on love, wisdom, and joy.

7) **Dhyana:** *Meditation.* Expansive emerging with the infinite omnipresent nature of Divinity.

8) **Samadhi:** *Bliss.* Absorption of Consciousness in the Self. Pure Awareness.

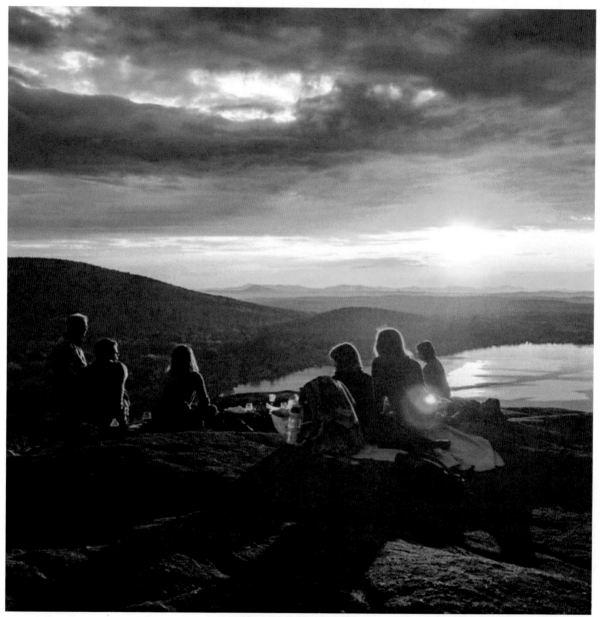

Life Internally and Externally

Yamas and Niyamas

All spiritual traditions encourage a life of ethics. The *Yamas* and *Niyamas* are the first two limbs in Patanjali's *Yoga Sutras* that outline the art and science of Yoga. They are the roots for the other Sutra levels of consciousness to grow. The Yamas and Niyamas represent the quality of one's inner dialogue, and they are the behaviors of enlightened beings. They arise spontaneously within the natural, harmonic flows of the web of life. They are non-sequential milestones on the spiritual path that support the refined inner exploration of body, breath, senses, and the mind.

Maharishi Patanjali describes the *Yamas* as being naturally in-line with the harmony of interconnection. When you are in flow and in accordance of the natural law of living from the level of the atman, you cannot act in harmful ways. The *Niyamas* ask, "How do you live, think, and act when no one is looking, yet you are your only witness?"

Yoga is not simply a physical discipline but rather encompasses multiple paths that are infused with rich philosophies – some theistic and some non-theistic. *The Yoga Sutras* are considered non-theistic, though the notion of Ishvara – another term for Divinity – is embodied.

Like the Noble Eightfold Path, the Yamas and Niyamas are guidelines to support a healthy and balanced life, bringing spiritual awareness into our social context. You infuse life into *The Sutras* by considering how each one resonates in your personal journey. You feel each Yama and Niyama expand within your heart and in places within your body, and you allow your emotions to guide your intellect and discern your path. These guidelines are not rules. They are gateways to examine your Authentic Self. The Yamas and Niyamas help you lead a life of conscious compassion, which is the essence of Yoga.

The Yoga Tradition is rooted in the concept of *ahimsa*, meaning non-harming of all living beings. Love begins within oneself, and if you love yourself, you can then see yourself in all beings and therefore can't harm another. It is the concept of *Namaste – I see myself in you*. Ultimately, there are two energies – Love and Fear. The Yamas and Niyamas support a life of alignment. This is the alignment of the heart and mind, the inner and outer living experience. This is a life of Love.

The 5 Yamas: Rules of Noble Social Behavior

1. Ahimsa   **2. Satya**   **3. Brahmacharya**   **4. Asteya**   **5. Aparigraha**

Guidelines for how you interact with the macrocosm of the outer world. The Yamas are social disciplines and restraints to guide you in relationships with others to claim peace with the world.

1. Ahimsa

Non-violence in thoughts, words, and actions. Awareness. Ahimsa is empathy in thought, word, and action to yourself, and therefore to other beings. Practice self-love, worthiness, compassion, love, understanding, and patience. The heart and mind are filled with love and compassion for all beings, eliminating violence. Lightness diffuses density.

Be aware of your inner dialog; how you appreciate yourself; and how you show appreciation toward others. Would you allow another to talk to you the way you inwardly converse with yourself? The way you allow both abuse and joy in your life is directly related to what you believe you deserve, seen through this inner dialog and personal belief system. Gandhi's life was based on the principle of Ahimsa, but he used boundaries as a potent tool. Internal and external boundaries are a key piece of Ahimsa.

2. Satya

Truthfulness; integrity in thoughts, words, and actions. Ability to distinguish observations from interpretations; knowing reality is comprised of selective attention and interpretation. Honesty in tapping into your feelings and allowing them expression. Owning feelings, clear communication, assertiveness, brave conversations, forgiveness, non-judging, letting go of masks. Knowing everyone has unique lenses on life. Truth, non-harming, love, and divinity are interconnected.

"The elf of the tongue needs the giant to control it." Honesty can be used as a weapon, so compassion supports the discernment of honesty where love is higher than truth. You practice Satya when love directs how you use truth. Ahimsa (non-violence) must be practiced with Satya.

Be aware that frustration and anger are not permanent; communicate honestly; discern where statements of truth are coming from and whether they are harmful; do the truths need to be said? How is Satya – truthfulness – played out in your life? Are you fully truthful in the seed of your thoughts, translating them through your words and all of your actions? Can truthfulness cause harm, and is it okay to cause harm if you are being truthful? How vulnerable do you feel to be totally truthful? Do you react or respond when others are not truthful with you, or do you ignore it? How have you evolved in your satya as you have aged?

3. Brahmacharya

(Originally translated as celibacy.) Moderation, channeling emotions, moderation in all things, self-containment. "Brahma" = Unity Consciousness "Acharya" = Pathway. Being in rhythmical flow with the universal elements, associated with Dinacharya. Connected to Source, using moderated energy of mind, intellect, speech, and body in ways that lead to centered and complete connection. Treating yourself and others with respect and seeing Divinity in all, honoring the fire of the spirit. All life is seen as an expression of Divinity.

Where could you be more moderate in your life? What (or who) can be considered addictions, energy vampires, etc.? Who/what is drinking from your cup rather than your saucer, and why are you allowing this to occur? Where do you feel these thoughts in the body?

Developmental Stages of Brahmacharya:
- ❖ Self-containment through moderate sexuality and diet
- ❖ No thoughts of past or future sense pleasures
- ❖ Freedom from attachment to pleasure
- ❖ Free from duality and the illusion that you are incomplete, causing inner peace
- ❖ Perpetual inner ecstasy, replacing outward focus of sensual/sexual energies

4. Asteya

Non-Stealing. Not coveting, not being jealous. Not stealing time or energy from yourself or others. If you attain what you want through honest means, you have no fear. If you attain what you want through dishonest means, you live with fear. Nothing outside yourself provides security and happiness.

How is Asteya, non-stealing, played out in your life? How do you steal? How do you allow others to steal from you? Consider non-stealing of time, joy, life, money, etc. Do your judgments (quiet or spoken) steal joy from others? How do you see Asteya being played out in the arenas of your daily life by various characters?

5. Aparigraha

Non-Possessiveness. Non-attachment to possessions, relationships. Generosity in thoughts, words, and actions. Simplicity. Fulfilling needs rather than wants. Create space so you see yourself and allow newness to holistically enter your life. Sattvic living, free of distractions from expectations and attachments around relationships, sex, food, and material possessions.

What are you taking for granted? What are you attached to? Are these things defining you, holding you in a pattern? How was this pattern learned? Do you agree that you can experience abundance by letting things go? How can you experience gratitude for your abundance? Where do you feel these thoughts in the body?

The 5 Niyamas: Rules of Noble Personal Behavior

1. **Saucha**   2. **Santosha**   3. **Tapas**   4. **Svadhyaya**   5. **Ishvara-Pranidhana**

Guidelines for self-observation and discipline of your microcosm, your internal world. The Niyamas harness energy generated from the Yamas to support peace within yourself.

1. Saucha

Purity in body, mind/thoughts, intentions, and actions. Clarity. Cleanliness in regard to good health habits and a clean and orderly physical environment, which influence thoughts. Practice tempered thoughts, words, and discriminations. Clear your external and internal energy to reveal your joyful nature and your desire to know the Self.

Are your choices consciously nourishing or unconsciously toxic/patterned? How are you influenced by the foods you eat and the weather? Does your mind and body hold onto the emotions you experience in books and movies, phone calls, and in your personal interactions with others? How do colors and your clothing styles influence your comfort and relaxation? Are you able to experience nature without a bombardment of worries and without technology? Do you take your personal opinions too seriously?

2. Santosha

Contentment, the fragrance of the present moment. Choosing love. Acceptance, gratitude, and joyfulness. Inner peace is independent of situation or external status. Accept what is and make the best out of everything. No mud, no lotus. Remaining balanced in success, failure, and adversity through the knowledge that the Universe does things for you, not to you. Discern and do not allow the behavior of others to affect your inner peace. "Accept that which you cannot change, change what you can, and have the wisdom to know the difference."

367

When you struggle within the present moment, you struggle within the universe. Santosha is the absence of the need to control, the absence of the need for approval, the absence of the need for power. What can you be appreciative of during discomfort? How can you tap into your strength and non-dominating willpower in the midst of feeling stuck or when facing a void? How can you find beauty and mystery in ordinary life? How can you honor the mundane and experience daily duties with reverence, transforming them into the extraordinary?

3. Tapas

Austerity. Discipline. Purifying Flame; Beacon of Light to the world. Inviting heat and fire to transform you mentally, emotionally, and physically, like a Phoenix, burning away the ego to reveal the inner Self. This joyful inner discipline and determination leads to outer joy with great enthusiasm for daily life. In this, you revel in the necessary sacrifices to ultimately support your spiritual journey. Dive deep, embrace courage, strength, and simplicity, and therefore embrace your dharma. Transformation is a pathway to higher consciousness.

Is your lifestyle disciplined by the biological rhythms of nature (Dinacharya)? How do you discern your words? Do you bring peace to yourself and others, without saying a word? Do you walk heavily or lightly upon the earth? Do you flit from idea to idea, never carving space to cultivate, fail, succeed, and learn mastery?

4. Svadhyaya

Looking inside through self-education, self-study, self-observation. Distinguishing knowledge and knowingness. Practice, reflect, meditate, refine. Find your own truth and value in understanding spiritual concepts, questioning everything. Expand your knowledge through reading inspiring texts, pondering, exploring, and discerning what feels true.

Explore your patterns. Does your security and does your joy come from a connection to spirit or worldly belongings? What sets you off? What elates you? Why? Where were these patterns learned? Do you make decisions based on your intellect or from your heart? Do you allow your truth to be expressed in your body/your intuition? Do you allow new ideas in and listen to other opinions, challenging yourself to change and face fears? Do you stand for your truths with compassionate strength?

5. Ishvara Pranidhana

Surrender to God. Surrender to Divinity, Light, the Energy of the Universe. Faith. This embodiment of Faith leads to sincerity, patience, and eternal energy to engage in your Practice. Let go of the riverbank and BECOME River Divine. Offer every moment to your inner and outer growth. By embracing your darkness, you can infuse it with Light, and thus have no shame nor fear of the dark. That is where your fertilizer resides for you to grow. Be real. Celebrate it All. Abiding in the faith that you are loved and supported by the Universe.

The classical tool of Ishvara Pranidhana is to nirodhah the mind with a mantra through the Japa Mala Practice. Remember, Ishvara is not affected by karma, and it is found in the name of the mantra. So, choose a mantra that represents God/Divinity to you. Also consider what other rituals can root you to the present moment or instantly connect you with Divinity. Are you expressing appreciation and gratitude each day, each moment? Are you tapping into the understanding that goodness arises out of what may be deemed negativity? Do you see Divinity in all? Or do you feel separate from Divinity? Can you embrace your 'dark side' and celebrate it? Is there light without darkness?

Patanjali's Limbs 3-8

3. Asana   4. Pranayama   5. Pratyahara   6. Dhyana   7. Dharana   8. Samadhi

After embodying the Yama and Niyamas, you sit and breathe, settling beyond the senses to find concentration. Meditation arrives, with the inner expansion of undifferentiated Bliss.

3. Asana

Asana's original meaning is "comfortable seated position." In the 15th century, asana began to shift from being a seat to being physical postures, later expanded and refined in the 20th century. In today's world, asana is still a means to support meditation, as asana poses make the body supple so that a comfortable, meditative seat is more accessible to achieve. Ultimately, asana means full mind-body integration, embracing the eternity of the present moment. Only after becoming more deeply established in your Being, which is living in harmonious spontaneity with the Yamas and Niyamas, can asana be fully effective.

4. Pranayama

Pranayama masters life force. It is the breath-body comprised of animating prana that flows throughout the universe. How fluid your prana flows affects the vitality of your body, mind, and spirit. If your prana is not fluid, exhaustion, fatigue, and dis-ease are likely. Blockages influence how one views reality, distorting the perspective as ego-based from your protective personality rather than spirit-based. Pranayama expands the state of awareness and is one of the most powerful tools of the Yoga Tradition. The conscious regulation of breath invigorates your pranic flow and harnesses your mind to be centered, present, and interconnected with nature and the whole cosmos.

5. Pratyahara

Pratyahara is temporarily drawing the senses inward to explore the subtle universe and universal elements within the physical form. This supports quieting the realms of consciousness into a more expanded, meditative state. "It takes the strength of controlling 10,000 horses to control the mind." Pratyahara is the first definition of Yoga, as originally explored in the Upanishads. The senses are called tanmatras and invoking them consciously better reveals how the world of Prakriti and the senses are patterned projections of awareness. Pratyahara is also a gentle practice of gratitude for the senses and is an invitation for nourishing, sattvic living. Pratyahara is also the premise for guided meditation and Yoga Nidra.

6. Dharana

Perception is both selective and subjective, based on the quality of pranic flow contained in what is represented through awareness. Dharana is concentration harnessed through attention and intention. Awareness of entering deeper levels of consciousness is both mentally acknowledged while also being *simply is*. Where the mind goes, prana flows, and the magic lies in the keen discernment and clarity of intention. Dharana is a sort of *drishti*, a focused gaze, and it is a means for developing concentrated intention for deeper meditation.

7. Dhyana

Dhyana is meditation; a deeper experience, witnessing being both within and beyond the world. At the center of the ever-changing dance of life is the witness self. Like the eye of a storm, the Authentic Purusha source is the witness to the Prakriti and the changes of life situations, relationships, desires, visions, feelings, and thoughts. The more meditation is explored, the easier it is to remain aligned in a world where the only constant is perpetual change.

8. Samadhi

Samadhi is the state of pure Awareness; of coming Home to your authentic Self. This bliss state is where time and space merge into the realm of eternity and infinity. The more Samadhi is explored, the more natural you experience all conscious realms of life from the lens of spirit. It is living a life with the essence of *Namaste – pure Love*. Life is Lila, a divine play, and all beings have roles and teach lessons to support the evolution of existence.

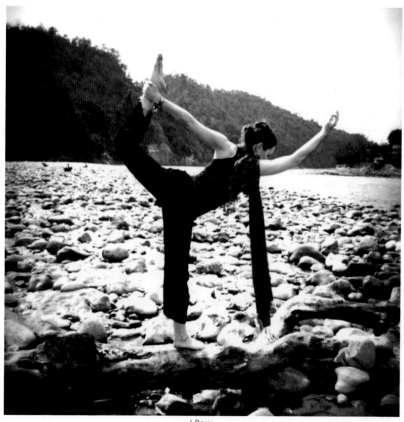

I Bow

Sthira Sukham Asanam, Yoga Sutras 2:46

Steadiness and Ease ~ AKA *The Sweet Spot* in Your Yoga Practice

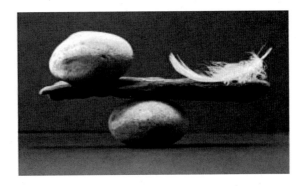

2.46 – Sthira Sukham Asanam
Asana is a steady, comfortable posture.

2.47 – Prayatna Saithilyananta Samapattibhyam
By relaxing effort and fixing the mind on the infinite (asana is perfected).

2.48 – Tato Dvandvanabhighatah
Thereafter, one is undisturbed by dualities.

When I am in a pose, I subtly shift my entire body on the inhale. In this precious moment, I examine if I am holding tension in my jaw or facial muscles, and I relax them. I consider if my balance is equalized in my footing and make adjustments as to how I press my body weight into the ball, heel, or sides of each foot, as I lift and spread my toes wide. I relax my shoulders, while lengthening my spine and crown. I ensure full engagement in my arms and fingers. I loosen my belly to breathe deep, allowing myself to take up space. On the exhale, I rest, embodying eternity as I relish the impermanence and beauty of the posture; the breath; the moment. I allow it to feel deliciously good.

The Yoga Meal

A Practice Honoring the Eight-Limbed Path

Yoga asks you to identify and take responsibility for how you receive energy and give energy. This begins by examining how you feed your body. You are encouraged to go slower than the fast-food nations we live in. A slow eating pace fosters deeper enjoyment of the foods we're consuming and provides a path to celebrate our cultures and communities through varied culinary arts. It honors the fostering of healthy plants and animals, supports local growers, and the list goes on. The Yoga Meal asks you to understand your place in the planetary ecosystem and take responsibility for your choices. The Yoga Meal also demands you change behaviors to be more conscious and compassionate, taking time to appreciate the blessing of food and its gift of the present moment.

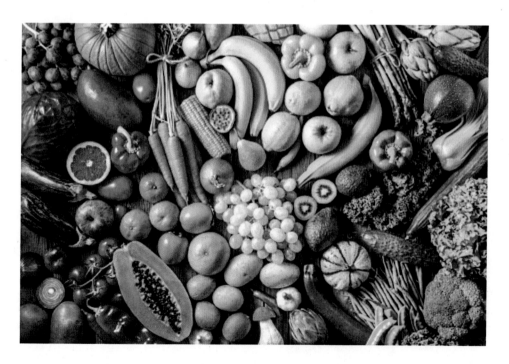

1) Yamas ~ Interconnection of Resources

- ❖ **Ahimsa:** *nonharming*
  Another's life energy your food. Consider animals, producers, and environment

- ❖ **Satya:** *truth*
  Finding who you truly are to support a healthy body.

- ❖ **Asteya:** *non-stealing*
  Buy responsibly- sourced food that dignifies people, animals, and environment.

- ❖ **Brahmacharya:** *moderation*
  Consider what is essential for nourishment.

- ❖ **Aparigraha:** *non-hording*
  Never take more than you need.

2) Niyamas ~ Ayurvedic Perspectives

- ❖ **Saucha:** *purity*
  Internal organs functioning with ease.

- ❖ **Santosha:** *contentment*
  Be comfortable in your own skin. What is medicine to you may be poison to another.

- ❖ **Tapas:** *austerity*
  Warm meals support the digestive fire.

- ❖ **Svadhyaya:** *self-study*
  Food feeds the heart! Know what heals you, physically and emotionally.

- ❖ **Ishvara-Pranidhana:** *surrender to Divinity in all things*
  Gratitude, gratitude, gratitude for your meal.

3) Asana ~ Posture

Cultivate patience and delight in your senses with each bite. How does it look, feel, smell, taste? Who can you share your meal with?

4) Pranayama ~ Breath Control

Take your time and don't rush your meal.

5) Pratyahara ~ Withdrawal of the Senses

What does your food remind you of? What emotions arise?

6) Dharana ~ Concentration

Make careful decisions of what you put in your body and understand with an invested intention of how you do so.

7) Dhyana ~ Meditation

Enjoy the sensations of chewing, smelling, tasting, and allow the food to become a part of you on a physical and emotional level.

8) Samadhi ~ Union

Your food becomes your body on a cellular level. What is not needed is eliminated. Ultimately, you can digest the universe!

Lead a Yoga Meal Awareness Practice

In a little paper cup, place a single cranberry, a piece of cholate, and a walnut to give to your participants. Encourage people to take time to smell, feel, and observe the intricate aspects within each food-object. Ask what stories and emotions are coming to mind?

*A glimpse into my first meal awareness practice:

I was drawn to the walnut. The walnut reminded me of my granddad and his beloved Sonora House in the Sierra Nevada foothills that he built for my grandmother; it smelled of sunlit oak leaves. As a very young child, Granddad taught me how to crack walnuts with a hammer, and how to have patience to retrieve its meat. I felt warmth, safety, and belonging in his presence. I felt the nourishing companionship of my brother and sister. I also felt mystery, as the walnut looks like a brain. (It is said that foods that look like a particular organ benefits that organ!)

Honoring feelings evoked by a few seconds of breathing and gazing at a food, supports your relationship with it.

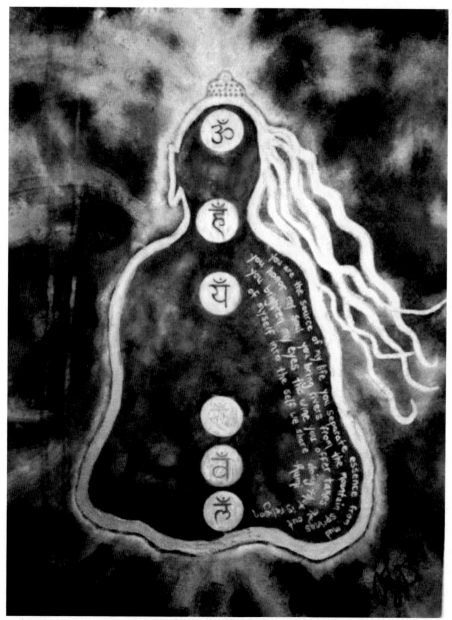

Within, painting by Lily Kessler

Reflection

Classical Yoga: Sacred Sutras, Sacred Promises

From the Eight-Limbed Path, match the letter with the correlating number.

1. **Pranayama**
2. **Dhyana**
3. **Ahimsa (Yama)**
4. **Ashtanga**
5. **Santosha (Niyama)**
6. **Pratyahara**
7. **Svadhyaya (Niyama)**
8. **5 Niyama's**
9. **Saucha (Niyama)**
10. **Satya (Yama)**
11. **Asana**
12. **Aparigrapha (Yama)**
13. **Ishvarapranidhana (Niyama)**
14. **Bramacharya (Yama)**
15. **Samadhi**
16. **5 Yama's**
17. **Dharana**
18. **Asteya (Yama)**
19. **Tapas (Niyama)**

a. **Outwardly Ethical**
b. **Contentment**
c. **Self-study**
d. **Truthfulness**
e. **Seated Pose**
f. **Cleanliness/Purity**
g. **Meditation**
h. **Non-attachment**
i. **Breath Control**
j. **Non-violence**
k. **Dedication, Heat, Austerity**
l. **Bliss-state, Absorption**
m. **Energy moderation**
n. **Surrender to Ishvara; God**
o. **Withdrawal of the Senses**
p. **Concentration**
q. **Non-stealing**
r. **Inwardlly Ethical**
s. **Eight-Limbed Path**

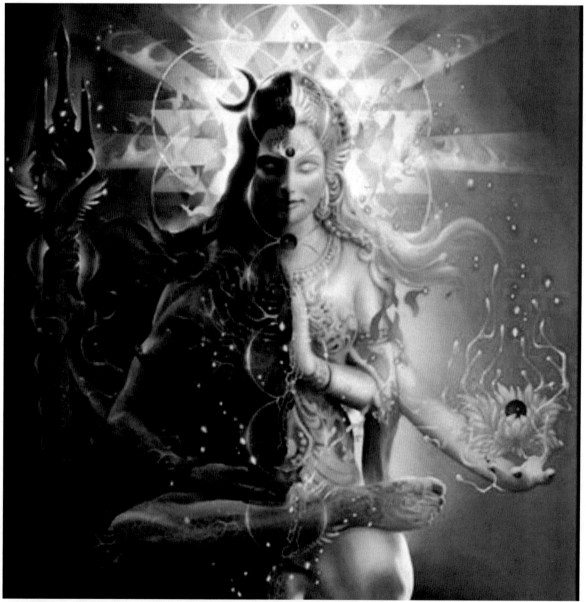

Balance

380

Chapter 10

Tantric Layers of the Self:
Hip, Holy & Huge

Historical Timeline

PRECLASSICAL YOGA ERA

INDUS-SARASVATI AGE: 6500-4500 BCE
- SANATANA DHARMA: "ETERNAL LAW"
- INDUS RIVER VALLEY & SEALS

VEDIC AGE: 4500-2500 BCE
- CONSCIOUSNESS EXPLORED
- VIBRATION OF INTENTION & CAUSATION
- CAUSE & EFFECT: MANTRA & KARMA

SAMKHYA YOGA: 8000-100 BCE
- REALITY EXPLORED: PRAKRITI/PURUSHA
- BODY'S CONSTITUTION: DOSHAS
- AYURVEDA

UPANISHADIC AGE: 2000-1500 BCE
- NON-DUALISM OF ATMAN/BRAHMAN
- DISTILLATION OF VEDAS
- MEDITATION

BHAKTI YOGA: 1000-500 BCE
- ADORATION
- HINDU EPICS / UNIVERSAL INSIGHTS
- 3 BRANCHES OF YOGA

BUDDHISM: C. 500 BCE-PRESENT
- INDIVIDUALITY / MONASTIC TRADITION
- MIDDLE WAY
- FOUR NOBLE TRUTHS / EIGHT-FOLD PATH

CLASSICAL YOGA ERA

CLASSICAL YOGA: 75 BCE-100 CE
- THE YOGA SUTRA'S OF PATANJALI
- EIGHT-LIMBED PATH
- HARNESSING THE MIND

ESOTERIC AGE

TANTRA: 600-1300 CE
- 6 + 1 CHAKRA SYSTEM
- WESTERN NOTION OF EMBODIMENT
- SUBTLE BODY (NADIS, CHAKRAS, ETC.)

HATHA YOGA: C. 1300-1400 CE
- MIND V. BODY
- HATHA YOGA PRADIPIKA
- ASANA / BREATH / BANDHAS / MUDRAS

RISE OF MODERN YOGA

SWAMI VIVEKANANDA: 1872-1950
- INFLUENCED RISE OF MODERN YOGA
- INTRODUCED YOGA TO THE WEST

SRI T. KRISHNAMACHARYA: 1891-1989
- YOGA'S EXPANSION
- FATHER OF MODERN YOGA
- MODERN CONTRIBUTORS

Chapter 10

Tantric Layers of the Self: Hip, Holy & Huge

1. Overview of Lecture

Chapter 10 explores the concept of Tantra: *tan-* (expansion) *-tra* (contraction) from a Western viewpoint. The focus is on the Streams of Prana called *the nadis*, the 6 + 1 chakra system with Western notions of embodiment concepts.

2. Learning Objectives: I will…

a) Understand the concepts of expansion and contraction and how they feel in the body
b) Distinguish the concept of Shiva and Shakti; masculine and feminine energies
c) Articulate the relationship between the Doshas, Koshas, Nadis, and the Chakras
d) Memorize the 6 + 1 chakra areas, and their names in Sanskrit and English
e) Recognize the chakra relationships to the Sushumna, Ida, and Pingala nadis

3. Pre-lecture Assignments

a) Read the chapter and become familiar with the Reflection questions
b) Daily Sadhana – Daily Personal Practice

4. Reflection: *found at the end of the chapter*

A Peek Into Tantra

The Tantra Tradition is not a part of Classical Yoga. The subtle body, energy work, chakras, and Kundalini are all exclusive parts of Tantric Yoga. In this tradition, every moment of life holds potential for awakening and liberation. Ultimately, Tantra seeks to empower people.

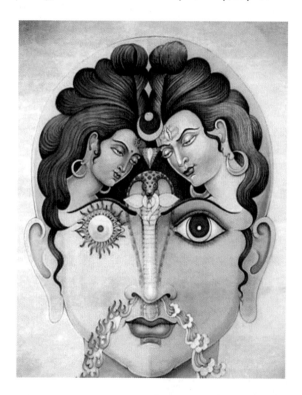

Tantra as a philosophy is not easily defined. The scope of the tradition is vast and contains contradictory practices and principles from both Hinduism and Buddhism. Tantra was and is an interreligious spiritual movement within Buddhism, within Shaivism (the religion of Shiva and Shakti), and in many other religions in South Asia, Southeast Asia, and East Asia. Tantra's first esoteric roots began developing around 100 BCE, around the time of *The Yoga Sutras*, and was a tradition by 500 CE.

The etymological meaning of *Tantra* means expansion (*tan-*) and contraction *(-tra)*. The contextual meaning of Tantra is to loom, warp, and weave like threads on a loom. The interweaving of traditions and teachings within Tanta are the interconnected threads within a text, technique, or practice. Tantric texts were originally poetic metaphors pointing to Oneness and Divine Love.

Tantric scriptures are called tantras, which is where the tradition gets its name from. The first tantra appeared around 500-550 CE, entitled (according to translation) as *The Hymns on the Reality Exhaled by God*. This text is massive and incredibly detailed, documenting something that was existing in oral transmission until it got so complex that it needed to be written. This is the first documented evidence of Tantra. Interestingly, this first text includes 50 physical poses in which you conform your body to the shapes of the Sanskrit alphabet. This is also the earliest information on physical poses in Yoga. As Tantric Yoga grew, however, this information was lost. Some scholars have attempted to reconstruct these poses, but it is not yet understood what they were. (Note, asana postures were not developed in depth until the 20th Century, with no relation to this Tantra.)

Tantra lineages teach there is the One that appears as three, and that is Shiva, Shakti, and the individual self. In other words, you are comprised of three aspects until you awaken into Oneness; so, it's non-dualistic. Another interesting semi-parallel of this trinity is found in Christianity, stating God the Father, God the Son, and God the Holy Spirit; three that are One.

The Hindu Tantric view is based on the concepts of *Shiva*, the masculine potential energy, and *Shakti*, the feminine, the manifested force of the Universe. Shiva provides the seed of potential, and Shakti provides the energy to differentiate and manifest energy into form. Shiva and Shakti are unified and can't exist without the other. They are considered non-dual.

Tantra postulates that you are undifferentiated consciousness, yet you need to see dualities for something to exist. The practice of Tantra allows you to see Divinity within yourself and within all life experiences. Everything is God, and Tantra leads you to experience your own Divine nature. This practice is a tightrope walk between the inward state of Shiva and the outward state of Shakti, resulting in a conscious life experience.

Do not let the behavior of others destroy your inner peace. ~ Dalai Lama

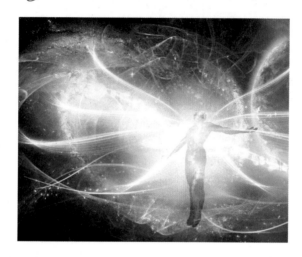

Principle Tantra Beliefs Include:

- ❖ God is found everywhere; non-dualistic
- ❖ There is no separation between you and God
- ❖ Everything is within you because you are the Universe
- ❖ Because you are the Universe, you are connected to all that is around you
- ❖ The Universe does things for you, NOT to you
- ❖ You are a spiritual being having spiritual experiences in a spiritual body
- ❖ Everyone and everything is from Divine Source
- ❖ All life is honored; all life experiences are considered holy
- ❖ The Universe is a manifestation that can be connected to and channeled through rituals
- ❖ Everything has the potential for you to experience divinity within your Self
- ❖ All you need is within you - you are the microcosm in the macrocosm
- ❖ You see, process, and digest experiences and information through the lens of the heart

Principle Tantra Practices Include:

- ❖ Supporting communion with the Divine through insight and intuition
- ❖ Experiencing the divine in daily life: silence, prayer; meditation; interconnection
- ❖ While in a confrontation, remembering you are Divine and human, and both are good
- ❖ Seeing dualities for something to exist; by seeing dualities, you can move beyond them to see how both are needed; one cannot exist without the other
- ❖ Using samskaras that contract and pull you away from your divinity to discover patterned ways of thinking that hold you back (the Klesha Avidya – ignorance)
- ❖ Cleaning the lens of your heart so you can see divinity within yourself, other people, animals, the natural world, and situations
- ❖ Not taking others' opinions/beliefs and making them your own
- ❖ Not responding through conditioned behavior (labels, family, culture, society)

Interferences to Your Divinity Include:

- ❖ How you process and digest information
- ❖ The conditioned patterns of behavior you grew up with and still maintain as belief-systems
- ❖ The 5 Kleshas – beliefs in limited power of action (mental and/or physical); limited knowledge (the limited ability to understand the vastness within yourself); desire (to be unique, special); limited time (the time it takes to digest and understand, feeling that there is always so much more to learn and understand); Karma (living under a delusion; fear of death).

387

Feelings and Emotions

Understanding the difference between feelings and emotions helps you tap into your psychology and allows you to take responsibility for your life. In society, the terms *feelings* and *emotions* are used interchangeably. However, there is a great difference in how feelings and emotions are expressed.

Your sensitive body is a storehouse of pent-up feelings that are fostered by an inauthentic society. *Chin-up. Buck-up. Don't change. Pretty girls don't cry. Real men don't cry. Turn that frown upside-down.* When feelings are unexpressed, even joyful feelings, they accumulate and become emotional hindrances. Your minds-eye, your perspective, becomes distorted by the power of unconscious emotions. You become a ghost, living in the past or in the future, with neither the energy nor consciousness of the beauty and simplicity of the present moment. In this vacancy, something else can move in to take up space within your tissues, such as disease.

Your feelings are a result of unpatterned behavior. When you allow an organic feeling to rise, with control and self-accountability, you remain clean, even in anger, agony, and adoration. Furthermore, when you recognize how your past patterns (emotional reactions) influence your present moment, you tap into and heal the layers of your life, distinguishing truth from illusion.

Truth is in the merging of the multidimensional layers of Self, comprised of mind, body, spirit. These are the koshas, known as the Energy Bodies.

They are influenced by your dosha.

Unpatterned Behaviors and Patterned Behaviors

Conscious	Unconscious
Response	React
Ease	Dis-ease
Present Moments	Past Experiences
Flowing	Stagnant
Expressed with Clarity	Expressed with Repression
Innocence	Destruction
Rational	Irrational
Personal Responsibility	Blame
"I feel" / "I need"	"You ___ ..."
Strengthens the Heart	Hardens the Ego
Union	Separation
Expansion	Constriction
Lightness & Energy	Heaviness & Dullness
Open	Repressed
Vulnerable	Defensiveness
Embraces Pain	Defense to Pain
Heaven	Hell
Relief	Physical Feeling of Discomfort

The Layers of Consciousness: The Koshas

A Traditional Perspective

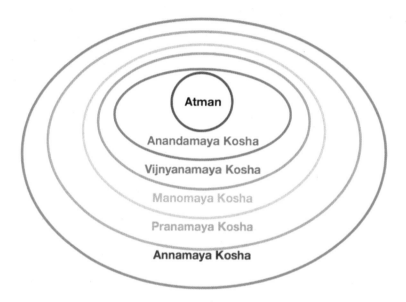

When answering the question "Who am I?", you discover that your 'Self' is the sum of five interconnected, energetic layers called the *koshas*, meaning layers or sheaths of the human existence. Koshas are the physical body, pranic body, mental body, wisdom body, and the spirit body. They are first described in *The Upanishads*; charted by Yogic sages over 3,000 years ago. Understanding them is a practical and profound tool that supports embodiment principles.

The koshas function as one holistic system, each as sensitive in their own way as physical skin. The health of these systems reflects the health of the physical body, formed by the compressed energies of the koshas. Together, all the sheaths comprise the landscape of the self; a subjective experience of being alive, as your energy reflects your perception of reality. The koshas open the universe within, so you may feel Yoga from the inside, cultivating and deepening your mind-body-spirit connection.

Annamaya Kosha – Physical / Food Sheath / Waking

The dense, physical body manifests Earth, Water, Fire, Air, and Ether and is related to the root chakra and earth element. Integrate this kosha by practicing body awareness through breath consciousness and asanas.

Pranamaya Kosha - Pranic Body / Dream Sleep

This kosha animates the physical body with breath and is related to the chakra system. Gunas are an expression of this kosha: Rajastic (dynamic), Tamasic (inactive), or Sattva (balanced). Practice Pranayama to develop deeper awareness of this kosha.

Manomaya Kosha - Mental & Feeling Sheath / Deep Sleep

This kosha represents the mind, personality, and the nervous system. It embodies a sense of separate self, including likes, dislikes, preferences, and avoidances, and it includes the five sensory organs. Practice Pratyahara, sensory awareness, to access this kosha.

Vijanamaya Kosha - Wisdom Sheath / Yogic State

This kosha represents intelligent consciousness, able to recognize that there is more to life than the wants of the ego/mind. Cultivate this sheath through Dharana and Dhyana (concentration and focus). Doing so deepens clarity and motivation and allows one to see larger perspectives to make sounder choices.

Anandamaya Kosha - Bliss, Spirit, Love Sheath / Integral Consciousness

This is the kosha of the Self, embodying unity consciousness and the interconnection of all beings. The ability to recognize the relationship of the Purusha self to the rest of the cosmos.

A Deeper Look at the Koshas

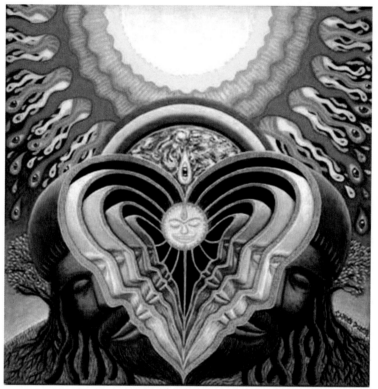

A Look at the Koshas

Physical & Extended Body - Field of Molecules

The extended, personal, and energetic body are linked to the environment which contains an endless supply of energy and information. Influenced by sound, sensation, sight, flavor, and aroma, with no distinct boundary between personal and extended bodies, which are in constant exchange

Annamaya Kosha ~ Physical Sheath (Doshas, Ayurveda, Asana)

- ❖ In balance when attentive to personal dosha and embodied through asana and diet

- ❖ Lifestyle linked with sattvic foods minimizing toxicity while maximizing nourishment

- ❖ 4 most sattvic foods revered by yogis: almonds, honey, milk, and ghee (only organic)

Pranamaya Kosha ~ Pranic, Life-force Sheath (Pranamaya, Nadis, Chakra System, Meridians)

- ❖ Govern flow of life force throughout the body

- ❖ Pranayama techniques designed to awaken and purify and increase holistic vitality and creativity

- ❖ 5 Seats of Prana in the Body: Head, Throat, Heart, Belly, Scrum

Subtle Body - Field of the Mind

Decisions are made by attempting to calculate the advantages and disadvantages. Integrates information based upon beliefs and feelings to come to a decision.

Manomaya Kosha ~ Mental & Feeling Sheath (Pratyahara, Prakriti, Emotions, Gunas)

- ❖ The mind is the repository of sensory impressions

- ❖ When you hear a sound, see a sight, feel a sensation, taste a flavor, or smell a fragrance, they are impressions on your waking awareness and your perception of reality.

Vijanamaya Kosha ~ Wisdom Sheath (Discrimination, Purusha, Intuition, Buddha)

- ❖ Distinguish the real from the unreal

- ❖ Real: that which cannot be lost

- ❖ Unreal: anything that has a beginning and an end to it

- ❖ Knowing the difference between the two is the essence of Yoga

Causal Body - Field of Pure Potentiality

Universal Domain: Deepest aspect of Being beyond time, space, and causality, giving rise to the manifest universe. All distinctions merge into unity, but this unbounded ocean of Being disguises itself in the sheaths of the causal, subtle, and physical realms. This deep, still, unbounded realm is the source and goal of Yoga – of life.

Anandamaya Kosha ~ Bliss/Love/Spirit Sheath (Meditation, Truth, Ecstasy)

- ❖ Most subtle, no judgment, pure presence

- ❖ You cannot perceive or measure this sphere of life, though it gives rise to your thoughts, feelings, dreams, desires, memories, and the molecules that make up your body and the material world.

- ❖ *Personal Domain*: Every individual has a personal atman with unique memories and desires that guide the course of life, and you must nurture your authentic gifts with attention and intention.

- ❖ *Collective Domain*: Living Story, the Hero's Journey, embodiment of living myths, deities.

If you want to change your life you have to change your daydreams.
Understand that what you see in the outside world reflects your inner
landscape - how you see it, it sees you. (That alone holds me accountable.)
So do your inner gardening, work to develop a sense of beauty, and
your spiritual light will shine into the world and be reflected back to you.
It's Yoga, Baby.

~ Lily Kessler

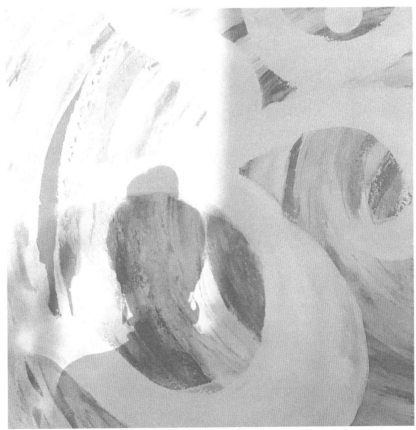

Here I Am, I Am Here

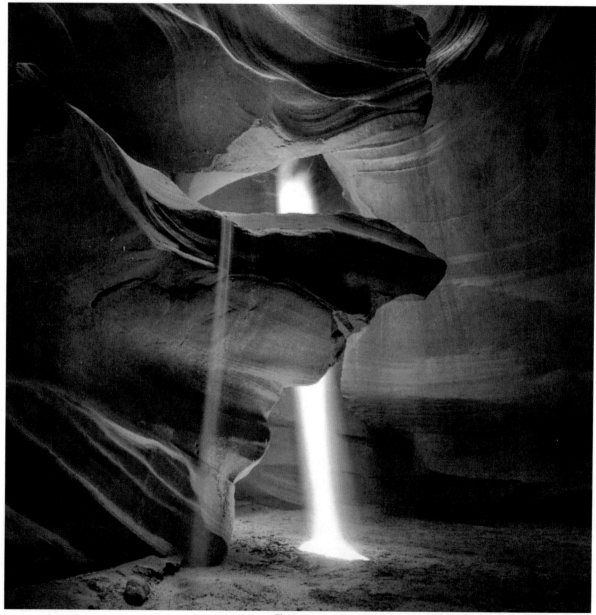

The Layers

396

The Layers

By Stanley Kunitz, written at 101 years of age

I have walked through many lives, some of them my own,
and I am not who I was, though some principle of being abides,
from which I struggle not to stray.

When I look behind, as I am compelled to look
before I can gather strength to proceed on my journey,
I see the milestones dwindling toward the horizon
and the slow fires trailing from the abandoned camp sites,
over which scavenger angels wheel on heavy wings.

Oh, I have made myself a tribe out of my true affections, and my tribe is
scattered! How shall the heart be reconciled to its feast of losses?
In a rising wind the manic dust of my friends,
those who fell along the way, bitterly stings my face.

Yet I turn, I turn, exulting somewhat, with my will intact to go wherever I
need to go, and every stone of the road previous to me.

In my darkest night, when the moon was covered
and I roamed through wreckage, a nimbus clouded voice directed me:
"Live in the layers, not on the litter."

Though I lack the art to decipher it, no doubt the next chapter
in my book of transformations is already written.
I am not done with my changes.

Toroidal Energetic Field and Koshas

Spherical consciousness means that your consciousness is bigger than your physical body, and this extended body is the true Self. Visualize that the soul is a bubble, and the body is a manifestation inside the bubble of the soul. The ego brain misidentifies the physical body as the true self rather than the extended soul-form, opposed to *who I am is in my brain, but my extended body is my true self.*

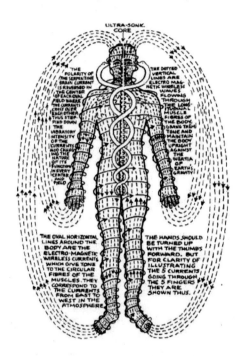

You are a bioelectric, biomagnetic being. A torus is a donut; a toroidal, energetic, unified field representing a process of how multidimensional energies dynamically move. A torus is a coherent field comprised of a central axis with a vortex at both ends. This toroidal donut, this center column, this *Sushumna*, this central channel flows straight though the physical form. Please note, the central channel is not the spine. It is in the center of the body, slightly forward of the spine, running from the crown of the head to the pelvic floor, where most people feel their most powerful emotional and spiritual experiences. The spine is considered a mirror, or a reflex, of the central channel. Therefore, some people experience Kundalini energy running up and down their spine.

The base of the central channel is the pelvic floor. Ancient Sanskrit texts state that both men and women have a yoni at the pelvic floor, with men's being energetic rather than a physical opening, symbolized by the downward pointing triangle just above the pelvic floor in the perineal body area. Earth energy can be drawn up through the energetic yoni to the Third Eye center. The heart chakra's position is in the center of the central channel. The point of the heart center is the center in all three dimensions: 1) between the crown of the head and the pelvic floor 2) between the sides of the body, and 3) between the front and back of the body.

Embody the 3 Points of the Root, Heart, and Crown in the Central Channel:

❖ (*Getting Yoga-weird...*) Place the middle finger of the left hand on the pelvic floor.

❖ Place middle finger of the right hand on the crown of the head.

❖ Sit up straight and intuitively feel the energetic connection between the two points running right through the middle of the body.

❖ Release your hands and continue to feel the connection.

Energy flows in one vortex, travels through the central channel, out the other vortex, and then wraps around itself to return to the first incoming vortex. All living flora and fauna, as well as natural phenomena's such as hurricanes and tornadoes, including planets and stars and galaxies, have toroidal energy systems. At the very center of a torus is a point of singularity of ultimate stillness. This is pure balance, *sattva*.

Ultimately, the human body is a spiritual body system designed to digest the Universe. This human bioenergetic system is a vehicle of expression, transformation, and expansion. The light or heavy energies you encounter are opportunities to create circuitry to align the flow of the torus. Your life experiences consist of circuit building to tune into the pure love frequency, and some consider that this is life's ultimate meaning. As an example, what once caused you friction may no longer have power over your mind and body. Connections were made. *Digestion of energies occurred.*

In every moment, you embody everything in the cosmos. You are informed and influenced by your surroundings as you simultaneously inform and influence those same surroundings. What trajectory of energy will you gift the universe? Ease or dis-ease?

The koshas are fields of energy that are influenced by life experiences. When you resist the integration of the energies you encounter, the torus becomes warped and out of alignment. The chakra system is influenced, and dis-ease is felt within your body, through various physical and mental manifestations. As you know, Yoga is about embodiment. The Practice hones inner awareness to identify where messages are coming from within the body so spiritual/emotional/mental work may be done. When you understand the root of dis-ease, you open space and larger perspectives for holistic alignment to take place.

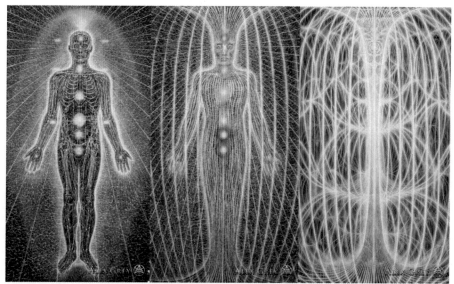

Images by Alex Grey / alexgrey.com

Alex Grey's images represent the three states of being:

1. The basic human template is seen in the LEFT image, bound in the body, identified with the container of this level of consciousness. The egg shape around the form is the toroidal field.

2. The MIDDLE image shows a more pronounced toroidal field of a fully awakened, enlightened being; Christ Consciousness. Awareness of self has shifted beyond the physical body.

3. The image on the RIGHT is a spiritual light-body where there is no physical form; no boundary of beginning and end; a pure connection in the weave of the universe itself.

When you see sacred geometric images, they can serve as your activation. You are, in effect, activated into higher dimensions and consciousness. I recommend you meditate on these images. While doing so, you are receiving more of the energy in your subtle layers that you can then begin to grasp consciously; it is a recoding and repatterning of your own energy field.

To meditate, sink into an image of sacred geometry, feeling the expansion of your Self inter-penetrating the whole field of matter around you. Extend your toroidal field grid through the walls, the floor, through the earth and air, through everything, bringing yourself into harmony with all.

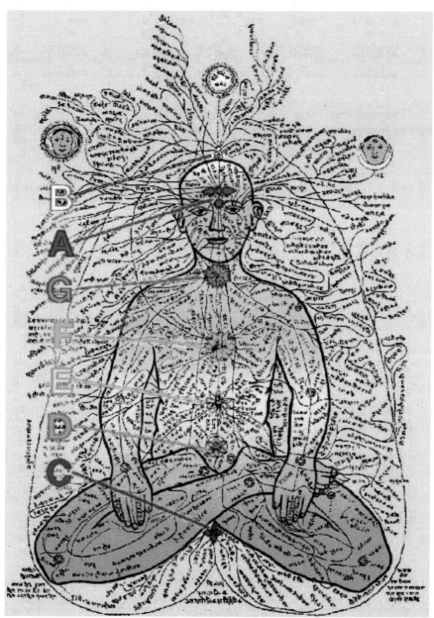

Nadis – Based on Ancient Image

The Nadis, Streams of Life

The Sanskrit word *nadi* derives from the root word *nad*, which means flow, motion, vibration. The nadis are the subtle energy conduits, or streams, in which prana flows throughout the body. The most ancient of tantric texts states there are 35,072,000 nadis which channel prana to every cell. (Today, 72,000 nadis is the accepted number.)

Nadis are very fine and subtle and are not tangible nor visible. For visualization purposes, you can imagine a network of nerves. Nadis are thought to be the first expressions of life within the womb. They are a whole network of extremely subtle tubes which branch out. Nerves, blood vessels, bones, muscles, and flesh then form around these channels. Your body is a perfect reflection of this network of luminous channels. Your own thoughts flow through these channels made of stuff as fine as sunlight. The quality of your thoughts either enliven or dull the pranic force of your chakras. In other words, the quality of your thoughts give rise to your reality.

The three principle nadis are the Sushumna, Ida, and Pingala. These energetic streams are comprised of both feminine and masculine qualities and merge into two main "rivers" – the feminine energy of *Ida* and the masculine energy of *Pingala*. The *Sushumna* is the central channel, located forward of the spine in the middle of the body. The Sushumna connects the Ida and the Pingala nadis.

Originating in the Muladhara Chakra at the base of the central channel are the *Ida* (the left channel) and *Pingala* (the right channel) Nadis, which alternate from the right to the left side at each chakra until they reach the Ajna chakra where they merge with Sushumna, the central channel, midway between the eyebrows at the third eye center. This meeting is called *Mukta Triveni*, liberated. When Ida and Pingala cross, they create the chakra centers. Nadis don't have a physical manifestation, yet Energy/Prana/Qi/Spirit moves through them.

Hatha means "forceful" in Sanskrit. *Ha* and *-tha* combine two powerful esoteric seed mantras.
Ha represents the solar qualities of Pingala; *-tha* represents the lunar qualities of Ida.

Ida ~ Meaning *comfort*. Left channel carries prana, front side of the body (yin), feminine, softer, white, cold, lunar nadi, nurturing by nature, controlling all mental processes, and is associated with the Ganges River.

Pingala ~ Meaning *tawny*. Right channel, back side of the body (yang), masculine, red, hot, solar nadi, stimulated by nature, controls all vital somatic processes, and is associated with the Yamuna River.

Sushumna, the Central Channel ~ *Meaning most gracious, quality-less, unprejudiced Witness.* This channel connects the root chakra to the crown center, balance, associated with the Saraswati River. Within the Sushumna, Kundalini energy moves upwards, running up the body from just below the Muladhara chakra through and beyond the Sahasrara Crown Center.

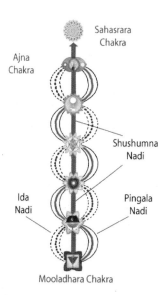

The Ida and Pingala nadis represent the duality of existence; masculine and feminine; Shiva and Shakti. The dualities of masculine/feminine, solar/lunar, yang/yin create existence and are needed by each other to exist. The integration of Shiva and Shakti is represented by *sattva*, or balance within the whole energetic field; alignment. If you are in balance, your awareness is heightened, your perception is expanded, and your life becomes heaven on earth.

Practice

Yoga makes space in the day for practice. Yoga makes space for prana in the mind and heart. Yoga makes space in the body tissues with breath. Breath, *pranayama*, invigorates and strengthens the current of prana which creates unity between the isolated chakras until they are united together, freely exchanging balanced energy, invoking wholeness rather than duality.

When you live inside a duality and use your ego to protect a self-imposed, self-limiting identity, you are disconnected. This is a mental space that doesn't associate with your body's conversations and sensations, therefore the flow of prana between the chakras is restricted. The outer world is limited through your judgments and emotions, or the lack thereof. When you drop back into your body through Yoga or other means, prana flows, and light expands throughout the koshas. You can then access truth and see your place in the world more clearly.

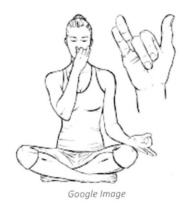

Google Image

To balance Ida and Pingala, practice **Nadi Shodhana**. Nadi Shodhana is the most universal form of Yogic breathing. The left nostril represents the feminine/lunar/cooling energies. The right nostril represents the masculine/solar/warming energies.

Practice this calming and aligning breath at the beginning or end of an asana or meditation practice. **This powerful, alternate-nostril breathing cleanses the nadis, purifies and balances the subtle**

405

channels of the body, and awakens the two hemispheres of the brain. Throughout the day, bring awareness to Ida and Pingala energies by noticing if the left or right nostril is more open (dominant) than the other while recognizing your mind-state at the time. Nostril dominance alternates approximately every 90 minutes. Ask yourself if you need more lunar (restful) or solar (active) energies? Remember, this harkens to the gunic energy of Tamas, Rajas, and Sattva.

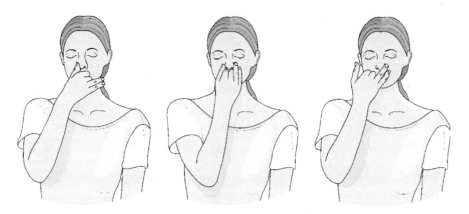

How

❖ Sit comfortably, strong in your spine and soft in your body.

❖ Gently close your eyes and exhale fully.

❖ Allow your left hand to rest on your knee with your thumb and index finger lightly touching.

❖ Take the thumb of your right hand and close your right nostril. *My personally preferred technique has my fingers pointed to the sky.*

❖ Inhale slowly and fully through your left nostril and hold your breath at the top of the inhalation.

❖ Your right thumb remains pressing against your right nostril, while your right pinky closes your left nostril.

❖ Only your right thumb releases to exhale from your right nostril. Your left nostril is still closed.

❖ Inhale slowly and fully from your right nostril.

❖ Close off your right nostril with your thumb.

❖ Exhale from your left nostril, lifting your right pinky.

❖ Repeat this alternating pattern for several more rounds, focusing your awareness on the pathway of your breath – up one side of your body (from your pelvic floor to the crown of your head), and back down the other side of your body (from the crown of your head to your pelvic floor).

Tips

❖ It is important that your breath remains slow, gentle, fluid, and relaxed throughout the practice.

❖ I don't usually count out loud during inhales or exhales to my class when I teach this technique, as counting causes anxiety for many people. However, you can use a silent count to establish a breathing pattern that you are comfortable with. For example, inhale to the count of four, hold for the count of four, exhale to the count of four. This count can be adjusted based on your comfort level.

❖ If you are feeling lethargic, close off your left nostril and breathe only through the right nostril to support the building of energy. If you are feeling aggravated, close off your right nostril and breathe only through the left nostril to support a calming energy.

Kundalini, The Source of the Universe

When you are ready in your spiritual practice and spiritual life to work through a specific knot, then the energy will get stuck to that point.

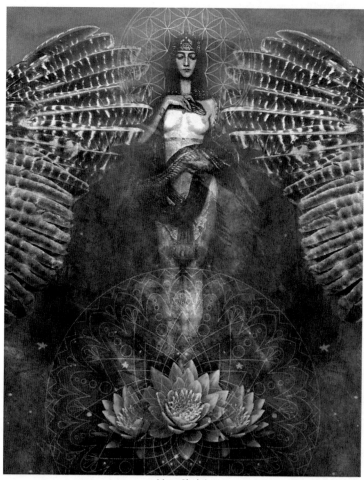

Mata Shakti

Energy is called Kundalini Shakti. The word *Shakti* means Power, Potency, and Goddess. *Kundalini Shakti*, the Goddess Serpent, is considered The Mother of the Universe, with an all-encompassing creative power which is the source of everything.

Kundalini literally means coiled power and has both a very broad and a very specific definition, depending on the context. In the original tradition, Kundalini refers to the phonemic power of mantra. This power is unlocked by lighting up different parts of the oral pallet with the tongue by speaking Sanskrit, which then lights up and activates different parts of the brain. Tone and intention are key here. Mantra, chants, or sounds can help activate certain channels, energy centers, or chakras in the body.

Bija mantras (pronounced BEEJ), also called *Beej Mantras*, means seed. *Bijas* are single syllable vibrating sounds endowed with great spiritual powers, and they are tools for expansion. They are like batteries of mantras, leveraging and activating prana and energy. When chanted with concentration and devotion, bija mantras fulfill the pure desires of the devotee.

For example, each chakra has a bija mantra, which reflects the power of the chakra itself, and is meant to activate that particular chakra along the central channel of the body, or the Sushumna. Kundalini can be awakened through the power inherent in these super-charged bija mantras, which are only found in the Tantric Tradition, except for the use of Om. Om is linked to Indian culture, Buddhism, Hinduism, and Jainism, and is not limited to Tantra.

The WHO: Expansion and Contraction

It is the nature of consciousness to contract and expand, again and again and again. Here, you experience yourself in two radically different ways. One is a limited, contracted, separate, individual existence. It can feel like agitation and confusion. The other experience is that of a mystical, expanded state where you understand yourself as a unified consciousness that fills the whole universe. It feels like being in integrity and alignment, regardless of the situation.

Belief in your own separation is the engine that amplifies contraction. Through the power of ignorance, *Maya*, energy can contract so much that it imagines itself to be an insignificant, unworthy, limited individual. This is illusion. Through spiritual insight and continued practice, the contractions won't be as extreme when they occur. But know that contractions must occur because they give rise to your expansion, and expansion is the path to liberation.

A very simplified and worldly example of expansion and contraction is consciously opening yourself up to be more patient with others around you. The contraction can come through a slow driver or being with someone who is agitating you, but they both offer opportunities for you to practice your patience with a mindset change. The contraction is the practice ground for integrating your expansion.

While in a contraction, feeling into the wisdom of your gut is key. When there is continued agitation or stagnancy in a contracted space, look at what you are attached to, what your ego identifies with, and what you are defending. <u>You</u> need to change, not the situation. The contraction is often the doorway into the Void of the Unknown; the beginning of a Hero's Journey.

The WHY: The Uchara Practice to Awaken Kundalini

Kundalini pierces and opens chakras through a practice called *Uchara* (*Uccara*). This is an upward push of energy in a traditional Tantric Meditation, with the highest aim of self-realization. Uchara means the utterance of a mantra.

Uchara raises a bija mantra through the central channel to the point of the physical palate. You move a living seed of sound through the subtle chakras into the headspace where it resonates. Depending on the specific practice chosen, this mantra is invoked in silence or through intonation. At times, the, energy may be moving smoothly, and at other times, it may feel knotted.

In practice, if you are raising the bija mantra up the central channel and it feels stuck somewhere, then you have found a *granthi*, or a knot. A *granthi* is a densification of psychic energy beneath any given chakra. It is made up of a network of *samskaras/vasanas*, which are impressions of unresolved past experiences of pleasure and pain, including trauma.

The WHAT: Varied Types of Kundalini practices

The Chakra Theory is comprised of varied histories and systems, which are lineage-dependent, each with different ways of working with the spiritual energy of Shakti.

One Kundalini System:

This is the Western 6 + 1 Chakra System known as the Seven Chakra System. Opposing pranic forces that circulate within the Ida and Pingala nadis are unified, awakening and guiding Kundalini from her coiled existence around the coccyx to rise up the Sushumna (the central nadi channel), energizing all chakras.

Two Kundalini System:

The Kaula Lineages are the transgressive left-handed, goddess oriented, radically non-dual lineages. Here, there are two Kundalini's in both the crown and the base. To descend or rise, they both need to be activated. The two Kundalini's become one.

Three Kundalini System:

Many spiritual traditions all over the world have three fundamental centers in common – the head, heart, and lower belly/base. These centers are where three Kundalinis reside. You must awaken the central power of your heart, squeeze/compress your lower power to ascend energy, and usher the descent of your crown's upper energy. The three Kundalinis meet in your heart.

The HOW

When you work with a knot, you work with *Nada Suchi*. This Sanskrit term literally means the needle made of mantric power. This is Kundalini energy that pierces knots using the sound vibration of a mantra. You focus your attention at the base of the blockage and vibrate tone there as strong as you can. This takes focused practice. Eventually, the granthi is pierced, and the flower of the chakra opens. Like the granthi, a physical flower has a dense structure of plant material at its base. When you make a flower garland in India, for example, you take a literal needle and thread and pierce the flower through the base. This is a metaphor of what is happening energetically when Kundalini moves.

PRACTICES

There are many different practices that honor the bija – from japa mala meditations to visualization meditations to chanting. Here are two bija practices to move Kundalini energy:

Heart Glow

❖ Visualize Pure Presence pouring into the crown of your head, giving rise to the whole universe. Summon this Pure Goddess Power down into your heart, using your breath. Infuse this energy with your sense of smallness and separate individuality.

❖ Hold your breath in this space. Mentally vibrate the mantra *Hreem*, or a bija mantra of your choice.

❖ *Hreem* is the bija mantra of goddess Bhuvaneshwari, an avatar of Parvati, Shiva's other half. Parvati is the divine feminine Shakti energy. It is believed to connect you to the energies of Shiva and Shakti, simultaneously.

❖ Hold your breath for as long as you can, without strain. As you release, you may experience an energetic surge up the central channel. Repeat.

Bija Chakra Balancing

❖ Begin by sitting comfortably. (I often meditate seated in a chair.) Make sure that you're able to sit up straight and tall and that your sitting bones are grounded, balancing your shoulders over your hips, your head over your shoulders, with your chin parallel to the earth.

❖ Close your eyes and breathe deeply into your body. Complete 3-7 full and complete breaths before continuing.

❖ Bring your attention and breath to each chakra location as you chant 3X the associated bija mantra for that location, as listed below:

  o **LAM - Red Root Chakra**
  o VAM - Orange Sacral Chakra
  o RAM - Yellow Solar Plexus Chakra
  o **YAM - Green Heart Chakra**
  o HAM - Blue Throat Chakra
  o **OM - Indigo Third Eye Chakra**
  o **Silence - Purple Crown Chakra**

❖ At your crown, feel your energy rise up and out of the crown, reaching upwards into the beyond. Stay here in silence for as long as you feel comfortable. Then slowly, bring your attention back down to each location through, moving through your crown, third eye, throat, heart, solar plexus, sacrum and then root chakra.

❖ Ground your energy down through your hips and/or your feet. When you're ready to come back into the room, slowly open your eyes.

Western Chakra System

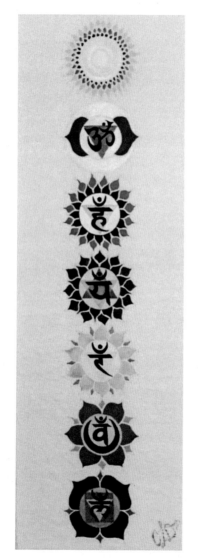

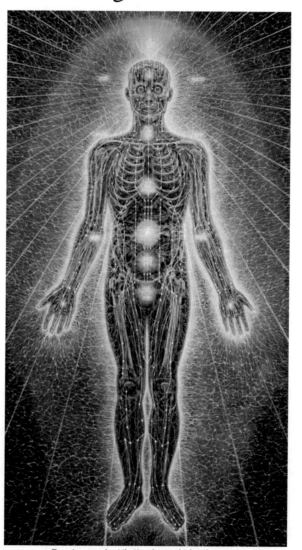

Two Images by Lily Kessler and Alex Grey

The 6 + 1 Chakra System

Chakras are compressed energy bodies within the koshas, which make up the physical, etheric, emotional, mental, and spiritual body. Information for the koshas is received in the gut because it is more sensitive and receptive than the brain. The gut receives billions of bits of information and feeds it to the brain. It is from this loop of information (from your gut to your brain and back and then repeat, forever repeating) that you create your perception of reality.

The theory of the subtle body and the energy centers, called the *chakras* (*cakras*), is from Tantra. The energy body is nonphysical and supersensuous and is experienced experientially through the energy centers of the chakras. In Sanskrit, the literal meaning of chakra is a 'spinning wheel or disc' glowing with light and harkening to celestial bodies.

The chakras can be thought of as more than just "spinning discs of energy" within your body. In fact, the chakras extend well beyond your body, including overhead and underneath you. They establish a toroidal field of energy that surrounds your physical body. They also represent "bandwidths" of energy that extend both within and outside of your physical body. Understanding the chakras helps you maintain both your internal integrity and balance, as well as your interconnectedness and balance with the world around you.

The energetic converging points of the nadis (channels, meridians) give rise to a particular chakra center. Chakra centers are focal points for meditation within the body, often visualized as shapes of energy frequency resembling lotus flowers or discs. There are many chakra system theories within the original tradition of Tantra. It is important to note that each of the many Tantric branches expresses a different chakra system, or more than one. Various lineages host practices anywhere from a three-chakra system to a five, six, seven, nine, ten, twelve, sixteen, or twenty-one chakra system, and more!

All chakra systems have three specific energy centers in common: the belly/sexual center, the heart center, and the crown center. Humans feel emotional and spiritual sensations in these areas, yet it is

415

also understood that these felt sensations are not related to the anatomy of the physical body. Rather, these sensations are the experience of the energy body, providing a *fluid reality* within the various energy centers. A common visualization associated with experiencing these energetic sensations is to ask, "Where do I feel this emotion in my body?"

Chakra systems are prescriptive. For example, a six-chakra practice embodies deity energy, a five-chakra practice internalizes the five-elements, and the three-bindu system opens your awareness of reality. Specific visualizations are given on subtle objects made of colored light, shaped in a particular way, activated in specific areas of the body, and/or enlivened with purposeful mantra.

The main purpose of the chakra system is to embody deity-energies through mantra at specific points in the energy body. The sounds of Sanskrit are offered to each of the petals of the chakras, and each. Each chakra is also associated with the Great Elements of Earth, Water, Fire, Wind/Air, Space/Ether. This is a practice called *nyasa*, which literally means "depositing" or "setting down" purpose-specific mantras on various parts of the body while silently chanting/feeling its sound during meditation. Ultimately, this is the ancient practice of healing through sound vibration, invoking the energy of a specific deity/energy, in a specific area of the body.

Geometric shapes associated with the chakras also belong to the Great Elements, not the geometry of the chakra itself. Earth is a yellow square, Water is a silver crescent, Fire is an inverted red triangle, Wind is a six-pointed star, and Space is a circle. These Great Elements are infused in seed-sounds. LAM is the seed-mantra of Earth. VAM for water, RAM for fire, YAM for wind, HAM for space, AUM for Third Eye, AUM for Crown.

The Seven Chakra System, more accurately called *the 6+1 chakra system*, has been present since the thirteenth century, based on a text called *The Sarada-tilaka*. In 1577, a man named Purnananda Yati provided an explanation of the six chakras based on this original text. In 1918, John Woodroffe interpreted Purnananda's translation, which gave rise to the Western notions on the subject, and therefore Western Yogic authors. This Seven Chakra System is considered Western occultism, which means that these notions are from a tradition that spans only decades, without the pedigree of centuries. (The term *the West* encompasses Euro-American understandings of Yoga, which is now also pervasive in India.)

Assigning a psychological state to a chakra as a lump-whole, in contrast to the original Sanskrit text stating *each petal of each chakra* is associated with a particular mantra/energy, began with Carl Jung in his book *The Psychology of Kundalini Yoga* (1932). Anodea Judith's *Wheels of Life* began other chakra associations, infused with psychology, colors, sounds, bodily and emotional functions, and levels of consciousness. Today, the Seven Chakra System has many contributors, and many associations and correspondents to gems, herbs, metals, planets, angels, Yogic paths, asana postures, essential oils, etc.

This tradition states that chakras are subject to imbalances, having depleted or excessive energy caused by samskaras, daily stresses, trauma, or internalized cultural values that are out of place with individual values. When balanced, you feel wholeness and a sense of alignment because *prana* (vital life force) is flowing. When high vibrational frequency is increased through various Yoga practices, this flow becomes easier to generate and maintain. Integration of your energy raises your creativity, heals your wounds, and allows the atman to be expressed.

The bulk of the original chakra system teachings are limited to scholars, yet some modern academics are strengthening this conversation in more public arenas. Yet, occultism does not negate the benefits of this newer Seven Chakra System. The point of Yoga practice is to embody and digest the universe, which is supported by this modern system. The world of Yoga is in a fascinating era, and the knowledge of its ancient roots will only amplify newer traditions as they develop.

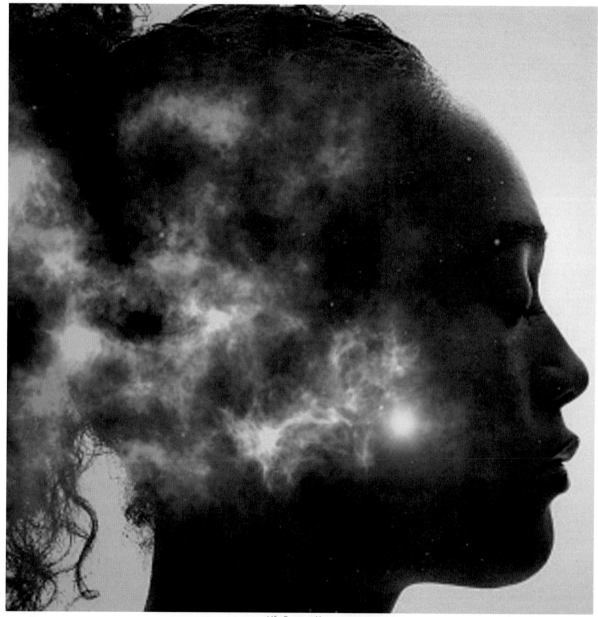

Life Force = You

418

Psychology and Chakras

I am not a demon; I am not in hell. I am not a victim; I'm not a hungry ghost, I'm not dependent on something outside of myself. I'm not an animal; I don't need to numb myself. I'm not just a human mind that needs information. I'm not a Titan; I don't need to be better than anybody, or achieve and accomplish. I'm not a god; I don't need to feel the attachment to be blissed out or in judgement all the time. ~ Christopher Wallis

Western Yoga Culture, along with the work of Carl Jung, has influenced the addition of the psychological states within the 6 + 1 chakra system. This contrasts with other Tantric philosophies, where mental narratives are not fed by the mind.

You are striving to go beyond your conditioned mind and your socially constructed identity and labels. This includes your psychology of experiencing yourself as an energetic reality; a complexification of light and power and energy, which is something much closer to your true nature.

The Western Chakra System gives you fodder to feed your mind-narrative, like psychological associations. Tantra Yoga teaches you that your Divine Self is significant, not your psychological state. However, understanding psychological aspects can be a key to self-understanding through embodiment principles which can lead to self-realization.

The closest information regarding psychological associations comes from Buddhist sources, naming six chakras relating to six realms. This is called the Six Realms of Existence. (Note that the term *realm* is not a plane of existence, but rather it is a psychological state.)

If you can see that you are fixated in a particular realm, you can be freed. In a meditation practice, you purify and transmute these twisted and distorted understandings of yourself by bringing attention and new energies to particular physical and subtle areas. Your True Nature is not any of these Six Realms. The Six Realms are, in fact, how you lose yourself, how you fail to recognize your true nature, by fixating on an aspect of your psyche which is not your essence-nature.

419

The 6 Realms of Existence

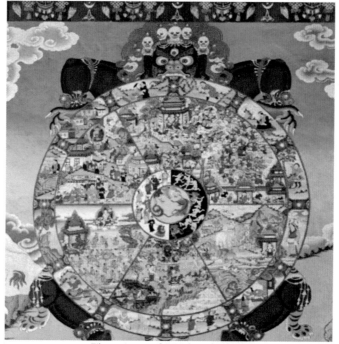

Tibetan Image of 6 Realms of Rebirth

Demon Realm, or **Hell Realm**, is the realm you believe in when you believe you have been unfairly wronged and victimized. You are filled with hatred for those who did you wrong. Send the energy of unconditional love to the Muladhara Chakra.

Hungry Ghost Realm is the realm you occupy if you constantly look outside of yourself for fulfillment, perhaps in terms of sex, money, power, achievement/recognition, the right spiritual teaching, the right partner, etc. Whatever you are looking outside of yourself for, hoping whatever it is will finally fulfill you, makes you feel as if you are a hungry ghost. In Indian stories, a form has a tiny neck and a huge belly, as they can never get enough. Send the energy of generosity to the Svadhisthana Chakra.

Animal Realm is the realm of being as an animal is, as it relates to laziness, dullness, ignorance, and numbing out behavior. This stems from ignorance on how to be happy. Send the energy of wisdom to the Manipura Chakra.

Human Mind Realm is localized in the heart center. In ancient India, thoughts and the mind were experienced in the heart. This is the realm of the lack of openness; wanting to have all the information first or know information better than others to have a sense of control or power. It is the critical and fearful parts of the self. It is the need to be seen and understood and to feel loved. How can someone know and understand you when you are still figuring out who you are? Instead, you know that every being is a divine mystery that you cannot comprehend. Send the energy of openness to your Heart Chakra. It is okay to open yourself up to unknowing (that you don't really know anything for sure).

Titan Realm is centered on pride and competition. The United States and the corporate world are in the Titan Realm. Send the energy of peace to the Vishuddha Chakra, soothing that aspect of yourself that must get ahead and be better than others.

God Realm, the **Deva Realm**, is the place you get trapped in by the fixation of your own specialness. You need to feel yourself as superior to others, attached to spiritual highs. This is a place of suffering, but you don't know you are suffering until a later time. Send the energy of compassion to your Crown Center.

You abide in your *True Nature* when you are not fixated on any one realm. When you recognize that YOU are none of these illusionary realms, you land in your essence-nature and love *what is*. You never shrink from what is given to you, be it the blessings or the work. You live in the present moment.

Do not be attached to what you do or who you think you are. Rather, be with what is and flow with what is in a natural, spontaneous meeting of moment after moment. *This is being clean and clear, open, and present, free of agenda, free of the need to justify yourself, willing to be with what is, whatever it is.* This is the natural state that is free of fixation.

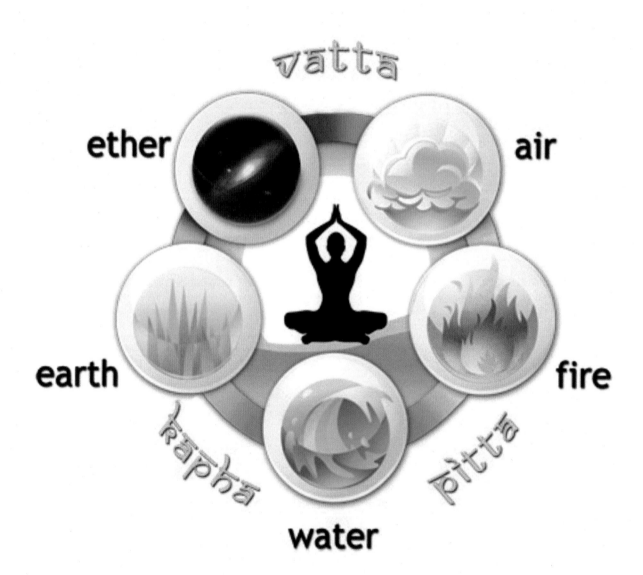

Bija Seed Mantras ~ The 5 Elements

❖ **Ether (space):** all encompassing, pure potentiality, light, subtle and clear
❖ **Air:** movement, change, light, mobile, clear, rough, and dry.
❖ **Fire:** transformation, hot, direct, assimilation, digestion, metabolism, sharp, fluid, penetrating
❖ **Water:** cohesion, protection, taste, heavy, wet, lubricating, cool, soft
❖ **Earth:** solid structure, form, grounded, stable, thick, dense, solid, hard, heavy, stable

	Space / Ether	Wind / Air	Fire	Water	Earth
Chakra	5th Throat Vishuddha	4th Heart Anahata	3rd Solar Plexus Manipura	2nd Sacral Svadhisthana	1st Root Muladhara
Sound	HAM	YAM	RAM	VAM	LAM
Sense	Sound	Touch	Sight	Taste	Fragrance
Organ	Ears	Skin	Eyes	Tongue	Nose
Motor	Vocal Chords	Hands	Legs	Reproductive Organs	Excretory Organs

Muladhara Chakra

First Chakra, Root Chakra, Base Chakra

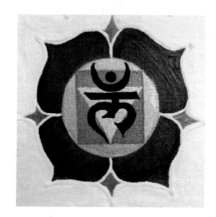

I am here; here I am. I belong. I have a right to be alive, happy, and free.

- ❖ **Location:** base of the spine, reigning bones, legs, feet, genitals, blood, teeth, kidneys, nails
- ❖ **Development:** womb-12 months
- ❖ **Relations:** self-preservation and physical safety, strength and vitality, survival needs, prosperity, I belong, I Am, truth, decision, commitment, defense
- ❖ **In balance:** emotional and spiritual stability, awareness, groundedness, connected to home/work, strong health, feeling 'at home' anywhere
- ❖ **Out of balance:** insecurity, anxiety, mental/physical lethargy, inability to be still, defensive

- ❖ **Element:** earth / smell
- ❖ **Color:** red
- ❖ **Bija Seed EARTH ELEMENT Sound:** LAM (can be used to bring Earth energy into any chakra)
- ❖ **Vowel Sound:** Uh
- ❖ **Musical Note:** C, 396 Hertz, liberates guilt and fear and energizes achievement goals
- ❖ **Pranayama:** Ujjayi, Apana Vayu breath with visualization of breathing from the heavens through the crown center and into the earth
- ❖ **Mudra:** Chinmaya Mudra, Gesture for Embodied Knowledge
- ❖ **Bandha:** Mula Bandha

Activated by gravity, invoking slow movements to anchor consciousness with easy rooted-balancing, leg stretches, and folds.

- ❖ **Recommended Asanas:** Easy Seated, Balancing Poses, Forward Folds, Mountain, lunges, leg stretches, Cat/Cow Variations, Knee-to-Chest, Locust, Plank, Side Plank, Downward Facing Dog, Goddess, Chair, Pyramid, Warrior 2, Half Moon, Tree, Yogi Squat, Boat, Butterfly, Plow, Pigeon, Hero's, Frog, Rabbit, King Dancer, Child's Pose

Svadhisthana Chakra

Second Chakra, Sacral Center, Wisdom Body

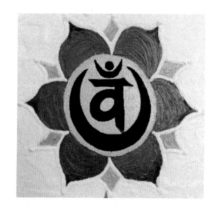

I feel Truth in my gut, and I abide by this wisdom. I flow through life like water.

- ❖ **Location:** just below the naval, reigning the pelvis, lower back, sex organs, bladder, prostate adrenal glands, fluid function, nervous system
- ❖ **Development:** 6-24 months
- ❖ **Relations:** sensuality, attraction, social connections, raw power, emotional identity, sense of self, self-gratification, creative potential, trust, sexuality, wisdom center, relationships, generating like and dislike

❖ **In balance:** creativity, joy, expression of feelings, desire, connection, go with the flow, trust, intuitive, trusts change and embraces transformation

❖ **Out of balance:** guilt, frustration, lack of connection, emotional instability, lower back pain

❖ **Element:** water / taste

❖ **Color:** orange

❖ **Bija Seed WATER ELEMENT Sound:** VAM (can be used to bring Water energy into any chakra)

❖ **Vowel Sound:** Ooo

❖ **Musical Note:** D, 417 Hertz, clears energetics of past events and facilitates transformation

❖ **Pranayama:** Deep Belly Breath, Apana Vayu and Vyana Vayu breath with visualization

❖ **Mudra:** Svadhisthana Mudra, Gesture of the Inner Dwelling Place of Balance

❖ **Bandha:** Mula Bandha

Activated by fluid, sensuous movements, deep and full breath cycles, lunges, and twists.

❖ **Recommended Asanas:** Boat, Pigeon, Downward Facing Dog, Lunge, Twists, Cat/Cow Variations, Eagle, Warrior 2, Warrior 3, Bow, Wheel, Locust, Child's Pose, Crow, Easy Seated, King Dancer, Plank & Side Plank, Chair, Pyramid, Rotated Triangle, Half Moon, Plow, Frog, Hero's, Tree, Yogi Squat, Knee-to-Chest, Goddess, Butterfly

Manipura Chakra

Third Chakra, Solar Plexus Chakra, Seat of 1000 Suns, City of Jewels

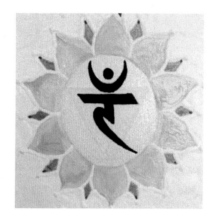

I reside in non-dominating willpower. I Am That.

- ❖ **Location:** solar plexus a finger height above navel, reigning the stomach, digestive system, muscles, diaphragm, lower back, pancreas, gall bladder, liver, spleen
- ❖ **Development:** 18 months – 4 years
- ❖ **Relations:** Sense of self, individuality, integrity, will power, ego identity, personal power, purpose, productivity, desire, emotional balance
- ❖ **In balance:** energy, effectiveness, spontaneity, self-will and personal power, autonomy, metabolism, identity, strong and clear boundaries, open to possibility, embracing uniqueness

428

- ❖ **Out of balance:** shame, fear, anxiety, need to control, oversensitive to criticism, stomach ulcers, diabetes, allergies, chronic fatigue, low self-esteem, need to control
- ❖ **Element:** fire
- ❖ **Color:** yellow / gold
- ❖ **Bija Seed FIRE ELEMENT Sound:** RAM (can be used to bring Fire energy into any chakra) **Vowel Sound:** Ah
- ❖ **Musical Note:** E, 528 Hertz, activates imagination, intention, intuition to 'see' a higher purpose
- ❖ **Pranayama:** Breath of Fire (Kapalabhati), Samana Vayu with visualization upward/downward breath
- ❖ **Mudra:** Vajra Mudra, Gesture of the Diamond
- ❖ **Bandha:** Uddiyana Bandha

Activated by energized limbs and torso with strong drishti to build prana,
Including balances, twists, and extended side stretches.

- ❖ **Recommended Asanas:** Balancing, Twists, Standing Side Stretch, Bow, Downward Facing Dog, Chair, Triangle, Lunges, King Dancer, Boat, Warrior 1, 2, 3, Locust, Plank, Side Plank, Extended Side Angle, Half Moon, Tree, Forward Folds, Bridge, Goddess, Lunge Twists, Pigeon, Camel, Crow

Anahata Chakra

Fourth Chakra, Heart Chakra, Unstruck, Unbreakable

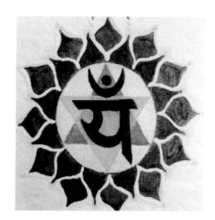

Namaste. The Universe loves me, and I trust life unfolds in my favor.

- ❖ **Location:** the center of the chest in heart space (heaven meets earth), reigning the skin, chest, hands, upper back, thymus gland, circulation, arms
- ❖ **Development:** 4 – 7 years old
- ❖ **Relations:** self-acceptance, service, forgiveness, zest for life, Divine Relationship, connects lower 3 chakras and upper 3 chakras, love for self, universe, others,
- ❖ **In balance:** loved, wise, stable, compassion, empathy, devotion, acceptance, faith, altruism, passion, balance, conscious lovemaking, nurturing

❖ **Out of balance:** grief, fear, discomfort, lack of compassion, lonely, unloved, fear of betrayal, codependency, shallow breathing, melancholia, high blood pressure, heart disease

❖ **Element:** wind (instead of air, as the nature of this element is mobility) / touch

❖ **Color:** emerald green / rose pink

❖ **Bija Seed WIND ELEMENT Sound:** YAM (can be used to bring Wind energy into any chakra)

❖ **Vowel Sound:** Ah

❖ **Musical Note:** F, 639 Hertz, activates cell communication, releases genetic and family trauma

❖ **Pranayama:** Viloma, Prana Vayu and Samana Vayu with visualization of upward/downward breath with full attention on the heart space. Inhale appreciation; exhale love and healing

❖ **Mudra:** Padma Mudra, Gesture of the Lotus

❖ **Bandha:** Mula Bandha & Jalandhara Bandha

Activated by opening the heart gate with backbends,
side stretches with the heart rotated upward.

❖ **Recommended Asanas:** Backbends, Camel, Puppy, Cobra, Humble Warrior, Mountain, Bridge, Bow, King Dancer, Triangle, Rotated Triangle, Crescent Moon, Sphinx, Fish, Supported Plank, Child's Pose

Vishuddha Chakra

Fifth Chakra, Throat Chakra, Manifestor Chakra

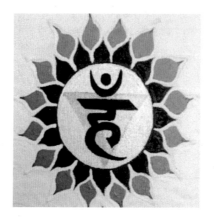

The quality of my thoughts and words creates my reality.

- ❖ **Location:** base of neck, reigning the throat, mouth, neck, jaw, ears, voice, lungs, airways, arms, hands, thyroid, parathyroid
- ❖ **Development:** 7 – 12 years
- ❖ **Relations:** contentment, self-expression, artistry, ability to speak and listen, ease in meditation, boundaries, imagination, source of communication, a key channel for your heart

❖ **In balance:** strong ability to listen/speak with discernment and clarity, eloquence in communication and body language, considering perspectives while rooted, fluent, clear

❖ **Out of balance:** lies, confusion, in-articulation, insecurity in self & spirit, perfectionism, blocked creativity, inability to communicate nor listen, neck ache, asthma, Thyroid issues

❖ **Element:** sound / hearing / focus

❖ **Color:** bright blue

❖ **Bija Seed SPACE ELEMENT Sound:** HAM (can be used to bring Space/Ether energy into any chakra)

❖ **Vowel Sound:** Ee (as in see)

❖ **Musical Note:** G, 741 Hertz, reveals possibility, harnesses self-will, and allows self-expression

❖ **Pranayama:** Ujjayi, Udana Vayu with visualization

❖ **Mudra:** Kali Mudra, Gesture of the Goddess of Spiritual Purification

❖ **Bandha:** Jalandhara Bandha

Activated by throat expanding movements paired with sound to move throughout/vibrate the body, with back bends allowing the throat to be exposed skyward OR the throat curled toward chest.

❖ **Recommended Asanas:** Backbends, Bridge, Shoulder Stand, Camel, Fish, Rabbit, Yoga Mudra, Plow, Child's Pose, Boat

Ajna Chakra

6th Chakra, Third Eye, Seat of Intuition

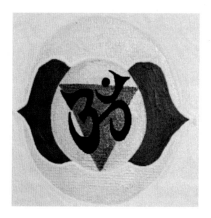

I listen to the truth in the wisdom of my body.

- ❖ **Pronounced 'Ag-ni-a' with a hard -g sound**
- ❖ **Location:** center of the brain, reigning the brow center, base of skull, ears, nose, sinuses, nervous system, pituitary and pineal gland, left eye, left brain
- ❖ **Development:** Adolescence – more conscious choices
- ❖ **Relations:** self-mastery, archetypal identity, self-reflection, perception, inspiration, sixth sense, inner vision, receptivity, source of insight, psychic information, imagination

- ❖ **In balance:** in-line with the Witness Self, psychic/intuitive, extraordinary phenomena, larger perspectives, freedom from attachment, charisma
- ❖ **Out of balance:** untrusting, muddled thinking, distracted, learning difficulties, closed to change or new ideas, frustrated by others and self, nightmares, headaches, poor vision
- ❖ **Element:** light / time
- ❖ **Color:** indigo / white
- ❖ **Bija Seed Sound:** Om, Aum
- ❖ **Vowel Sound:** mmm
- ❖ **Musical Note:** A, 852 Hertz, pierces personal illusions and allows insights into motives and agendas
- ❖ **Pranayama:** Alternate Nostril Breath (Nadi Shodona), Udana Vayu and Vyana Vayu with visualization
- ❖ **Mudra:** Trishula Mudra, Gesture of the Trident
- ❖ **Bandha:** Mahabandha

Activated by openings to support internal seeing, while flushing the prana within and through all chakras with visualization and breath work.

- ❖ **Recommended Poses:** Child's Pose with forehead on mat, Downward Dog, Fish, Head-to-Knee, Yoga Mudra, Eagle, Head Stand, Shoulder Stand, Plow, Handstand, Puppy, Yoga Mudra, Folds, Bow

Sahasrara Crown Center

Thousand-Petal Lotus

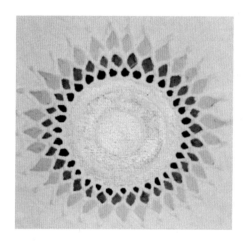

I am always One with All.

❖ **Location:** crown of skull, reigning central nervous system, skin, pineal gland, cerebral cortex, right eye, right brain

❖ **Development:** search for meaning, see multiverse

❖ **Relations:** thought, Universal identity, self-knowledge

❖ **In balance:** bliss, empathy, magnetism, wisdom, death of the body, release of karmas, meditation, transcendence, mental connection to everything

- ❖ **Out of balance:** depression, confusion, obsessive thinking, chronic exhaustion, epilepsy, Alzheimer's
- ❖ **Element:** ether / thought
- ❖ **Color:** violet or white
- ❖ **Bija Seed Sound:** none
- ❖ **Vowel Sound:** nngg (as in 'sing')
- ❖ **Musical Note:** B, 963 Hertz, enables direct experience of holistic Divinity
- ❖ **Mudra:** Ananta Mudra, Gesture of Infinity
- ❖ **Bandha:** none &/or Mahabandha
- ❖ **Pranayama:** Breath of Bees (Brahmari), Vyana Vayu, Prana Vayu, Apana Vayu with visualization

Activated by poses that support the release of attachment and increase the awareness of presence and fully consciousness experiences.

- ❖ **Recommended Asanas:** Meditation, Rabbit, Savasana, Fish, Wide-Leg Forward Fold, Head Stand, Child's Pose

Tying It Together:
A Summary of the Building Blocks of the Energetic Body

GUNA + DOSHA + KOSHA + NADIS + CHAKRAS = YOUR UNIQUE REALITY

Your physical body and your unique perception of reality is a part of an interactive energetic system that includes the gunas, doshas, koshas, nadis, and chakras. Each system supports your holistic alignment, from your condensed form to your subtle bodies.

Introduced in Samkhya Philosophy, combinations of the gunas influence your perspective of Reality, which is comprised of Prakriti (the universe). The gunas are the energies of tamas, rajas, and sattva. Particular guna combinations give rise to the three doshas of Ayurveda.

The three doshas are pita, vata, and kapha. Each of the doshas are directly associated with the natural elements of earth, wind, fire, water, and ether, existing in various combinations. Every life form and object are influenced by the gunas in this realm of Prakriti. Doshas reveal aspects of your life where you need to find balance; *opposite energies heal, same energies exacerbate.*

The koshas are the field of Lila, in which the concept of individual reality is explored. The koshas define the five energetic layers of consciousness, including the physical, spiritual, mental/emotional, wisdom, and bliss layers. Your consciousness extends well beyond the limits of your physical body, which is supported by, and interacts with, the energetic layers and attributes of your subtle bodies. Here, samskaras are created or transformed.

The degree of fluidity between the bliss body and the mental and emotional kosha layers informs the pranic flow of the nadis. The enteric layer of the koshas is the chakra system.

Chakras digest countless bits of information fed by the kosha/nadi relationship. Resulting feelings of how experiences are digested not only give labels to the experiences, but also alters the central nervous system into the modes of *fight or flight* or *cleanse and restore*. To support chakra alignment, the right use of the mind is to understand that holistic growth and healing can be found in every experience, regardless of its resulting label and emotions. **You are larger than these aspects.**

The practice of Yoga and meditation invites consciousness into each moment, into each situation, for growth opportunities. You then respond, not react, to the energies that surround, inform, and support you. You understand and accept that life does things *for you, <u>not</u> to you.* You know experiences arise when you are energetically prepared to meet them, ready to explore your blind spots, and transform into your more aligned and rooted Self.

Universe loves me so much, things are done for me, not to me. This is the mantra that I live my life by every single day. It is also initially difficult to live by, especially when I am in the process of embracing transformation. But the more I show up for the mantra and open into its vast possibility, the more the truth of it shows up for me.

First, I need to note that it is vital to allow myself to feel what I feel. I allow myself to feel sadness, hurt, anger, confusion, and experience ALL of my feelings when they arise. Also, I don't share this mantra when I am supporting another person. I would invalidate his or her feelings and would be insensitively, spiritually abusive. The key is not to bypass what arises within your emotions or your body. Only after the initial storm of emotions have subsided will this mantra have the possibility to open you to higher perspectives that promote even greater healing and additional possibilities.

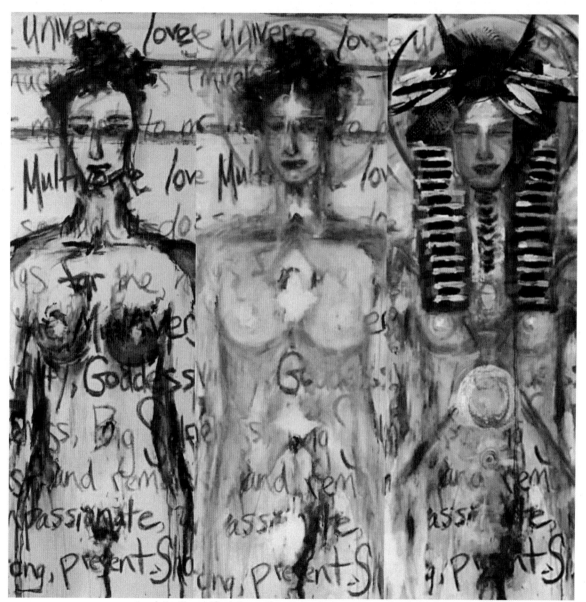

Involution Toward Evolution, self-portrait painting sequence by Lily Kessler

This is my self-portrait; an image comprised of three pictures of the same painting.

The image on the left was born on a day when a piece of news brought me to my knees. I painted my emotions after scratching this sacred mantra into the canvas with pastels. I was scared, saddened, and infuriated. This artistic expression was an intentional practice to acknowledge the moment, though I knew that the image would transform when I digested the energies.

In the coming months, I healed by obtaining new perspectives and boundaries.

The final image was completed after my first experience in Egypt, complete with gold-leaf, iridescence, and sacred symbols. Within myself, I integrated my sorrows as my steppingstones to growth. My circle at this stage in my life was complete.

441

Ancient Realignment Tool for Embodiment

Subject / Object

Stories which arise in your life experiences are made of perceptions, thoughts, beliefs, and attachments that influence chakra alignment, and even the definitions of your reality. These stories, positive or painful, become cheap imitations of Home. People defend their pain and stories infused with pain. To integrate the energies within any story, you must dismantle the story (Object) to bring awareness back to the physical sensations within the body (Subject).

Life is experienced through *Subject/Object*. Tuning into where you feel your emotions within your physical body is called *embodiment*. Keeping yourself focused on your inward energies is considered staying on *Subject*. Tuning into your physical embodiment sensations is your biggest tool to bring you back into alignment; a *sattvic state of being*. Self-empowerment is taking full responsibility for feeling what you feel without blaming another person for 'making' you feel that way.

The ego, conditioned behaviors, belief systems/labels, are based on *Object*. This is a dispersal of energy that focuses on the outer material/physical world. Object is represented by Prakriti, where all beings and situations are teachers to support your spiritual growth. To claim freedom, the reasoning mind, aka *the protective personality*, must unattach from the story.

The WHAT

Feel the location of the emotion in your physical body (the seed) and consciously breathe along the Central Channel into this place. Energy is activated in this place, and with breath, you are moving the shape of energy and dispersing it into a neutral state. Ultimately, understanding and feeling into these activated places increases self-connections, which create Self-wholeness. This also strengthens intuition; feeling into the truth and gut of the body.

Day to day, moment to moment, the practice is to stay *on Subject*; staying present and internally focused on your core. *Remaining on Subject* keeps you story-free and self-accountable for your own emotions.

442

There is no room for victimhood, only opportunities for reflective growth given by *a teacher*. Remember, **all beings are your teacher, and you are a teacher to all beings**. Every living being and situation are teachers who give you opportunities to digest lessons, find ease in navigating situations that arise, and to simply grow in consciousness.

The EXAMPLE

When forming my 300-hour Yoga Training Program, I asked a teacher, who was a specialist in her field, to teach for me. She couldn't do so, as she was under contract with another studio. So I found another teacher who could fulfill the role I needed. Simple enough.

Not so. This teacher became vindictive after I hired another person for the position. She sent an email to her student-base telling them that my studio was not a studio founded in integrity. *Integrity is important to me, to say the least.* The moment I read her email my body began to shake and my heartrate soared. I immediately reached out to a friend to vent before I contacted a lawyer to inquire about slander.

While I shook with astonished rage, my friend said, "Lily, you *are* out of integrity." I about fell to my knees in shock. Then she added, "You continue to do things you don't want to do and continue to work with people you don't want to work with. So, yes, you are out of integrity."

So I did my Yoga. I recognized the teacher who offended me actually offered me an incredible gift through her jealousy. Her message - and the story that was created from it - had a powerful momentum that captured my attention. She revealed to me that I was leaking my lifeforce into places and people that didn't serve me. I finally saw with clarity that I needed to build boundaries, clean slates, and sever ties to ensure I personally stood in solid integrity to reflect the sanctuary of my beloved Yoga studio. It was about the energy of *integrity*, but the story (object) shifted when I focused on myself (subject).

Once I breathed deep into that 'activated' space to anchor myself, things naturally flowed differently. It takes humility to see how you could have handled things differently. It takes strength to lean-in to learn what message needs revealing. Yet this is how you regain your power and heal your life.

443

Practice Subject/Object

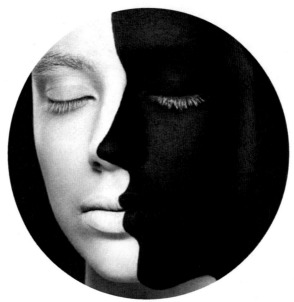

Subject/Object

1) Dismantle the spin of the story.

2) Bring yourself back home to Subject (you), not Object (other) through visualization/breath embodiment practices to move the energy. ***You are feeling energy,*** and this knowledge is known from the higher perspective of Purusha's intelligence.

Emotions are energies, and this knowledge is known from the higher perspective of Purusha's intelligence. When you feel what you feel, bring yourself back into your body (Subject/Inside: self, spirit, soul, and breath), not into a story based on another (Object/Outside: people, worries, social media, etc.), through breathing into where you feel the emotion land in your body. Breath moves and stabilizes energy. Exploring and harnessing emotions are opportunities to deepen authenticity.

444

Duality. Me and you.
Light and dark. Bad and good. Love and fear.
Pleasure and joy. Blame and acceptance.
Ultimately, Yoga is the merging of these dualities.
This requires recognition of the great Both/And;
Extinguishing labels by acknowledging
them to claim equanimity.

~ Lily Kessler

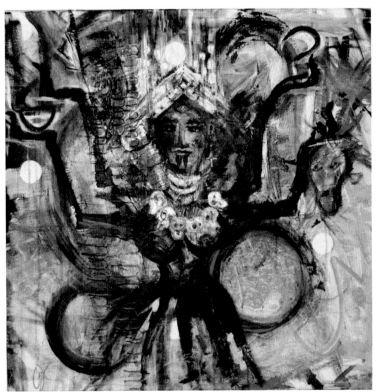

Sister Kali, painting by Lily Kessler

445

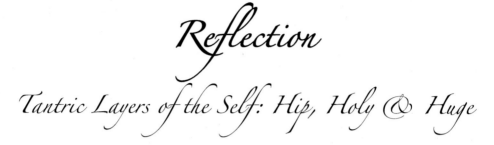

Reflection

Tantric Layers of the Self: Hip, Holy & Huge

1) In your own words, explain the relationship between the koshas, the nadis, and the chakras, and how they define your interaction with the world.

2) For your own personal review, please complete the following.

   Circle the two definitions appropriate for each term:

   Shiva is – masculine / feminine

          potential force / manifested differentiation

   Shakti is – masculine / feminine

          potential force / manifested differentiation

3) There are _____ nadis in the human body. There are three major nadis.

   Where they cross, they create a _____.

4) Describe the attributes of both the Ida Nadi and Pingala Nadi.

5) What is the physical location and name (both English and Sanskrit) for each chakra?

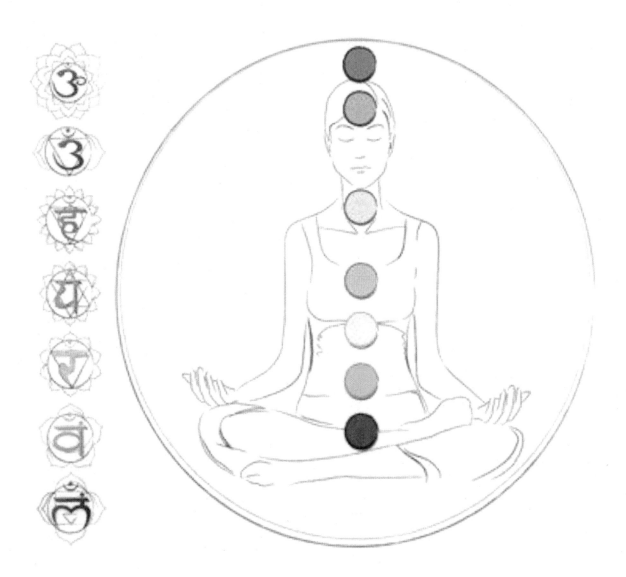

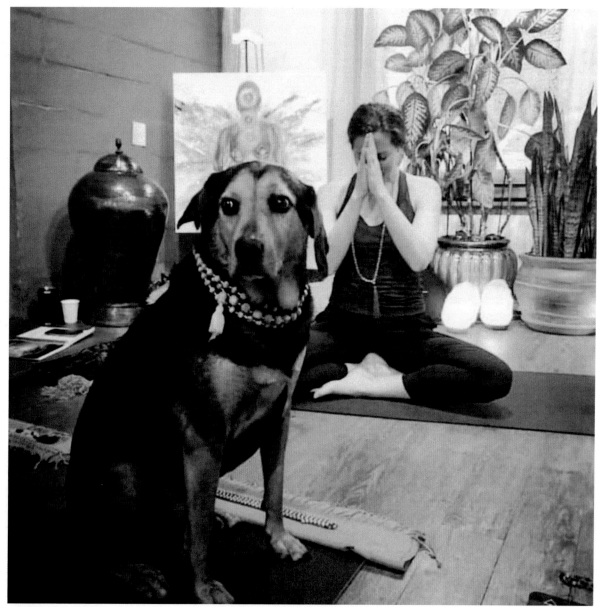

Western Yoga

Chapter 11

The Arrival:

Hatha Yoga and the Growth of Modern Asana

Historical Timeline

PRECLASSICAL YOGA ERA

INDUS-SARASVATI AGE: 6500-4500 BCE
- SANATANA DHARMA: "ETERNAL LAW"
- INDUS RIVER VALLEY & SEALS

VEDIC AGE: 4500-2500 BCE
- CONSCIOUSNESS EXPLORED
- VIBRATION OF INTENTION & CAUSATION
- CAUSE & EFFECT: MANTRA & KARMA

SAMKHYA YOGA: 8000-100 BCE
- REALITY EXPLORED: PRAKRITI/PURUSHA
- BODY'S CONSTITUTION: DOSHAS
- AYURVEDA

UPANISHADIC AGE: 2000-1500 BCE
- NON-DUALISM OF ATMAN/BRAHMAN
- DISTILLATION OF VEDAS
- MEDITATION

BHAKTI YOGA: 1000-500 BCE
- ADORATION
- HINDU EPICS / UNIVERSAL INSIGHTS
- 3 BRANCHES OF YOGA

BUDDHISM: C. 500 BCE-PRESENT
- INDIVIDUALITY / MONASTIC TRADITION
- MIDDLE WAY
- FOUR NOBLE TRUTHS / EIGHT-FOLD PATH

CLASSICAL YOGA ERA

CLASSICAL YOGA: 75 BCE-100 CE
- THE YOGA SUTRA'S OF PATANJALI
- EIGHT-LIMBED PATH
- HARNESSING THE MIND

ESOTERIC AGE

TANTRA: 600-1300 CE
- 6 + 1 CHAKRA SYSTEM
- WESTERN NOTION OF EMBODIMENT
- SUBTLE BODY (NADIS, CHAKRAS, ETC.)

HATHA YOGA: C. 1300-1400 CE
- MIND V. BODY
- HATHA YOGA PRADIPIKA
- ASANA / BREATH / BANDHAS / MUDRAS

RISE OF MODERN YOGA

SWAMI VIVEKANANDA: 1872-1950
- INFLUENCED RISE OF MODERN YOGA
- INTRODUCED YOGA TO THE WEST

SRI T. KRISHNAMACHARYA: 1891-1989
- YOGA'S EXPANSION
- FATHER OF MODERN YOGA
- MODERN CONTRIBUTORS

Chapter 11

The Arrival: Hatha Yoga and the Growth of Modern Asana

1. Overview of Lecture

Chapter 11 explores Hatha Yoga: *ha* (sun) – *tha* (moon). Symbolisms of the deities are discussed, as well as exploring the historical development of Hatha Yoga and its contribution to modern-day asana. Some of the key individual contributors responsible for this transformation are examined, as are different lineages in this ever-evolving Yoga Tradition.

2. Learning Objectives: I will…

a) Learn the historical context of Hatha Yoga and how it translates to Modern Yoga
b) Identify the key players of Modern Yoga (Swami Vivekananda, Swami Krishnamacharya)
c) Articulate how and when *the asana movement* came to the West

3. Pre-lecture Assignments

a) Read the chapter and become familiar with the Reflection questions
b) OPTIONAL: Hatha Yoga Pradipika
c) Recommended Films:
   ❖ *Enlighten Up: A Skeptic's Journey Into the World of Yoga*
   ❖ *Awake: The Life of Yogananda*
d) Daily Sadhana - Daily Personal Practice

4. Reflection: *found at the end of the chapter*

Hatha Yoga At-A-Glance

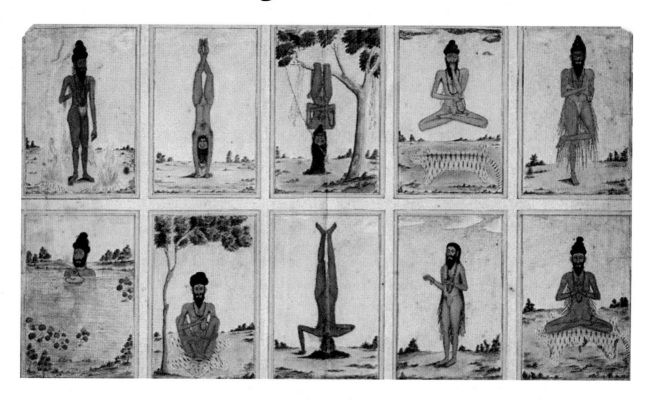

Hatha Yoga began in the 1500's. *Ha-tha* literally means sun-moon, harkening to a Yoga of balance. *Hatha* can also be translated as willful. Hatha Yoga is considered *Raja Yoga*, meaning Royal Yoga, which leads one to experience a high state of consciousness known as *Samadhi*, the bliss state. Unlike modern day's Hatha Yoga, the traditional practice was not geared toward physical fitness. Various methods were seen to purify the body to liberate the mind by awakening the subtle energy of *Kundalini* (the serpent Goddess/Shakti) within a meditative state.

The original, forest dwelling yogis of the first ashrams, before the time of Buddha and beyond the Patanjali era, believed that stopping the wheel of rebirth meant overcoming their physical incarnation. Therefore, extreme physical practices were used to create the meditative state necessary for awakening. The body was seen as impure and in need of being cleansed for a connection to the divine to occur.

Here is a 3rd Century description from *The Mairtayaniya Upanishad*: "Venerable, in this ill-smelling, unsubstantial body [which is nothing but] a conglomerate of bone, skin, sinew, muscle, marrow, flesh, semen, blood, mucus, tears, rheum, feces, urine, wind, bile, and phlegm—what good is the enjoyment of desires? In this body, which is afflicted with desire, anger, greed, delusion, fear, despondency, envy, separation from the desirable, union with the undesirable, hunger, thirst, senility, death, disease, sorrow, and the like—what good is the enjoyment of desires?"

Pranayama and bandhas were explored to expel impurities. Extreme twisting poses were developed to rid body of toxins. Aspects of Vedic health were explored: flame gazing, vomiting, cleansing the nose (neti pot), enemas, swallowing a cloth then pulling it back out. With this, some practitioners were seen as demonic with super strength, often hired as mercenaries because they were able to move beyond the limitations of the physical body and tap into the different spheres of consciousness.

Yet it wasn't until Tantra, still underground in the fourth to sixth centuries, that non-dualist insight took hold, meaning that if there is only Spirit, then all of creation, including the human body, is a manifestation of Spirit and is therefore sacred. Scholar Georg Feuerstein stated, "Instead of regarding the body as a meat tube doomed to fall prey to sickness and death, they viewed it as a dwelling place of the Divine and as the cauldron for accomplishing spiritual perfection."

It wasn't until the *Siddha* (perfected) movement within Tantra that you get elements that would coalesce into Hatha Yoga. In their quest for supernatural powers, the "Diamond Body" or *vajra deha* was explored. This is a Tantric term used to describe the process of refining both the physical body and "energy body" through the practices of Hatha Yoga.

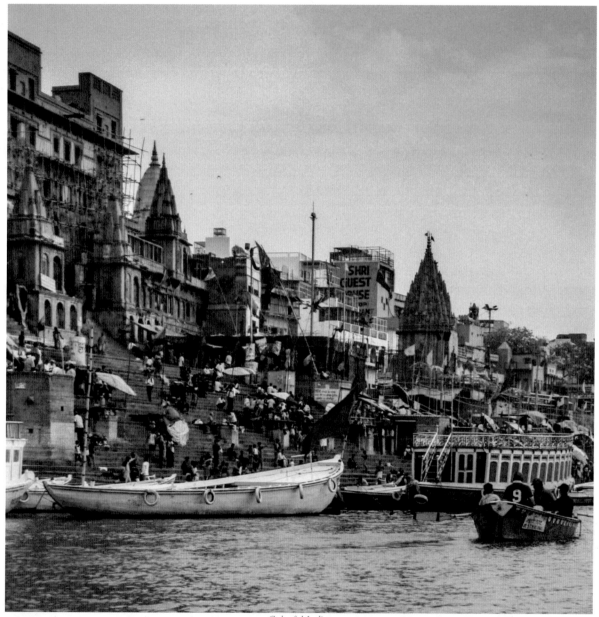

Colorful India

454

To achieve a Diamond Body, Yogis developed the postures (*asana*), breathing exercises (*pranayama*), energy seals (*mudra*) and purification techniques (*shat kriya*) of Hatha Yoga. Traditionally, Hatha Yoga is said to have originated with Matsyendra Natha and Goraksha Natha in the 9th or 10th Centuries CE. And it was kept secret. As the lore of asana development goes, even when texts were finally written about Hatha Yoga, many centuries after its inception, readers were admonished to keep it secret, still.

Circa 14th Century, a primary text called *The Hatha Yoga Pradipika*, written by Swami Swatmarama, was developed. It is Hatha Yoga's oldest surviving seminal text. The word "*pradipika*" means to cast to light. *The Hatha Yoga Pradipika* sheds light on the practice of Yoga. It consists of four chapters: asana, pranayama, mudras, and samadhi. It was inspired by various texts of the time as well as Swatmarama's personal experiences and was meant to be a guide for sannyasins, spiritual renunciates who wished to eradicate desire.

The Hatha Yoga Pradipika describes and reveals the intimate relationship between Hatha Yoga and Raja Yoga. It teaches about balancing the polarities of chakras through the means of asanas, mudras, bandhas, nadis, pranayama, and through purifying practices - all of which foster the awakening of Kundalini.

Asana came to mean a Hatha Yoga posture sometime in the 9th or t0th century. Asana wasn't further developed until the 20th Century.

The Hatha Yoga Pradipika begins with a chapter called *Asana*. It explains, "Being the first accessory of Hatha Yoga, asana is described first. It should be practiced for gaining steady posture, health, and lightness of body."

The Original 15 Postures

1) *Svastikasana* - auspicious posture

2) *Gomukhasana* - cow face posture

3) *Virasana* - hero posture

4) *Kurmasana* - tortoise posture

5) *Kukkutasana* - cock posture

6) *Uttana karmasana* - intense tortoise posture

7) *Dhanurasana* - bow posture

8) *Matsyasana* - fish posture

9) *Paschimottanasana* - intense West side stretch posture

10) *Mayurasana* - peacock posture

11) *Savasana* - corpse posture

12) *Siddhasana* - a seated pose known as "accomplished pose", done by pressing the heel of the foot against the perineum and gazing between the eyebrows

13) *Padmasana* - a seated pose in which the hands are clasped together and the chin is placed against the chest

14) *Simhasana* - seated pose on the knees, with the mouth open and the gaze at the tip of the nose

15) *Bhadrasana* - like bound ankle pose with the ankles pressed into the groin and the hands clasped around the feet

Though *The Hatha Yoga Pradipika* is considered the oldest surviving text on Hatha Yoga, two other primary texts include *Shiva Samhita*, and *Gheranda Samhita*. Regarding asana, *The Gheranda Samhita* says, *"There are 8,400,000's of Asanas described by Shiva. The postures are as many in number as there are numbers of species of living creatures in this universe. Among them 84 are the best; and among these 84, 32 have been found useful for mankind in this world."* In these three seminal texts of Hatha Yoga, more than half are seated, and Tree is the only standing pose. (Note, there is no mention of sun salutations, standing postures, nor head or handstand postures.)

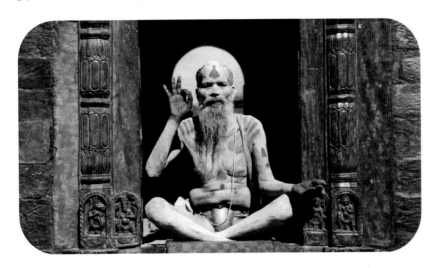

Most of the asana poses known today came through Krishnamacharya's lineage. He passed away in 1989. Sri Krishnamacharya taught B.K.S Iyengar, Pattabhi Jois, T.K.V. Desikachar, Indra Devi, and other Yoga masters, who are very briefly explored in the following pages.

Anne Cushman states, "Here's something to remember about Yoga poses: people made them up. Some of them were made up a long time ago—hundreds or even thousands of years. A lot of them—including many that we think of today as "classic" Yoga poses—were invented by Indian yogis in the early part of the 20th century. Some were imported from places as diverse as YMCA exercise classes and Swedish gymnastics—and then given Sanskrit names. Some were invented as recently as last week. There is nothing inherently sacred about any of the postures that you'll see arching and twisting on Yoga calendars. What makes them sacred is the way we inhabit them."

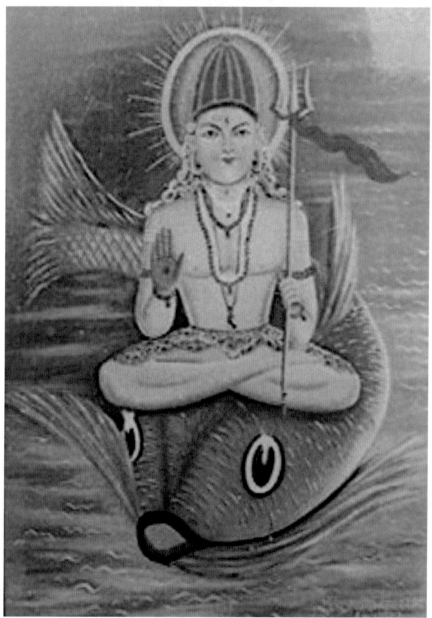

Shiva Imparting Knowledge

Hatha Yoga Mythology

There will always be variations in the story of Yoga, including a large range of dates. But the story itself is based on actual evidence. Always be flexible, not rigid, in "this is how it has to be". That said, there are set ways in a particular order like the Eight-Limbed Path and the Yoga Sutras that have proven to be pathways to liberation.

Matsyendra and his student Goraksha are considered the founders of Hatha Yoga, and Swami Swatmarama is the student of Goraksha. However, the two founders have taken on mythological dimensions. Matsyendra is known as Avalokiteshvara, a bodhisattva of compassion in Buddhist-Nepal. In India, he illustrates the metamorphosis that human beings are capable of through the radical transformation that Yoga offers. In one myth, the infant Matsyendra is thrown into the ocean because his birth has occurred under inauspicious planets. Swallowed by a giant fish, he overhears Shiva teaching Yoga to his wife, Parvati, in their lair at the bottom of the ocean. He emerges as an enlightened master from the fish's belly after spending 12 years exploring the practices of Yoga.

Matsyendrasana is the deep twist familiar in a modern-day Yoga practice and is one of the few asanas described in *The Hatha Yoga Pradipika*. "Twisting poses symbolize revolving the front body, or what is conscious, to the back body, the subconscious." American Yoga College's Rama Jyoti Vernon says, "They bring light into darkness and the dark to light, a process essential to Yoga."

Matsyendra's chief disciple was Goraksha. According to legend, a woman prayed to Shiva for a son and was granted ashes to eat to ensure a pregnancy, but she threw the ashes on a dung heap. Twelve years later, Matsyendra visited this blessed woman, who confessed that she'd thrown the ashes away. Matsyendra visited the dung heap, and he found a 12-year-old boy who was a perfect Yogi, having practiced *sadhana* (ego-transcending spiritual practice) since birth. Matsyendra named him *Goraksha*, meaning cow protector. *Gorakshasana* is where the heels of the feet are brought to the front and kept near the navel, with various modifications. Ultimately, the two stories symbolize how the Yogi is inspired by the part of you that is the rejected child. The practice reveals your innermost heart and allows you to claim your life in truth.

459

Swami Vivekananda

Introduces Yoga to the West (1863 - 1902)

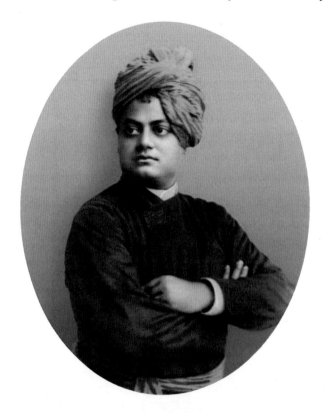

Yoga was first represented to the West by Swami Vivekananda. He is best known in the West for his speech to the 1893 World's Parliament of Religions in which he introduced Hinduism to America and called for religious tolerance and an end to fanaticism. Born Narendranath Dutta, he was the chief disciple of the 19th-Century mystic Ramakrishna and the founder of Ramakrishna Mission. Swami Vivekananda is also considered a key figure in the introduction of Vedanta, Hinduism, and Yoga to the West.

Swami Vivekananda's Welcoming Speech at the Parliament of the World's Religions
Chicago, September 11, 1893

Sisters and Brothers of America,

It fills my heart with joy unspeakable to rise in response to the warm and cordial welcome which you have given us. I thank you in the name of the most ancient order of monks in the world; I thank you in the name of the mother of religions, and I thank you in the name of millions and millions of Hindu people of all classes and sects.

My thanks, also, to some of the speakers on this platform who, referring to the delegates from the Orient, have told you that these men from far-off nations may well claim the honor of bearing to different lands the idea of toleration. I am proud to belong to a religion which has taught the world both tolerance and universal acceptance. We believe not only in universal toleration, but we accept all religions as true. I am proud to belong to a nation which has sheltered the persecuted and the refugees of all religions and all nations of the earth. I am proud to tell you that we have gathered in our bosom the purest remnant of the Israelites, who came to Southern India and took refuge with us in the very year in which their holy temple was shattered to pieces by Roman tyranny. I am proud to belong to the religion which has sheltered and is still fostering the remnant of the grand Zoroastrian nation. I will quote to you, brethren, a few lines from a hymn which I remember to have repeated from my earliest boyhood, which is every day repeated by millions of human beings:

"As the different streams having their sources in different paths which men take through different tendencies, various though they appear, crooked or straight, all lead to Thee."

The present convention, which is one of the most august assemblies ever held, is in itself a vindication, a declaration to the world of the wonderful doctrine preached in the Gita:

"Whosoever comes to Me, through whatsoever form, I reach him; all men are struggling through paths which in the end lead to me."

Sectarianism, bigotry, and its horrible descendant, fanaticism, have long possessed this beautiful earth. They have filled the earth with violence, drenched it often with human blood, destroyed civilization and sent whole nations to despair. Had it not been for these horrible demons, human society would be far more advanced than it is now. But their time is come; and I fervently hope that the bell that tolled this morning in honor of this convention may be the death-knell of all fanaticism, of all persecutions with the sword or with the pen, and of all uncharitable feelings between persons wending their way to the same goal.

(As made available online in the public domain)

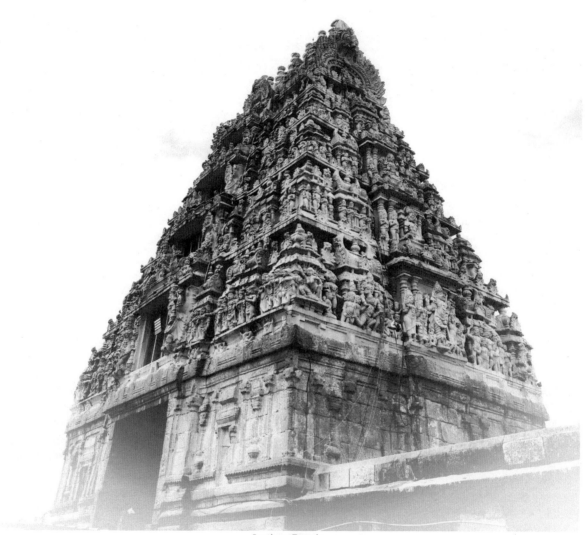

Southern Temple

462

Swami Vivekananda's Closing Speech at the Parliament of the World's Religions
Chicago, September 27, 1893

The World's Parliament of Religions has become an accomplished fact, and the merciful Father has helped those who labored to bring it into existence and crowned with success their most unselfish labor.

My thanks to those noble souls whose large hearts and love of truth first dreamed this wonderful dream and then realized it. My thanks to the shower of liberal sentiments that has overflowed this platform. My thanks to this enlightened audience for their uniform kindness to me and for their appreciation of every thought that tends to smooth the friction of religions. A few jarring notes were heard from time to time in this harmony. My special thanks to them, for they have, by their striking contrast, made general harmony the sweeter.

Much has been said of the common ground of religious unity. I am not going just now to venture my own theory. But if anyone here hopes that this unity will come by the triumph of any one of the religions and the destruction of the others, to him I say, "Brother, yours is an impossible hope." Do I wish that the Christian would become Hindu? God forbid. Do I wish that the Hindu or Buddhist would become Christian? God forbid.

The seed is put in the ground, and earth and air and water are placed around it. Does the seed become the earth, or the air, or the water? No. It becomes a plant. It develops after the law of its own growth, assimilates the air, the earth, and the water, converts them into plant substance, and grows into a plant.

Similar is the case with religion. The Christian is not to become a Hindu or a Buddhist, nor a Hindu or a Buddhist to become a Christian. But each must assimilate the spirit of the others and yet preserve his individuality and grow according to his own law of growth.

If the Parliament of Religions has shown anything to the world, it is this: It has proved to the world that holiness, purity and charity are not the exclusive possessions of any church in the world, and that every system has produced men and women of the most exalted character. In the face of this evidence, if anybody dreams of the exclusive survival of his own religion and the destruction of the others, I pity him from the bottom of my heart, and point out to him that upon the banner of every religion will soon be written in spite of resistance: "Help and not fight," "Assimilation and not Destruction," "Harmony and Peace and not Dissension."

(As made available online in the public domain)

Swami Krishnamacharya

Father of Modern Yoga (1888 - 1989)

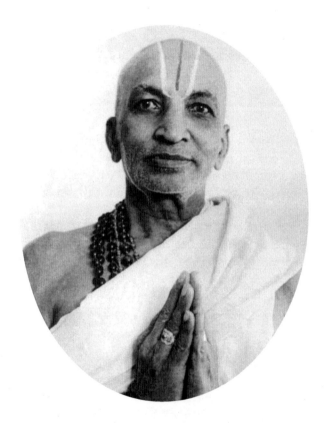

Swami Krishnamacharya is known as the Father of Modern Yoga. He was a very orthodox Brahman, a great pundit, and a great scholar. His contribution to the lineage is largely reflected within the modern-day asana practice that is understood by most as the embodiment of Yoga. Krishnamacharya's famous disciples are responsible for the spread of Yoga's popularity.

It is said that Krishnamacharya was a descendent from a revered 9th century Yogi. When he was five, his father initiated him into the Yoga Tradition through Patanjali's Yoga Sutras, which ignited his internal fire and passion to understand the philosophies of Yoga.

Though farfetched to many, Krishnamacharya is said to have received guidance, instruction, and his wealth of Yogic knowledge through a vision that came to him from his forefather, Nathamuni. This vision imparted vast wisdoms from a lost 14th century text named *The Yogarahasya, The Essence of Yoga*. Krishnamacharya is said to have memorized and transcribed this text, never asserting it to be his. He gave credence to his gurus and their gurus for all of his acquired knowledge. Krishnamacharya believed that Yoga belonged to God, and he was a messenger.

Krishnamacharya continued to seek knowledge of classical philosophies, receiving various degrees in philosophy, music, and psychology. He studied under one of the remaining Hatha Yoga masters, Sri Ramamohan Bramachari. Under guidance, Krishnamacharya studied and mastered the Yoga Sutras and Hatha Yoga in seven years.

Public attention was required to popularize the dying tradition of Hatha Yoga and the repression of other cultural riches. Krishnamacharya went on to patronize Hatha Yoga through lecture and through the demonstration of his highly developed *siddhis*, his supranormal Yogic abilities. His siddhis included clairvoyance, levitation, bilocation and astral projection, materialization, and having access to memories from past lives ... to name a few.

Even though Krishnamacharya lived in extreme poverty for years, he continued to teach and share the values of Yoga. The ruling family of Mysore, who championed the revitalization of Indian culture, financed him to spread his knowledge, healing arts, and counsel within and out of the palace for two decades. While on frequent Yoga "propaganda tours", teaching students ranging from British soldiers to maharajas, Krishnamacharya established a *Yogashala*, or Yoga school, in the palace's gymnastic hall, catering to young boys.

Krishnamacharya's palace shala was close in proximity to the bodybuilding gym of Yogananda Pramahansa's brother, Bishnu Charan Ghosh (who taught asanas to Bikram Choudhury). Here, asanas were developed and practiced. Drawing from Hatha Yoga, Indian wrestling, and gymnastics, movements were developed to build physical and mental vigor through breathing and meditative concentration. Poses were developed based on Yogic philosophies such as twisting to activate energy centers and animal poses to honor interconnection with nature. Sequences of primary, intermediate, and advanced asanas were established, and students were grouped according to their capabilities.

Two styles developed that enabled Yoga to embrace all students: *Ashtanga Yoga* (which required more athletic skills) and *Iyengar Yoga* (which used blocks and straps, so that even physically limited patrons could learn and heal through Yoga). Today, there is a fusion of the two different styles. Props are often used in many classes to help participants feel the energy of a pose. Additionally, Krishnamacharya also broke down the gender barrier, teaching a woman, Indra Devi, who took Yoga to Hollywood.

Krishnamacharya was successful in cultivating an official Indian Tradition based around asana. This led to his first book of Yoga written in 1934: *Yoga Makaranda, The Nectar of Yoga*. This book became the foremost series about Ashtanga Yoga, arriving in the West forty years later.

When you are bound,
the Beloved comes in the form
of the master.
When you are free,
the Beloved comes in the form
of the devotee.

~ Mooji

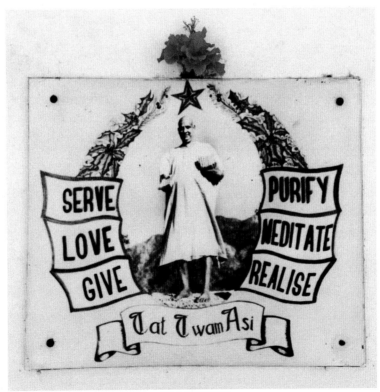

Ashram Blessing

Christine Lily Kessler

Modern Asana Yoga Contributors

APOSTLES, POPULARIZERS & STYLES

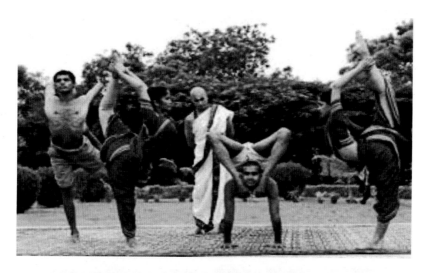

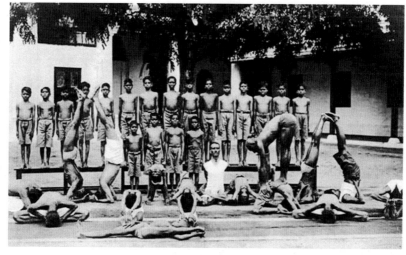

Indra Devi

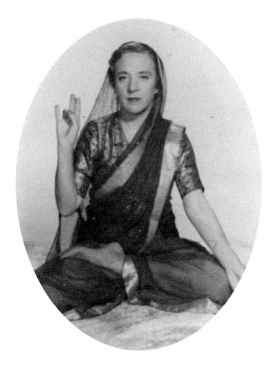

Divine Rain is considered the Mother of Western Yoga. When someone was passionate to learn, Krishnamacharya was passionate to teach. Born Eugenie V. Peterson, Devi persevered and rose above every given challenge that threatened to break her will. She proved to be an exemplary student and was the first woman to be taught Yoga in a centuries-old patriarchal tradition. Today, 80% of Yoga practitioners in the West are women.

Devi wrote the best-selling book on Hatha Yoga, *Forever Young, Forever Healthy,* and she founded the first school of Yoga outside of India. Devi was influential in convincing government leaders that Yoga was not a religion. She also attracted Hollywood stars, which cemented Yoga as culturally acceptable. Classes were based on Krishnamacharya's breathing and meditation philosophies and asana series, but Devi designed the arching flow that you see in many of today's classes.

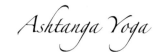

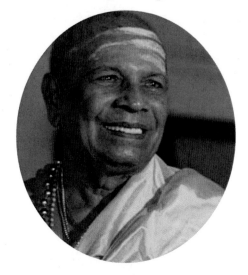

Founded by K. Pattabhi Jois, known as fierce and compassionate, and strict and loving. Ashtanga emphasizes *vinyasa* (the flow from one posture to the next). There is a set of postures in which each asana connects with the next in a continuous, flowing movement, linked by the use of constant *ujjayi* (breathing), *bandhas* (energetic locks) and *drishtis* (gaze). This intense vinyasa practice produces *tapas* (heat), which detoxifies and cleanses the body. There are a total of six Ashtanga Yoga sequences, to be learned in succession, after the mastery of the previous sequence. Traditional Ashtanga Yoga classes are taught *Mysore-style*, in which students lead their own practice. Many other Vinyasa-style Yoga Systems have been developed from Ashtanga Yoga, including "Vinyasa Yoga" and "Power Yoga."

Krishnamacharya created a series of poses. In the 1930's, his student, Pattabhi Jois, took the series into stages of further development. Jois emphasized vinyasa. This is Ashtanga Yoga, which became popular in the West in the 1970's. Jois branded the series, but poses were added as time progressed and the series evolved. Jois wasn't the only person teaching the series in Mysore. He had American students who were dedicated to bringing his teachings to the United States, and in time, Ashtanga and Pattabhi Jois became well known.

Iyengar Yoga

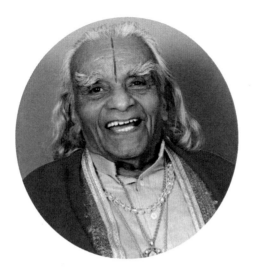

B.K.S. Iyengar is the father of Iyengar Yoga, a widely recognized Hatha Yoga style. Iyengar Yoga is a type of Hatha Yoga focusing on the correct alignment of the body, making use of straps, wooden blocks, and other objects as aids to achieving the correct postures. His Ramamani Iyengar Memorial Yoga Institute is in Pune, India. It emphasizes precise physical alignment. Because of the attention to detail, the pace of the class tends to be slow to moderate, and postures are repeated and held – a physically challenging workshop style class. Clear levels are also emphasized for safe and definite progression. This method incorporates therapeutic techniques, which are built upon once the student attains proficiency, one pose at a time.

Iyengar was a student of Krishnamacharya. Physically, he was the opposite of Pattabhi Jois and was physically disabled, weak, and ill until his twenties. Krishnamacharya worked with Iyengar for many years and altered the practice to accommodate his student's physical needs. Together, they worked to manipulate and support the flow of energy to encourage health through the use of props, which healed Iyengar's body.

He is responsible for making asanas accessible to a wide range of people, and he is known as the great translator of Yoga movements. You may thank him for allowing Yoga to be accessible to all people with the use of props (blocks, straps, etc.). Before Iyengar, Yoga was passed down one-on-one from master to student. Now Yoga is taught in public arenas.

Sivananda Yoga

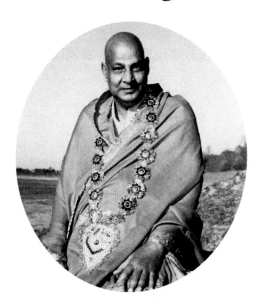

Sri Swami Sivananda created a five-point method of practice: proper exercise, breathing, deep relaxation, a vegetarian diet, and positive thinking and meditation. Classes follow a standard format, which includes breathing, sun salutation, the 12 classic Yoga postures, relaxation, and chanting. His teachings are: Serve, Love, Give, Purify, Meditate, and Realize. He has ashrams and teacher trainings around the world. His home-turned-museum is in Rishikesh, India.

Self-Realization Fellowship

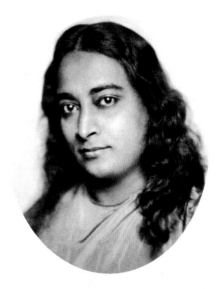

Paramahansa Yogananda was a great emissary of Yoga in the West, sharing inspirations and teachings in America through his Self-Realization Fellowship. "You realize that all along there was something tremendous within you, and you did not know it." He believed that Yoga could be found in all scriptures and was the essence of all religions.

Self-Realization Fellowship was founded in 1920 in the spirit of embracing all diverse cultures and people around the planet. Paramahansa Yogananda made available the universal teachings of Kriya Yoga, the sacred science of meditation and the art of balanced spiritual living. At its heart are advanced techniques of meditation that, with devoted practice, lead to a state of inner stillness that enables one to realize infinite potentiality in an everlasting atman.

These meditation teachings embody Yoga philosophies that support beauty, nobility, and the divinity of the human spirit.

Expansion and Quickening

Yoga is about how you cultivate your inner world. That includes what you tell yourself and how well you see how the universe works in your favor. Yoga creates a different perspective from being a victim to being empowered, which is a gift of the Universe. Yoga is the cultivating of the mind to get out of the state of the protective personality.

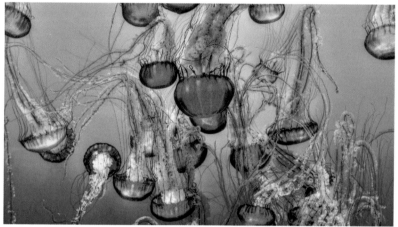

Expansion Contraction

After the Feast, the Rest. After the Expansion, the Quickening. Living in Feast - in Expansion - is tasting the essence of Divinity. Holding space for lessons to be integrated and reflected upon is the Rest. The Quickening is receiving and integrating the experience.

A Yoga practice will change over time, and that is a given. It must. Great peace and new growth will be had when you are able to admit things that were once interesting to you have been replaced by something new. This ebb and flow is the most natural cycle of the universe.

On the mat, you cultivate your relationship with Expansion and Quickening. Transitional movements from pose to pose offer the opportunity to cultivate an awareness of time and place; it's the journey, not the destination. Here you breathe and visualize and move your body and energy with intention. You integrate the process by sinking into the inner stillness of the pose itself through drishti and breath. That is also the purpose of Savasana – the Quickening.

Expansion and Quickening are simultaneously occurring in different cycles in various arenas within your life. I embrace this process with the mantra, "Who am I? I don't know." I am learning to get out of my own way, to bust down my inner walls and old belief systems, so I may rest in the understanding that my heart is an engine of bliss, and my brain is an instrument of deep wisdom. Yet like the snake, skin must be shed, again and again and again. You must die thousands of times to live.

When I lived in Washington, D.C., I was a ravenous, Yoga junkie. My social life was largely based around trainings, workshops, and retreats that I enjoyed alongside other vulnerable and inspiring seekers and teachers. I found Yoga to be healthy and sexy and edgy. I fell madly in love with Bhakti rituals, explored the sweet *bhav* of sattvic living, and embraced an elegantly nonchalant bohemian grunge.

As a Yoga teacher, I spent immense energy inventing dance-like flows and forming the perfect playlists. After all, this is what was hip and packed a classroom. This is what made you popular on the circuit. This was YOGA, baby! *Right?*

A series of wild and serendipitous events, however, scooped me from my cosmopolitan nest and landed me in Middle-America. My once-ravenous nature of outward Yoga exploration began to Quicken. The seeds that were planted and cultivated during the past decade of Expansion began to grow roots. I became immersed in the mindful, inward analysis of traditional, conventional, and religious ideas, as well as those of the esoteric, mystical, and revolutionary. I found deep delight in books, quiet meditations, and in authoring a book for my Yoga Trainings. *Years of exploration led to integration, integration, integration.*

Admittedly, I embrace change more than most people. I find great excitement in trying new things, *in living some and learning some*, to reinvent barrier-less inner and outer landscapes. The understanding that I am comprised of both nothingness and everything-ness is my practice of faith. Faith, *Sraddha*, is not only my given spiritual name, it also represents the foundation for my wild affair with life and God. Again and again, I surrender my life to be a blank canvas in which to explore terror and freedom. Change is both the foundation of Expansion and the foundation for Quickening. Both/And.

At this time in my life, my Yoga is my ability to breathe and discern and Quicken what I have learned. I outwardly hold space for others, so I may expand my inner space. I strive to understand my relationship with perception and reality, diving beneath a mountain of jargon that holds simple and essential tools to support my Awakening. I honor my body's wisdom to navigate decisions based on *the visceral feeling of Expansion and Quickening*. I have deep faith that the Universe loves me so much that things are done for me not to me, so when old patterns of attachment bubble to my mind's surface, I see an opportunity to transmute them. My Practice encompasses equally a Yoga mat and a vacuum, an overflowing inbox and the navigating of a new business, as well as donning my gardening gloves and pouring and enjoying a big pour of wine … or two (or sometimes, bourbon).

I have learned that it takes courage to admit change is needed to claim who you are, here and now, rather than settle for what you once were or who you are expected to be. At this time in my life, my Practice is to hold space for my lessons to settle. I vertically receive, deepening my understanding of Authentic Self and claiming my role as a teacher.

During the day do not do one thing while thinking about another.
Thought and action must be unified - no thought be permitted
without reference to action or intended action, and no action be performed
without intention. By this practice all day long the mind and body are
taught to act together, without any waste of physical or mental energy.

~ Ernest Wood

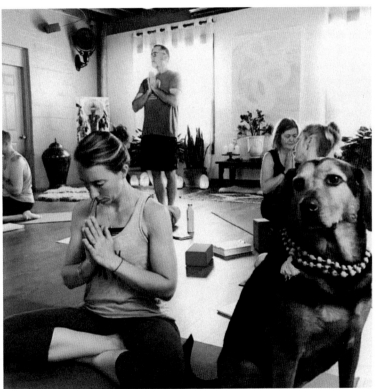

Intention

Reflection

The Arrival: Hatha Yoga and the Growth of Modern Yoga

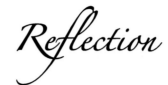

1) *Chicago, 1893. Parliament of the World's Religions is fraught with mistrust, and the representing parties are prepping to return home. Swami Vivekananda speaks to a restless crowd, and in a matter of seconds, he neutralizes the atmosphere with his opening words, "Sisters and Brothers of America." He introduces Hinduism and Yoga to the West.*

   a) You have been introduced to the vastness of Yoga in the previous chapters. Share what Yoga means to you AND describe how Yoga has the power to be a change-agent in the world. The answer may be one in the same.

   b) What will your role be in this change? What message do you have to offer?

2) Create a Prayer Stick for your sacred space. Directions are on the following page.

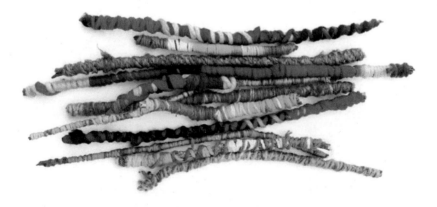

Prayer Stick

For eons, prayer sticks have played a significant role in spiritual rituals, especially in the Native American and Wiccan traditions. They are vehicles to communicate with Divinity. Prayers can be petitions, visions, and/or hold gratitude. Prayer sticks can harness intention and invoke blessings. Essentially, they carry the vibrational energy of their creator. They may hold both prayers and blessings.

How to create a prayer stick:

- ❖ Find a tree that has special meaning to you.

- ❖ Acquire a stick from the tree that is about an inch in diameter, being forked or straight.

- ❖ It should be about as long as the length of your arm from elbow to fingertips.

- ❖ Sit and meditate with your stick, saying/singing prayers, mantras, and blessings as you begin your creation.

- ❖ On thin strips of paper, write your prayers.

- ❖ Wrap your prayers around your stick.

- ❖ Wrap strands of yarn, fabric, leather strips, beads, etc. around your prayer stick.

- ❖ I recommend wrapping in layers to create different layers of textures and colors.

- ❖ Make sure your stick has at least one feather on it, ideally one that you found on a walk or one that has special meaning to you.

- ❖ Strands of shells and beads can be integrated.

- ❖ Metal and stones should not be used, unless 'called' to do so. Be very intentional.

- ❖ Place your stick in a significant place in your home to infuse its blessings into your life.

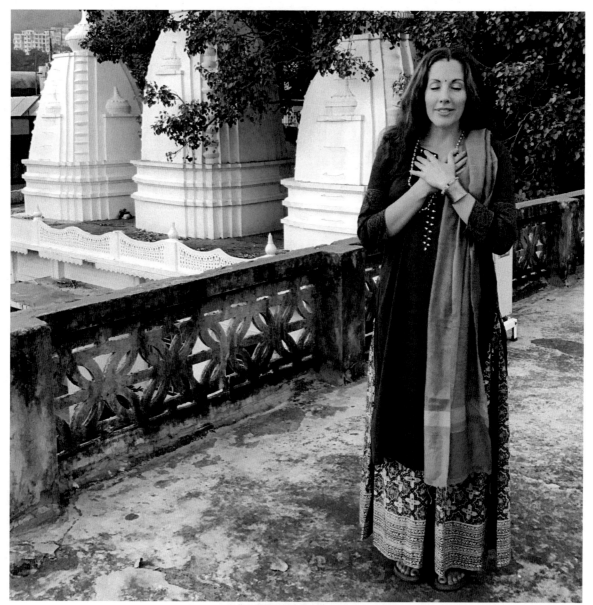

India, a Home of my Heart

Chapter 12

Final Thoughts:
The Art of Living Yoga

Smile with the flowers and green grass.
Play with the birds and the deer.
Shake hands with the ferns and twigs.
Talk to the rainbow, wind, stars, and the sun.
Converse with the running brook and the waves of the sea.
Develop friendship with all your neighbors, dogs, cats, trees and flowers.
Then you will have a wide, perfect and full life.

~ Swami Sivananda Saraswati

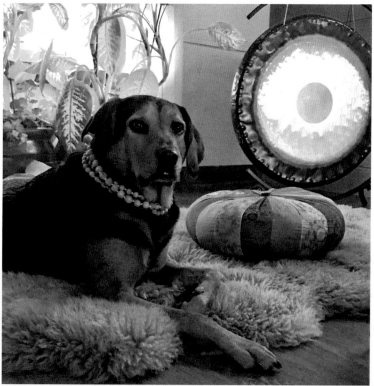

Shanti's Shala

Chapter 12

Final Thoughts: The Art of Living Yoga

1. Overview of Lecture

Chapter 12 is a summary of Yogic concepts, explores leadership discernment, and the embodiment of Yoga in everyday life. Attention to both the physical feeling and location of emotions are examined, indicating new opportunities for personal growth, as well as questioning current life patterns. How to connect with the Authentic Self is concluded with thoughts exploring consciousness and truth, and how to merge and equalize the dualities of Fear and Love within everyday living.

2. Learning Objectives: I will...

a) Articulate which tools I've learned that help me embody new perspectives and change
b) Recognize that emotions are doorways to liberation
c) Continue my exploration of self-accountability in my thoughts, words, and actions

3. Pre-lecture Assignments

a) Read the chapter, there is no Reflection
b) Daily Sadhana - Daily Personal Practice

Leadership Discernment

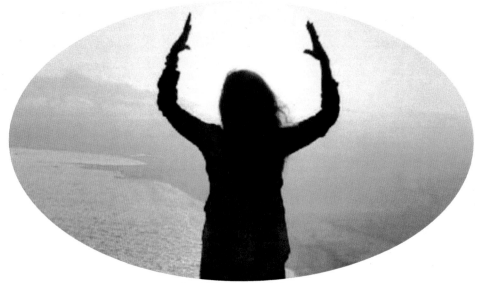

Own Guru, Nazca Lines, Peru

Our need to follow a leader should never come before our need to follow ourselves and do what is right for us.

Today, we have an unprecedented number of self-proclaimed gurus and cult-like dynamics in and around the world. In every arena across the diverse spectrum of spiritual/woke/religious communities and political/corporate groups, fundamentalist attitudes are growing. Fundamentalism works on inventing a past that never existed and then invoking a false nostalgia for it, largely void of any sophisticated analysis of the tradition.

Your identity, your Essential Self, is unique and sacred. You don't need altering and you should never be altered. It is dangerous to look for another person or group of people to give you an identity. Anyone

484

who tells you otherwise does not have your best interests at heart. If someone can alter your identity, you then fit into a mold of their making, and that's when abuse can happen.

Identity abuse happens when you are told not to trust your intuition and the wisdom of your body. Identity abuse happens when you are shamed for taking care of your needs, or for asking questions. Identity abuse happens when the guru's message is, "If it feels wrong, it's really right."

This is not something that happens only in fundamentalist groups.

When a leadership position is backed by numbers, financially and otherwise, identity can become confused. At its worst, leaders who lie about and assault other groups of people, and/or other belief systems, often defend their damning claims through 'false news' that defends their agenda, regardless of actual truth.

When your interest is pulled towards a message or leader, discernment is key. Leaders/gurus who abuse power separate people from their own needs and from their own identity. They divide them from their families and communities with messages of spiritual hierarchy and the fear of being forsaken, spiritually or socially. We see this in churches, politics, and ashrams, alike.

"I only want to be around conscious people." It is unfortunate how often I hear this phrase in some Yoga circles. This message is a mask of the protective personality, not a compassionate soul nor leader.

Surround yourself with people who accept you for who you are now, not who you could become; not what you could do for them. A true guru, or leader, or teacher, is one who values diversity, interconnection, and feedback, and encourages communication, education, and discernment. There is freedom to come and go without shame.

- ❖ **Show up as you are *now*.**
- ❖ **Take what serves you and leave what doesn't. An inspired leader will understand that.**
- ❖ **You are your own guru. You embody everything you need and seek; Yoga reveals *Your Self*.**

Weaving Concepts: Embodiment of Consciousness

How? An Awareness Experience

Inhale and pause. Feel your body stretch and expand from the inside. Fully exhale and relax. Relax your jaw. Put a little smile on your face. You are alive. Become the 'Experiencer' of the experience. Look at the colors in front of you. See the complexity of hues and textures that are before you. Notice the exchange of light, and tone, and detail. Notice what is touching your skin and the comforts within your body; focus on those places that reside in ease and health. Give thanks to these areas. Now notice the taste in your mouth and contemplate what part of you is truly experiencing taste. Welcome yourself into calm satisfaction as a gateway to peace and tranquility. You are collecting yourself; pulling yourself into the present moment from being a ghost to the past or a ghost to the future. When you reside with your breath, you release your conflict. You become aware of being alive in the space in and around you.

Diving Into the Now

Every moment is pregnant with *Grace* so you may transform and be the *Phoenix Rising*. Only by residing in the present moment can you experience what it truly means to be alive. Otherwise, you live in a sort of limbo, confused, ghost-like state; this is living in a Story from your own mind-stuff. Only through your direct experiences, insights and intuitions, can you claim a conscious existence. Only you can pave your own path. If you follow another's path, you stray from your potential. You may certainly gain inspiration and learn lessons from others, but your journey is for you, alone. You must tame your own inner jungle by bushwhacking your own way to carve your own path. Only you can do this.

Direct experiences offer opportunities to explore both conscious and the unconscious tendencies. Different people carry different labels, and therefore each person you meet can be a teacher to you in some capacity. Experiences provided by these teachers support you so you may see what you were once blind to - your dark side, and your strength and beauty. Only when you come to an understanding of all your pieces and parts, you may experience *moksha*, liberation.

Within the yoga and spiritual community, one concept that can sway out of balance is the notion that it is not "spiritual" to feel anger. Energies that feel like shame and numbness are created from blocking feelings of anger, frustration, and rage. When you tap into your emotions and understand where and why they come from, you are fully tapping into the intelligence of your spirituality. Emotions are doorways into exploring layers of your Self. Emotions are golden opportunities to ask yourself, "Why do I feel this way? What does this feeling remind me of? When did I first feel this emotion in my life?" The deeper you dive into self-inquiry, the more you bring yourself *Home*.

The Opportunity

When you *feel* butterflies, the *charge*, or twangs of emotion, the Universe is speaking to you. Know that your feelings are simply bits of energetic information arising so you can better navigate a situation. When you feel shut down or feel "rubbed the wrong way", awareness of your feelings is something quite wonderful to celebrate. However, your patterned way of thinking may forgo this opportunity if it sticks to your entrenched story, or samskara/vasana. Programmed stories arise to justify feelings. The ego loves spinning this same old tale again and again, and these stories can become a part of your identity, causing limitations, and hindering new perspectives from gaining traction. In this, many people identity with Victimhood, and will defend this self-imposed label until their dying day.

The Universe is offering you an opportunity to embody new perspectives each day. You have ample opportunity to look at a situation and move your internal energies through practices of breath work and body movement to integrate these emotional charges and neutralize them. Why? So a situation doesn't become a story that has power over you. Awareness of breathing into the present moment and recognizing if you reside in the energies of *Love* or *Fear* is key in this process.

You must be willing to self-examine and question whether you are stuck in a pattern of expectations. This is Jnana Yoga, necessary in self-study and honest self-responsibility. It demands that you look beyond your story and see how this pattern has shown up in your life, and why.

The Universe continues to offer experiences and relationships until you break your patterned way of thinking, speaking, and reacting. The moment you move from a *knowingness* (truth known in the head) to an actual *understanding* (truth felt in the heart and gut) is the moment you begin to Awaken into a new reality of your own making. The universe loves you so much it will present you with what you need to grow and move on. You will continue to confront the same challenges, time and time again, lifetime after lifetime, until you accept transformation.

Danger. I can't. They're wrong. I'm offended. No. Run away.

That's not my responsibility. I can't do this.

When you live in a story of your own creation, your ego-self is masterful at justifying *why* you are limited in the way you are. The ego-self points fingers of blame outside of yourself. Yet everyone you encounter and every experience you embrace is a teacher offering an opportunity for growth. You have rigid systems in place that you are not even aware of that have protected you from suffering, but innately cause suffering.

For example, I have been married three times and would be married another three times if I didn't acknowledge my stagnant patterns. I had a choice to really look at myself when I was on the brink of yet another divorce. I found myself pointing a finger of blame at situations that caused unhappiness, but I looked down and saw my other fingers pointing back at me. So, I *leaned into* my internal discomforts and fears and saw that all my other relationships had the same message for me all along. My protective personality rejected the message the Universe was trying to reveal until I hit my rock bottom.

There is potential of tremendous beauty by hitting rock bottom. It is a place of suspended animation. It is a place that shatters masks. In this place, there are options to live and thrive, to live and be a martyr, or die. I explored every one of these options and decided my inner world was indeed worthy of freedom.

My Hero's Journey began, and I peeled back event after event until I saw the raw truth of who I was and why. I saw my unworthiness was born through futile people-pleasing which made my life very unsatisfying and false, but I thought it kept me safe. For many years I was looking for a guru or a perfect husband to tell me I'm special and then do the inner work for me; to save me from myself. My Inner Guru was waiting to be uncovered.

On one Hero's Journey, I discovered my supposed greatest weaknesses were actually the source of powerful empathy and compassion. *Namaste. I see me in you. I understand suffering through my own experience. I understand you are suffering your own experience. I understand there is a way out. I see you. I feel you. I am you. You are me.*

The greatest strength of my heart and my life-message was birthed from the fertilizer of my own *shit,* which helped me refine and grow with eloquence. And I don't need anyone else's shit - I have enough! So I try not to take on anyone else's problems; I support them when I can if they meet me half-way, but I don't carry them. Carrying someone is not a true expression of Love, it is enabling patterns to continue.

On Life, Potential, and Liberation

The microcosm of the body and the macrocosm relationship of the Universe/Absolute are one in the same. You are the Universe and the Universe is imprinted on and within your body. You can experience everything in the universe by yourself without a church, or temple, or pilgrimage because spiritual possibilities are already within you. There is no point to renunciate anything because you hold the ashram-forest within. You are Divine.

Your daily experiences honor the exploration of your unconscious and support you in the confrontation of your *dark side.* You must acknowledge, explore, and make peace with your 'shadow' side for *moksha,* liberation, to occur. This is where compassion is born.

What holds you back from liberation is your limiting beliefs of your potential. You are stuck in predictable behaviors, judgments, and thinking processes - patterns of thought and action. If something clashes with your perception, it is considered *wrong.* Instead, when something clashes - rubs against your norms - it is an opportunity to explore another way of living that may serve you and the world more authentically.

A traditional view of limitation and ignorance is based on the concept of the Kleshas, as seen in Buddhism and the Yoga Sutras. You mistake the impermanent for the permanent. You mistake the pure for the impure. You mistake pain for pleasure. You mistake the self as the Self. You attach yourself to belongings, to people, to ideas and compare yourself and others through these attachments. You have an aversion to being challenged out of your comfort zone. You fear change and death. You have patterned mechanisms subconsciously ingrained within you with false notions of protection.

These mechanisms are unexplored voids within your consciousness called *samskaras* and *vasanas*. These are patterned ways of thinking and living. These are the *issues in your tissues* and enslave you in how you identify with the world. Vasanas follow you from life to life. The universe offers you various teachers and experiences so you may fill in your vasanas by leaning into and learning from lessons, gaining new awareness of Self. All fears and ignorance can be overcome with the practice of action, awareness, and appreciation, which are all keys to liberation.

Ignorance can be overcome with the practice of awareness and action. Ignorance can be diminished, and liberation will be had the more you embrace qualities of your Divinity. As patterns are peeled away one layer at a time, you will be amazed at how these patterns drive your life!

The quality of how you see the world gives rise to the quality of how you manifest your potential. The quality of how you manifest your potential gives rise to the quality of how you see the world - *Both/And*. The discernment of how you think, speak, and act opens the door for you to experience the present moment, fully aware and alive. The Path of Neutrality, which is a path to enlightenment is the awareness in seeing God/Interconnection in everything, even in what otherwise might be deemed hideous and evil. This practice demands you to ask, "Is there another perspective? Can larger insight and compassion be cultivated?" Yes and yes. When you consciously look for Divinity in every aspect of life, you can see more clearly your true identity and experience a full life without haunting patterns.

To break a habitual pattern or an addiction, the practice is to identify gaps that the habit/addiction strives to fill. When you are aware of this, not only will you reveal find great personal strengths, but you will also find a greater sense of wholeness. Yet if you fall back into a pattern, you shouldn't feel guilty or shamed. If you reside in the energy of self-victimhood, your life is stagnant and lived by the protective personality. Instead with Yoga, you celebrate that you have gained insight to navigate and improve upon a situation if and when it arises again. You move on. Always moving forward in your journey is the practice toward consciousness.

PRACTICE: *An example of shifting daily patterns is exampled through engaging in gossip. You literally choose to close your mouth and do not engage, even though your mind may want to explode with a juicy story. Gossip is neither helpful nor kind. Don't waste energy with those who engage in it or be ready to stand firm to be the change and alter the trajectory of the group energy. Patterns and addictions, such as gossip, are futile ways to avoid the truth of seeing yourself as you truly are.*

(inhale) And. (exhale) Now.

And. Now (... another moment). And. Now.

On Consciousness and Valuing the Senses

When you know where your feet are on the earth and you are rooted in breath and discernment, you are conscious. Conscious thoughts and conscious actions are necessary to empty your life of false impressions. Emptiness amplifies your spiritual path toward universal unity and wholeness. This emptiness is not to be feared. This is not an emptying of personality and uniqueness. Rather, your personality is free to be authentic and to tap into the bliss of pervasive Divinity that you might otherwise be blind to when you are full of patterned impressions. This is discernment.

When conscious, you step outside of yourself and see how you are a part of the whole. You see how all people's actions are a part of the whole. Once you are awake to this, you have a great responsibility.

You are sensitive to all things within your personal space and in the global environment. You weigh your actions to see if they support the freedom and the betterment of all life, because all life forms reflect yourself. You take on the role of a mother and a father to the world. If you see a need, you act. *Act for action's sake, not for the fruits of your action.* You live alert, empathetic, and fully conscious in the present moment. You see beyond the present and feel how your interconnectedness is like the conductor in an orchestra. You choose what tune will be played and how. Ultimately, Earth is your spiritual playground.

Heaven, *Tejase*, is available to you in the here and the now. Breathe in with expanded awareness and step into it. Harnessing your senses with the breath brings you to the fleeting, sacred present moment of consciousness so you may holistically experience Divinity within and beyond. If you focus your lens of life to see what is before you without the patterned story, you become capable of embodying bliss. When you revel in the five senses, you are connecting to the Universe itself.

Some traditions warn against taking refuge, sanctuary, in the senses. Rather, senses are viewed as illusory ropes that bind the atman to the world, stemming from a defiled body that is only to be purified and transcended once it dies. Yet harnessing the senses with the breath brings you to awareness so you can holistically experience Divinity within and beyond!

Consciousness takes vulnerability, and vulnerability is the greatest act of courage any life form can embody. When you are conscious, you are receptive to all life experiences; to all the beauties and the horrors that you have experienced. Receptivity of consciousness moves you from being a puppet to becoming a curious witness to *Lila*, the grand play of life. New experiences are no longer narrated or threatened by the voice of your ego that once so easily hypnotized you into a false reality based on past experiences. You see how your *Great Story*, based in ego's reality, was a sham. Yet there is tremendous value in that alone! You now understand how each moment of your life has provided stepping-stones, not stumbling blocks, toward the development of your consciousness. You see and *feel* yourself in all life forms. You may even feel the energy-story of inanimate objects. You are now able to navigate and alter energy.

On Energies of Love and Fear

There are two energies in this world - Love and Fear. A neutral way to view these energies is through the lens of experiences being *light* and *heavy*. Nothing is good and nothing is bad. All energies are support personal refinement. You know from your experiences that unfulfilled expectations can be viewed as disrespectful or uncaring, and this can feel like suffering. This is the energy of Fear. No living creature wants to feel unworthy, undesired, not seen, and not heard. Fear-energy tells you that unfulfilled expectations reflect your unworthiness. Many people suffer from this very example. Peace begins within, so does jealousy and hatred. Understanding that Fear is the underlying root of these afflictions is a way to step into compassionate Love energy. You must always, always, always be willing to remain fluid and forgiving in your thinking with yourself, and in turn, with others. Be willing to empathize with others in their choices, whether they be saviors or murderers.

When I was a child, there was a breaking story on the news of a mother of five who drowned each of her children. The country was appalled that this quiet, religious woman would do such a thing. Demand for the death penalty overshadowed uncovering the reasons why her mental illness led her to such an act. I was ripe to develop a judgment and pattern based on the reaction of the people around me.

I remember sitting with my grandmother, Nika, in her sunlit kitchen, waiting for her opinion, and she gave it to me stone-faced. Her words became etched in my soul the moment they left her lips, "I feel so, so sad for this woman. She was alone raising those children. She had no help from her husband or her church because she had to look perfect and live her perfect life as a perfect mother. I feel so sad for her. What mother has never questioned wanting to kill her own children? I have felt that." My grandmother went into a story that shared a piece of her fierce loathing of motherhood when she felt overwhelmed to the point of no return. Yet she did return. She understood that she was lucky to do so and saw herself clearly in the defeated eyes of a murderer and felt compassion for this fellow soul.

I sat stunned. My beloved grandmother had the potential of being a murderer? Of course she did. I did too. I knew it then and I know it now. I fell so in love with my grandmother at that moment and I saw her for the woman she was. She was dynamic, honest and raw. She was the most beautiful goddess I ever laid my eyes on because she experienced her life in connection with others.

493

This is the courage and insight it takes to live in the current of Love. You see yourself in all beings. You are the embodiment of Compassion. There is no greater expression of love than that of compassion.

I am not justifying the atrocious acts that this world endures. I am advocating understanding the root causes of them so you can be empowered to choose to respond, not react. How do you respond? You must *be for* something, not against something. You must be for peace, not against war. Do you see the difference? This energy of *flow* propels the world forward in a particular trajectory, rather than trying to stop the trajectory of another energy, which is impossible. You must discern and change the inner and outer landscapes that fuel hatred. You will never be able to stop fear and hatred in its tracks.

This leads to the contemplation of attachment and desires; samskaras and karma. When you are attached to the negative and the positive alike, you are not in control. Again, you must consider the essential quality of Purusha, the Absolute Witness Self. It is void of story, receptive to the Divine, not sterile and lonely. The Authentic Self is void of the energetic though-hook, which pulls on fleeting emotions and desires. It is void of limited categorization but resides in understanding of the whole picture, and the whole picture encompasses the spectrum of the Human Condition, both the objective and subjective aspects.

On the Authentic Self

The Authentic Self, Purusha, Atman, is purity and interconnection in its true essence. The definition of Maya is "illusion", essentially embodied within all limiting concepts. Maya is like the sun. The sun obstructs the view of the stars, yet the stars are always present, even when you can't see them.

Maya obscures your understanding of your vast potential. Ultimately, your life is not your own. From the moment of your birth, your parents and your 'tribe' color how you identify with who you are. This tribe supports your likes and dislikes, your acceptances and prejudices, your joys and fears. Your samskaras, beliefs, and limited thinking are justified by your parents and tribe. This is the Human Condition. There is no one to blame for your limitations, yet it is the quest of Humanity to transcend them; to rise above the base-norm to identify your higher Self and live authentically. Living authentically is to live a life of vulnerability. This is a courageous path of consciousness. Vulnerability questions the 'why' in all things. "Why do I feel this way?" "What is the reason for this response, this outcome?" You must question who you are and feel secure in *not* knowing. Life is *The Great Unfolding.*

When you think you 'know' who you are, you embody a sense of stagnancy. You have climbed out of one box, so to speak, and have fallen into another one. *I am a yogi. I am a Christian. I am a mother. I am a vegetarian. I vote…* Though many of the hats people wear are healthy, they can also cause separation from others. These boxes are breeding grounds for righteousness and cults. Always question and be aware of the subtle judgments you place on your choices and the choices of others.

To break free of the notion of *who you think you are* so that you may *step into who you may become,* you must break free from the limits of your understanding. By seeking reasons as to *why* you are the way you are, and why you think the way you think, you amplify your self-understanding. As you better understand yourself, you better understand the world and the limitless possibilities it offers, as everything is an opportunity. A mantra may be, "The Universe does things for my growth and betterment. *Even this.*" And the practice is surrendering to attachments while striving to find a larger picture of understanding. And even in that, letting go of any attachment of even finding an answer to your questions. It's a paradox.

My acupuncturist, Melissa, drove home this point. I have been seeing her for years, and I always feel rejuvenated after our session together. One day as I was leaving, she said, *"Lily, you come here with your baggage and you leave it outside the door. But when you leave, you pick it up again. Kick that shit off my steps and never look back at it."* One day (after years of work) I effectively did because I was ready. But then more baggage arose that I had to deal with, but it was easier to navigate because my patterns were now revealed. I was on to my ego's vicious game of survival. Again and again I had to lean in with love and tell myself that I would survive the Great Purge of Patterns that shook me to my core. This Purge still comes when least expected, but I welcome it now as pure growth.

So, every moment truly is pregnant with Grace. When I serve my heart, I serve others. If someone is offended with my decision or choice, I am their teacher to help them grow, no matter what. I don't serve myself or others by serving out of obligation.

On Becoming Zero AKA Unity and Oneness

Your experience of everyday senses gives rise to pleasure, which is a resource for attaining totality and satisfaction. When you cultivate pleasure without grasping, you gain joy. Joy is evergreen and allows contentment as you encounter good and bad conditions. If you deny yourself joy and pleasure, you deny your connection to spirituality; the greatest unifying gift to all of humanity.

Here is the key to understanding unity. As you empty yourself of preconceived notions and recognize holy spirituality, interconnectedness, and sentient qualities in all living beings, you see yourself in all lifeforms and empathize with their joy and sorrows. Seeing yourself in all beings and seeing Divinity in all beings, you will surely taste the sweetness of Unity. Unity has no qualifications of who is accepted in and who is not. All animals and plant life alike are bound within Unity. With this insight, new perspectives arise within daily living and choices for consumption on all levels.

Ultimately, your heart is your mirror to the world. Consider for a moment what you may feel when you are driving late to a meeting and you are "stuck" behind someone going the speed limit! In this moment, the practice is to feel and recognize when you are out of alignment, and speak and act in accordance to fairness and helpfulness. You must be willing to stand firm with grace and not allow your precious energy to be taken, nor allow yourself to be swept away in another's energy or another's enthusiasm. In this practice of discernment, life-long patterns may emerge. For example, you may find you seek belonging in a group, or you seek control over people. Once these patterns are identified, you can make decisions that amplify and support the quality of your inner alignment.

With practice, life becomes a manifestation of how Self is reflected, giving credence to the power of consciousness. The more you practice, the easier life will be. The more intuitive you will become. You become more holistically beautiful because your energy will radiate a healing, conscious presence. All things you once craved will no longer have power over you. Life will be lived in ease rather than dis-ease.

Where the mind goes, prana flows. If you see yourself and others as transcendentally beautiful, with the potential of being a sanctuary for all beings, and if you see yourself as pure, strong, and capable, Life becomes a living puja; you delight in the senses as God would delight in the senses. Life becomes an expression of wonder. You then begin to live a vertical life of Connection, changing from the outside-in as well as changing from the inside-out. Both are necessary for growth.

A Final Thought: The Spectrum

Every person and animal on the planet embodies a spectrum - the yin and yang of life. This spectrum is home to your universal energy. How your life is lived within the spectrum determines the ratio of how Love and Fear energy is exhibited. You may find great comfort in a friend, a lover, or a spouse. When that energy shifts, you will re-categorize where that person is on that spectrum. For visualization purposes, they may shift in your life to a brighter spectrum or a darker spectrum.

If someone's behavior disturbs your inner peace, it's an opportunity for you to lean into the experience and incorporate the lesson that is being offered to you. It is important to hold space for people when your peace is threatened. Every person's decisions and inter-personal actions stem from a patterned place in a spectrum. Each part of this spectrum is in line with either Love or Fear.

For example, someone may seem very negative in your life and you have decided they have done you wrong. You choose to either distance yourself, speak your truth, or clash your righteousness against theirs. You must understand that two rights do not make one right. You must also understand each of you have unique perspectives along individual spectrums that simply are not matched. In turn, another person may view your behavior as being just as offensive from their spectrum's perspective. If you remember that your viewpoint is focused on a small piece of another's inherent spectrum of possibility you will remain free from attachment to behavior. You will forgive because you will see yourself in them. Even though your unique story may ask you to cringe when a particular person walks into a room, pull yourself out of this story, and understand that another person's heart lights up with tender joy when they see the same face. See and feel through another's eyes and heart. You are them. They are you.

Ultimately, know your life has led you to this very moment. The universe does things to support your potential-growth, and sometimes it takes time to gain larger perspectives to understand why things happen. Yet having faith is the strongest and bravest way of living that a human being can embody.

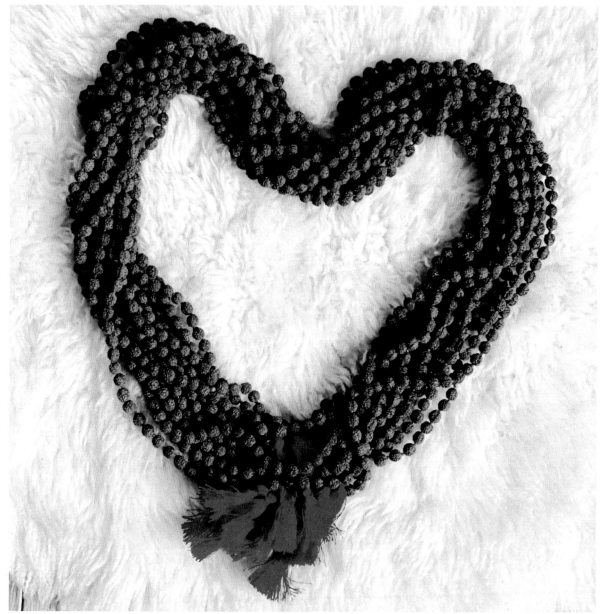

Mala Beads - gifts for my students upon the beginning of Yoga teacher training

For a New Beginning
By John O'Donohue

In out-of-the-way places of the heart,
Where your thoughts never think to wander,
This beginning has been quietly forming,
Waiting until you were ready to emerge.

For a long time it has watched your desire,
Feeling the emptiness growing inside you,
Noticing how you willed yourself on,
Still unable to leave what you had outgrown.

It watched you play with the seduction of safety
And the gray promises that sameness whispered,
Heard the waves of turmoil rise and relent,
Wondered would you always live like this.

Then the delight, when your courage kindled,
And out you stepped onto new ground,
Your eyes young again with energy and dream,
A path of plenitude opening before you.

Though your destination is not yet clear
You can trust the promise of this opening;
Unfurl yourself into the grace of beginning
That is at one with your life's desire.

Awaken your spirit to adventure;
Hold nothing back, learn to find ease in risk;
Soon you will be home in a new rhythm,
For your soul senses the world that awaits you.

Glossary

Moving Beyond the Jargon

Absorption: no separation of Self & Divine, Seeker & Sought are the same, unity will Everything

Advaita: non-duality

Ahimsa: Yama of the Yoga Sutras, non-harming, generosity of the heart toward self & others

Ananda: bliss

Anahata: 4th chakra of the heart center, balance, connection

Ajna: 6th chakra of the third eye, intuition, connection, link head to heart

Aryans: *Noble Ones* who migrated to Ganges from the Indus-Sarasvati Civilization

Asana: 3rd limb of the Yoga Sutras originally meaning *seated*, now modern-day physical postures

Ashram: holy home of a spiritual leader, monastic community, a home for religious retreat

Ashtanga Yoga: eight-limbed path of Patanjali's Yoga Sutras, a modern-day asana lineage

Asteya: Yama of the Yoga Sutras, dedicated in not stealing (time, energy, etc.), generosity & honesty

Atman: Pure Consciousness of the soul, Atman is Brahman, as first seen in the Upanishads

Aparigraha: Yama of the Yoga Sutras, non-attachment, non-possessiveness

Avidya: ignorance

Ayurveda: the Science of Life

Bhagavad Gita: *Song of the Lord,* teaches Bhakti Yoga, Karma Yoga, Jnana Yoga, Dhyana Yoga

Bhaj: share

Bhajan / Kirtan: a group of worshipers who chant or sing name of deities or mantras

Bhakti Yoga: Yoga of Devotion, love

Bodhi: awakened, enlightened

Brahman: Ultimate Reality, God Force, Potential, as first seen in the Upanishads

Brahmacharya: Yama of the Yoga Sutras, energy moderation & channeling emotions

Buddha: awakened, enlightened, representing Compassion & your true nature

Chakra: Wheel of Light, Energy Center, 7 major chakras

Chaitanya: One who is conscious; consciousness (mantra/practice)

Deva: *shining one*, male deity

Devi: *shining one*, female deity

Dharana: 6th limb of the Yoga Sutras, concentration

Dharma: life purpose, reality, Authentic Truth

Dhyana: 7th limb of the Yoga Sutras, meditation

Dhyana Yoga: path of meditation to be absorbed in Knowledge

Dosha: mind Body Constitution, Ayurvedic body type as seen in *pitta, kapha, vata*

Drishti: meditative focal point

Duality: Divinity & Self are separate from the other

Dukkha: suffering, unfulfillment

Gayatri Mantra: *Mother of the Vedas*, mantra of protection, healing, clarity

Guna: quality of living as seen in tamas, rajas, sattva

Guru: meaning *Remover of Darkness*, a term for a spiritual teacher

Hatha Yoga: element of Raja Yoga, emphasizing physical aspects of transformation

Hindu Trinity: Brahma/Creator, Vishnu/Preserver, Shiva/Destroyer

Ida Nadi: Feminine / moon / cold / blood / left nostril

Ishvara-pranidhana: Niyama of the Yoga Sutras, dedication to the Lord/Source, Divinity in All

Japa: yoga practice with recitation of mantras, may be done with a mala

Jivanmukta: one liberated while living

Jnana Yoga: Yoga of Wisdom/Knowledge of Self

Kaivalya: detachment yet also Oneness

Kali: Goddess of Time/Destruction, fierce aspect of the Divine

Kapha: dosha of structure & fluidity, water & earth elements

Karma: cause & effect

Karma Yoga: Yoga of Self-less Service

Kleshas: 5 binds that hold the soul from Moksha, seen in Buddhism & Yoga Sutras

Koshas: sheath/ Layer of the Self & Existence

Kriya Yoga: Yoga of Technique

Kula: spiritual community

Kundalini Shakti: Goddess Serpent located at spine-base, as seen in Tantra & Kundalini Yoga

Mahabharata: sacred Hindu epic embodying the *Bhagavad Gita* & Indian Philosophies

Mahabhutas: Great Elements found in all physical creations (ether, air, fire, water, earth)

Mahatma: great soul

Mandala: sacred geometry

Manipura: 3rd chakra of the sacral center, non-dominating will power, seat of Self

Mantra: sacred sound/phrase to evoke blessings, change, peace, protection, etc.

Mantric Causation: vibrational energy to evoke change as first seen in the Vedas

Maya: illusion that masks the Divine

Moksha: liberation from the cycle of samsara

Mudra: hand or body gesture invoking energy retention, meditation, etc.

Muladhara: 1st chakra of the root center, stability, security, *my gig*

Munis: name of first group of yogis as seen in the Vedas

Nada: union through sound

Nadi: subtle energy channel through which energy flows in the body; 72,000 'rivers' of energy

Nadi-Shodhana: Alternate Nostril Breath, channel clearing & energy balancing

Niyama: 2nd limb in Yoga Sutras, how you interact with yourself, moving into the microcosm

Non-duality / Non-dualism: Divinity & Self not separate

Ojas: vitality

Om: ultimate Vibration, the sound of Self/Source/Universe

Patanjali: mythological composer of the Yoga Sutras representing your ultimate potential

Pingala Nadi: Masculine / sun / hot / right nostril

Pitta: dosha of transformation & metabolism, fire & water elements

Prakriti: composed of the three gunas, nature, as seen in Samkhya Philosophy

Prana: Vital Breath, life force of the body & spirit

Pranayama: 4th limb of the Yoga Sutras, breath of life force controlled

Pratyahara: 5th limb of Yoga Sutras, withdrawal of the senses

Puja: ritual worship in a home or temple

Purusha: the Witness Self, Potential, as seen in Samkhya Philosophy

Raja Yoga: Royal Yoga, a yoga integrating Jnana Yoga, Bhakti Yoga, Karma Yoga & Kriya Yoga

Rajas: guna of change, action, energy, movement, creativity

Rishi: seer, sage

Rta: Vedic, universe can be manipulated through proper rituals & mantras, karma foundation

Sadhana: spiritual practice & discipline

Sahasrara: 7th chakra of the crown, enlightenment & transcendence

Samadhi: 8th limb of the Yoga Sutras, bliss state, enlightenment

Samsara: cycle of birth, death, rebirth

Samskara: pattern, subconscious impression related to past experience

Samkhya Philosophy: meaning *number*, everything in the universe has Divine Order

Sanatana Dharma: paths are many, Truth is one

Sangha: monastic tradition, community of like-minded thinkers

Santosha: Niyama of the Yoga Sutras, dedicated to contentment in the here & now

Sama: equal

Samadhi: Purusha integrated with Prakriti

Saucha: Niyama of the Yoga Sutras, dedicated to cleanliness, purity, refinement of inner & outer Self

Satsang: gathers of people seeking truth, Community, Practice

Sattva: guna of balance, harmony, purity, light, Being-ness

Satya: Yama of the Yoga Sutras, dedicated to truth & integrity of thoughts, words & actions

Sanskrit: *Language of God*, *Hanging Gardens*, Mother of Indo-European languages

Shakti: 'feminine' Power & Energy of ultimate Reality (wisdom, right action, awareness, intention)

Shala: spiritual home, sanctuary, place where yoga is practiced

Shanti: peace

Shishya: student

Shiva: masculine/potential force, ancient monotheistic God-representation, Adi Yogi

Siddhi: yogic supernatural powers

Sushumna nadi: central pranic nadi along the spinal cord, through 7 chakras

Swami: a certain order of monks

Svadhisthana: 2nd chakra of the sacral center, emotions & sexuality

Svadhyaya: Niyama of the Yoga Sutras, dedicated to self-study, analyzing inner & outer worlds

Svarupa: knowledge of one's individual form of the self, essential nature, lovely, wise

Svarupadhyana: meditation on realty; one's own essential nature

Tamas: guna of inertia, darkness, materiality, heaviness

Tantra: expansion/contraction

Tapas: Niyama of the Yoga Sutras, discipline, purifying heat, austerity

Tejase: sparkling, full of light & radiance, divine luminosity

Three Jewels: Buddhist Tradition, Eightfold Path of Wisdom, Ethical Conduct, Mental Discipline

Upanishads: knowledge distilled from the Vedas literally meaning *to sit near*

Vasana: sub-conscious or latent tendencies in one's nature

Vata: dosha of movement & change, wind & space elements

Vedas: books of knowledge asking *what is the soul*

Vedanta: 'Higher Inquiry' & Indian Philosophy

Vidya: Removing ignorance

Vijnana: act of an integrative living experience with knowledge of the highest form

Vishuddha: 5th chakra of the throat center, speak & see truth, discern

Yajana: Vedic fire ceremony, external ritual

Yama: 1st limb of Yoga Sutras, how you interact in the world, the macrocosm experience of Self

Yoga: union, conscious awareness, skill in action, connection to all: Divinity, Self, Other

Yugas: four ages to each cycle of preservation.

- ❖ 1st Cycle: everyone follows their dharma
- ❖ 2nd Cycle: 75% of people follow their dharma
- ❖ 3rd Cycle: 50% of people follow their dharma
- ❖ 4th Cycle: the planet's current cycle, 25% of people follow their dharma then destruction will come bringing in another Golden Age

A Note From the Author

I loved the way my grandmother, Nika, would talk in her West Texas accent. "What are you reading, now? Is it *progressive*?" Nika was a natural feminist who loved to learn and who bravely questioned social norms and belief systems, which remains one of the biggest gifts she taught me, along with the value of traveling the world.

In my early years, I was an avid reader and poet, yet, after being labeled with a learning disability, it wasn't until graduate school that I learned to write. The weight of this label ('learning disabled') taught me great empathy and compassion, and my first career was dedicated to teaching creatively in an out-of-the-box classroom in the public schools of the Washington, D.C. area. This is the time when I was first introduced to the rich tradition of Yoga. Sixteen years later, I found myself teaching Yoga in these same schools to both fellow teachers and children. What I witnessed opened me to dedicating my life to the Yoga Tradition, where I expanded into a global classroom.

It first started in the sanctuary of Pure Prana Yoga Studio in Alexandria, Virginia. I can still viscerally remember the smell of sunshine on wood floors, Yoga mats and incense, and when the windows were opened, roasted coffee from the shop below, with hints of car exhaust wafted through the air. It was intoxicating.

I originally began Yoga solely to burn calories, but then *a bread trail of gifts* started to appear in my daily life. This ancient, living thing called Yoga started to connect me to something timeless; to something good and powerful; wild yet disciplined; kind and supportive; formidable and fierce.

"Are you ready to transform your life?" my teacher, Natasha, asked upon me applying for Yoga Teacher Training. I honestly thought that question was the most arrogant one I had ever heard. Ironically, I now ask the same question of my students because I know, from first-hand experience, that you must be ready on some level, as you enter your own, unique, free-fall of faith into the Yoga Tradition. Here, you humbly learn to trust that you alone are your own guru.

From my first training, Yoga history intrigued me and beckoned me to lean-in more, but the internet was still growing and knowing where to start was overwhelming. So, I began to read book after book. I began to make travel a priority. I began to write. I began to teach what I thought I understood. Importantly, I wanted to face, head on, the cultural appropriation that was severing Yoga from its roots, as well as call out the hypocritical bigotries which are socially and culturally taught in the name of God or Guru. This energetic passion was instrumental in the creation of this book.

It is an honor for me to birth *The Art of Living Yoga*. I never set out to write a book, yet these pages are a portion of a refined version of my original Yoga Teacher Training Manual. Additional stories and information are woven within my online lecture series to make this knowledge come alive, as history reflects what is brilliant and living in the here and now.

Yoga is about holistic interconnection, and it is an agent to change the world to a planet of peace and tolerance. An internal wellspring of kindness can emerge in the midst of personal refinements, which are Yoga's by-products.

My mother said, "You have power, so use your power for kindness." And I say this to you, too. *You have power. Use your power for kindness.* Together we are in this wild, awe-inspiring, terrifying, joyful, messy, perfect, colorful journey and expression of life. So, let's be kind to each other.

Blessings to you.

With Love ~ Lily

Connect with me on Facebook/Instagram at: Christine Lily Kessler
LilyKessler.com

Christine Lily Kessler

Gratitude's

I kiss your heart. You are That.

I honor all my teachers, from beloved scholars to beloved students, and I humbly offer *The Art of Living Yoga* as my life's work… thus far.

I have gained deep inspiration from my first teachers who initially welcomed me into the Tradition, and then nurtured me as I expanded my interests. Thank you, Anne Harrison, Kathy Judd, Brittanie DeChino, and Jessica Silverman Hesprich. Additional studies and collaborations include Don Jorge Luis Delgado, Dr. Sue Morter, Christine Eartheart, and Yulia Azriel, with additional studies from Dr. Brene Brown, Dr. Edwin Bryant, Dr. Judith Hanson Lasater, and so many others.

I kiss the hearts of those who encouraged me to write this book, supported me along this journey. wish to thank D. D. Scott, my editor, for her invaluable advice, and her divine gritty-grace and confidence in this work; Carolyn Varvel for her thorough, creative, and literary critique of the book's structure, and for her kind wisdoms and personal support; Elliana Eleftheriou, who generously read the draft and offered refined insights to support philosophical verbiage; Iva Nasr, my colleague and friend, for her exquisite attention to detail, and our shared adoration of this Mystical Dance of Life; Eve Sizer and Charity Serdahl, my lifelong friends, for their unwavering presences in my life as truth holders; Marilyn Sue Dolan, my mother, for her integrity and elevated perspectives in our daily calls; Kim Loebe, my sister, for her endless patience while offering backrubs, garden breaks, and wine as encouragement; Shanti Roo for helping me align my thoughts on our meditative walks; 'my favorite' Tuesday Morning Yoga friends for keeping me accountable and walking by side these many years; my family for their extraordinary magic that delights my heart and soul; Michael Kessler, my beloved husband, for his dedication to walking his talk, and his innate belief in me; and to the land, ancestors, and cosmos.

I see you and I love you.

About the Author

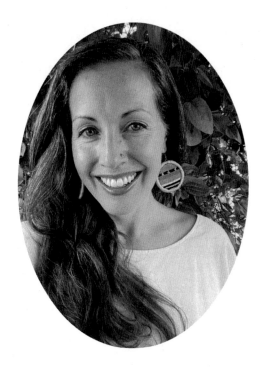

Christine Lily Kessler, E-RYT, EdS, and Adjunct Professor at Butler University, is fascinated by the facets of the ancient, living Yoga lineage. Her studies and peace-teachings honor the people, cultures, and roots of these vast traditions.

Lily believes Yogic Insights offer greater interconnection, equality, and peace for the world through exploring embodiment principles that activate full human potential. She draws from her 16 years of experience as a public-school teacher and specialist, inspiration from lifechanging awakenings, and her personal passion to foster authentic and safe community conversations that delve into exploring conscious and subconscious patterns of cultures and the world environment at large.

Lily is the founder of both Nourished Heart Yoga & Training and Blooming Life Yoga Studio & School. She has developed and led Yoga Alliance Certified 200- and 300-hour Yoga Teacher Trainings. In addition to her own schools, Lily has cofounded an international Yoga Training, and has been a guest presenter for over 30 certified Yoga programs within the United States and worldwide.

Lily has been welcomed to participate in Vedic pujas, invited to private ceremony with the Lakota Sioux, has been initiated within Mystic Orders, and continues to learn from other cultures and traditions. Seeing beyond the jargon and sharing similarities within people and places is a part of her lifelong peace effort. Lily is an Energy Codes® Master Trainer, Reiki Master, B.E.S.T. and Spiritual B.E.S.T. Practitioner, Relax & Renew® Certified, YoKid® Certified, and Yoga Nidra Certified. Lily is an artist and a global retreat leader, focusing on spiritual journey experiences to India, Peru, Costa Rica, and Spain.

Humbly, it is Lily's life's calling to make Yoga's vast and tangled roots accessible and recognizable in everyday life, as she, herself, is in the thick of her own learning and refinements.

Namaste.

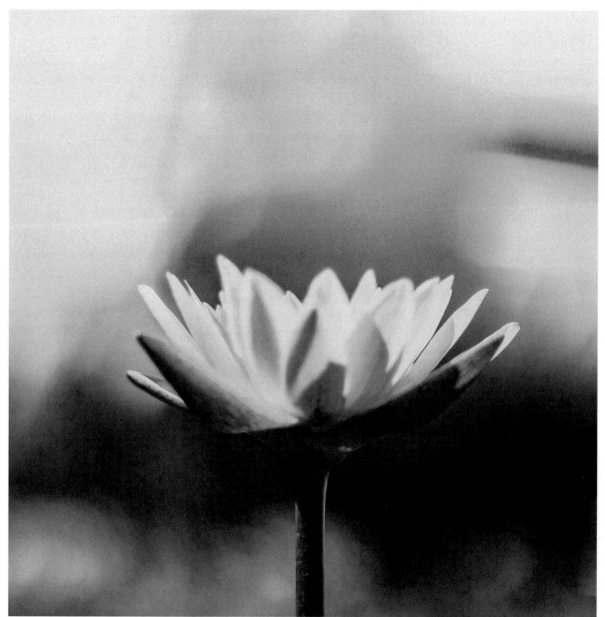

Begin Again